ANNUAL REVIEW OF GERONTOLOGY AND GERIATRICS

Volume 14, 1994

ANNUAL REVIEW OF

Gerontology and Geriatrics

Volume 14, 1994

Focus on
Assessment Techniques

M. Powell Lawton, Ph.D.
Jeanne A. Teresi, Ed.D., Ph.D.
VOLUME EDITORS

SPRINGER PUBLISHING COMPANY
New York

Springer Publishing Company, Inc.
536 Broadway
New York, NY 10012–3955

93 94 95 96 97 / 5 4 3 2 1

ISBN 0-8261-6496-X
ISSN 0198-8794

Printed in the United States of America

Contents

Contributors

Glenn Affleck, PhD
Department of Psychiatry
University of Connecticut School of Medicine
Farmington, CT

Marilyn S. Albert, PhD
Department of Psychiatry and Neurology
Massachusetts General Hospital
Harvard University Medical School
Boston, MA

Carolyn M. Aldwin, PhD
Human Development and Family Studies
Department of Applied Behavioral Sciences
University of California, Davis

Frances M. Carp, PhD
The Wright Institute
Berkeley, CA

Gary T. Deimling, PhD
Department of Sociology
Case Western Reserve University
Cleveland, OH

Pamela W. Duncan, PhD, PT
Center for Health Policy Research Education
Duke University
Durham, NC

Sherry L. Dupuis, MA
Department of Family Studies
University of Guelph
Guelph, ONT

Dolores Gallagher-Thompson, PhD
Older Adults and Family Center
Stanford University School of Medicine, and Geriatric Research, Education, and Clinical Center
Veterans Affairs Medical Center
Palo Alto, CA

Linda K. George, PhD
Department of Psychiatry
Duke University Medical Center
Durham, NC

Douglas Holmes, PhD
Research and Development
Hebrew Home for the Aged at Riverdale
Riverdale, NY

Mary Grace Kovar, DPH
National Opinion Research Center
Washington, DC

Renée H. Lawrence, PhD
Polisher Research Institute
Philadelphia Geriatric Center

M. Powell Lawton, PhD
Polisher Research Institute
Philadelphia Geriatric Center

Michael R. Levenson, PhD
Human Development and Family Studies
Department of Applied Behavioral Sciences
University of California, Davis

Rebecca G. Logsdon, PhD
Department of Psychiatry and Behavioral Sciences
University of Washington Medical Center
Seattle, WA

Roger C. Mannell, PhD
Department of Recreational and Leisure Studies
University of Waterloo
Waterloo, ONT

Alison T. O'Brien, BS
Department of Psychiatry and University Center for Social and Urban Research
University of Pittsburgh

Nancy A. Pachana, PhD
Harbor Medical Center
University of California, Los Angeles
Torrance, CA

Patricia A. Parmelee, PhD
Polisher Research Institute
Philadelphia Geriatric Center

Karen S. Rook, PhD
School of Social Ecology
University of California, Irvine

Richard Schulz, PhD
Department of Psychiatry and University Center for Social and Urban Research
University of Pittsburgh

Stephanie Studenski, MD, MPH
Center on Aging
University of Kansas Medical Center
Kansas City, KS

Howard Tennen, PhD
Department Of Psychiatry
University of Connecticut School of Medicine
Farmington, CT

Jeanne A. Teresi, EdD, PhD
Hebrew Home for the Aged at Riverdale
Columbia University Center for Geriatrics and Gerontology
New York State Office of Mental Health
New York, NY

Linda Teri, PhD
Department of Psychiatry and Behavioral Sciences
University of Washington Medical Center
Seattle, WA

Larry W. Thompson, PhD
Older Adult and Family Center
Stanford University School of Medicine, and
Geriatric Research, Education, and Clinical Center
Veterans Affairs Medical Center
Palo Alto, CA

Connie A. Tompkins, PhD
Department of Communication Disorders
University of Pittsburgh

Alex J. Zautra, PhD
Department of Psychology
Arizona State University
Tempe, AZ

FORTHCOMING

ANNUAL REVIEW OF GERONTOLOGY AND GERIATRICS

Volume 15

John E. Morley
Editor

Nutrition

Introduction
JOHN E. MORLEY

Epidemiology
DOUGLAS K. MILLER

Nutrition and the African American
MARIE B. BERNARD

Food and Aging: An Anthropological Perspective
SUSAN V. HOPPER

Social and Psychological Aspects of Nutrition
PATRICIA M.K. MORLEY

Diagnosis and Management of Protein Energy Undernutrition
JOHN E. MORLEY

Nutrition in the Nursing Home
DANIEL RUDMAN

Vitamins and Aging
LARRY E. JOHNSON

Exercise
ROGER J. MCCARTER

Cholesterol and the Healthy Senior
RAHMAWATI SIH

Introduction

M. Powell Lawton
Philadelphia Geriatric Center

and

Jeanne Teresi
Hebrew Home for the Aged at Riverdale
Columbia University Center for Geriatrics and Gerontology
New York State Office of Mental Health

This volume of the *Annual Review of Gerontology and Geriatrics* is the first in the series that is devoted to assessment. Although the emphasis is on accessibility of useful measurement information, the book begins in this chapter with an attempt to anchor such knowledge within a conceptually meaningful and directing framework. The editors feel that the subject matter of assessment flows from a larger view of what is worthwhile to assess. Further, the manner in which assessment of older people is performed is derived from both general measurement theory and from hypotheses as to how general or how age-specific some aspects of measurement practice should be. Thus, the content of assessment constitutes the focus of this introduction. Chapter 1 then anchors the assessment topic to some more general aspects of measurement theory and the issue of age specificity.

The authors adopted the following definition of functional assessment: "An attempt to evaluate the most important aspects of the behavior, the objective, and the subjective worlds of the person through standardized methods that can be applied by people with a wide variety of backgrounds and training" (Lawton & Storandt, 1984, p. 258). The criteria implied in this definition became the beginning point for the structure of the volume. A few compromises occurred along the way, such as including ratings made by physicians (chapter 2), trained design professionals (chapter 14), or physical therapists (chapter 4). The book was designed to enable a researcher to assemble a group of core indicators for most of the possible characteristics by which one might wish to describe older people in the most efficient way. Using such measures would allow the researcher either (a) to describe a subject population in the broadest terms or (b) to measure the personal and environmental context against which a more in-depth inquiry into one aspect of gerontology might be interpreted.

Several extremely useful treatments of the assessment of older people have been available for some time (Bowling, 1991; Kane & Kane, 1981; Mangen & Peterson, 1982; McDowell & Newell, 1987; Stewart & Ware, 1992). The present volume is intended, first, to update a rapidly-changing state of the art of assessment technology. It is intended to be useful by providing information regarding the content and psychometric characteristics of the measures, but it does not reproduce the instruments themselves. The potential user can call upon readily available reference citations and directories for information on how to obtain the instruments, a number of which are commercially published. This volume differs from others in its conceptual emphasis. Our conviction is that theory is needed to determine what should be assessed and how it should be assessed. Therefore, all authors were asked to begin their chapters with a conceptual definition of their assessment domain anchored to a statement of that domain's similarities to and differences from other domains.

Each chapter presents a selective review of the major measures in the topical area being addressed. Each author was asked to discuss the strengths and weaknesses of various measures and to make recommendations regarding the appropriate uses of the most important or most used instruments within the topical area. Such critiques are inevitably subjective, and the recommendations must, therefore, be interpreted cautiously.

AN OVERALL FRAMEWORK FOR ASSESSMENT

The volume as a whole, as well as each chapter, has tried to place all assessment within a larger conceptual framework. Such a framework provides both a way of organizing assessment and a way of identifying what needs to be assessed. This framework is discussed in greater detail elsewhere (Lawton, 1986).

One of the criteria for defining functional assessment is that measurement should be performed in an evaluative manner, that is, in a framework that asserts (with a few exceptions to be noted) that the attribute being assessed has a desirable-to-undesirable dimension. The first editor's conception of "the good life" represented an attempt to define quality of life in all-encompassing terms—certainly not to specify every possible facet of quality of life but at least to provide a framework within which all such facets could be located (Lawton, 1983). Four sectors were suggested to provide such a framework: Behavioral competence, objective environment, perceived quality of life, and psychological well-being (See Figure I.1). Although the four sectors are related to one another, none can be

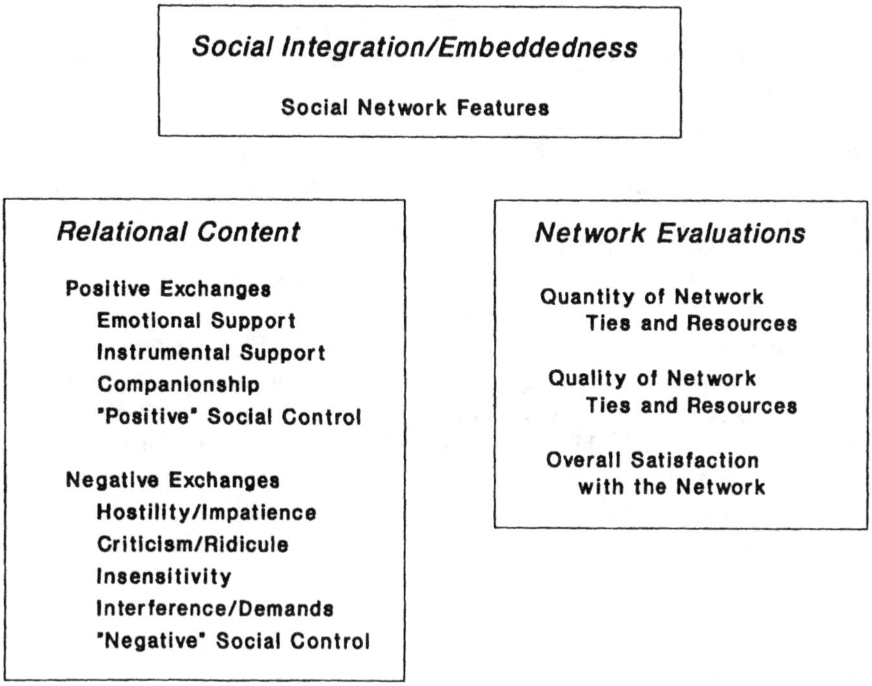

Figure I–1 Model of quality of life.

Reprinted with permission from M. P. Lawton, *The Genontologist*, 1983, *23*, 349–357. Copyright, Gerontological Society of America.

totally subsumed or predicted by combinations of the other three. It is asserted explicitly that well-being in any sector can constitute a human goal whether or not attaining that sector-specific goal elevates quality of life in any other sector.

Behavioral competence is the evaluated quality of behavior in domains that by normative social judgment are thought to be necessary for adaptation to the external world.

Objective environment is the measured quality (by physical, social normative, or consensual standards) of all that lies outside the skin of the person.

Perceived quality of life is the person's subjective evaluation of the adequacy of the separate domains of life and roles in life.

Psychological well-being is the subjective evaluation of the total quality of the self and the overall way the self relates to the world.

The definition of functional assessment asserts that a complete picture of quality of life may be ascertained only if both objective and subjective criteria are used in the total assessment battery.

Behavioral competence and objective environment are directly observable by others and therefore theoretically capable of being evaluated by social normative or physical criteria, in the absence of any evaluation by the subject. In contrast, perceived quality of life and psychological well-being are intrinsically subjective judgments on the person being evaluated. Like the objective indicators, they may of course be evaluated by an observer, but with greater risk error. Both the objective and subjective perspectives are necessary because each gives meaning to the other. Although an individual's subjective view is essential to defining what is right for that person, we must also know the objective properties of person and environment in order to plan for people in the aggregate.

It is suggested that each sector has an internal structure, which in turn is what determines the dimensions that may be evaluated by formal assessment techniques. Lawton (1983) suggested such a structure for behavioral competence, a hierarchy of domains whose arrangement was based on complexity. Complexity in this sector was defined as the increasing involvement of different levels of the human system, from the microbiological level to the macrosocial level, on which we place biological health, functional health, cognition, uses of time, and social behavior. As the behaviors to be evaluated become more complex, there is increasing influence of both personal preference and social or cultural factors in the processes resulting in their evaluation by the subject.

No dynamic structure has been derived for objective environment. Lawton (1970) suggested, however, that environment might be considered in five major groupings: (a) The *personal environment*, the world of one-to-one and significant relationships; (b) The *small-group environment*, networks composed of more than two people who maintain one-to-one relationships with one another and with the target person while exhibiting internal dynamics determined by the network rather than purely by the individuals; (c) the *suprapersonal environment*, the aggregate or modal characteristics of the people in physical proximity to the target person; (d) the *social environment*, which includes social and cultural influences on the person exerted through mechanisms such as government, the law, economic forces, norms, values, or social institutions; and (e) the *physical environment*, which represents all that may be counted, measured in centimeters, grams, and seconds, or perceived in the same way by multiple observers with high consensus. Much of the content of environmental psychology has dealt with evaluations at each of these levels, although no multidimensional assessment instrument has sought to encompass each of these domains systematically.

In the sector of perceived quality of life, although virtually any domain might be assessed, a limited number of such domains have been viewed as most important by the major investigators in this area (Andrews & Withey, 1976; Campbell, Converse, & Rodgers, 1976). Some examples are the judged quality of (or satisfaction with) domains such as marriage, family, job, housing, neighborhood, what one does in spare time, friends, and so on.

Finally, although psychological well-being has been a heavily researched sector of the good life, its internal structure is not apparent. One way to conceive this sector is to divide well-being into positive affect, absence of negative affect, and a cognitive sense of life satisfaction (Burt, Wiley, Minor, & Murray, 1978). However, general mental health, self-esteem, morale, and ego strength are only a few of the other constructs that fall loosely into this general sector of psychological well-being.

Despite the difficulties involved in attempting to organize each of these sectors into meaningfully structured domains, simply specifying them does allow us to identify many of the most important domains. The quadripartite structure of the sectors enables one both to locate existing measures for some domains and simultaneously to recognize that no measures exist for others.

THE SCOPE OF THE VOLUME

Although this volume's emphasis is on the concepts and content of assessment, virtually every chapter alludes to methodological issues in measurement. The book begins with Teresi's overview of some measurement issues, including the central question regarding how age-specific our measurement concerns should be.

A key issue is the extent to which a particular construct shares meaning across age groups. Does the construct change in definition across the age spectrum (e.g., leisure, some aspects of the environment)? Is the domain one that relates only to a particular subgroup of individuals (e.g., caregiver burden), or is the construct relatively invariant across age cohorts (e.g., some personality traits)? To what extent do age and correlates of age influence assessment? Assuming that the definition of the construct does not change across age groups, how are measures affected by such factors as cognitive dysfunction, frailty, age-related response bias, and educational level?

Although some constructs are relevant across the age span (their definition does not change), their measurement may be affected by prevalence. Certain health problems are more germane to older cohorts than to younger age groups. Response sets (possibly associated with age) may affect reporting of depression, pain, social relationships, and life events. Rater bias may play a role as well; for example, raters have been found to rate older people as more functionally impaired than equally disabled younger individuals (Fisher, 1993). Rater perceptions also play a role. For example, the slackened jaw characteristic of some older people may affect ratings of affect.

Manifestations (indicators) of some constructs may be different for different groups. For example, the types of disturbed behaviors associated with dementia are different from those associated with schizophrenia. Communication or perceptual difficulties associated with age may affect measurement of some domains (e.g., cognitive impairment). Other age-associated conditions (frailty, cognitive disorder) may result in floor and ceiling effects for certain measures (gait and balance, cognitive measures).

The substantive chapters are grouped roughly into sections dealing with behavioral content (chapters 2 through 8), intrapersonal processes (chapters 9 through 13), and ecological processes (chapters 14 and 15). The concluding chapter 16 is devoted to measures that incorporate all three types of content.

The behavioral section roughly corresponds to the domains of behavioral competence posited by Lawton (1983). In chapter 2 Lawton and Lawrence anchor their conception of health within Lawton's quadripartite schema for quality of life, demonstrating how rough are the generalizations that attempt to distinguish between behavior and intrapersonal processes. Although "objective" and "subjective" aspects of health represent a useful distinction, and physical health requires operational distinction from mental health for heuristic reasons, the boundaries are tenuous. In their discussion of health as a measurement issue, Lawton and Lawrence lean heavily on facets of health defined empirically by investigators. Their message is that few of these facets are mutually redundant; some additional information is afforded by using a measure tapping each facet. The investigator must be aware of the areas of overlap and nonoverlap that characterize any particular pair or group of measures and must match conceptual goals with an instrument whose focus is relevant to those goals.

Chapter 2 also positions in the overall model of health important subaspects of health that are given separate treatment in this volume: functional impairment (chapter 3), gait and balance (chapter 4), and pain (chapter 13). Of all the indicators of health status, the quality of performance or independence with which important daily activities are performed have been the most ubiquitous. Activities of daily living (ADL) are not only relatively easy to measure, but they constitute highly useful predictive measures regarding future state. Kovar and Lawton, in chapter 3, takes on the task of reviewing this area, simultaneously attempting to move ahead the state of the art. They begin with an important distinction that influences the form of all assessment instruments: whether the purpose of assessment is clinical or epidemiological. The power of ADL assessment for epidemiological and service-planning purposes is great. The chapter reviews the history and uses of assessment in the epidemiological mode, as well as some important issues in the technology of this branch of assessment. Especially noteworthy is the emphasis on the World Health Organization's conception of health and its place in overall quality of life (see also Lawton & Lawrence, chapter 2). The social-contextual locus of health in the pathway from disease to impairment to disability to handicap is a model that should guide health researchers far more than it presently does.

It is also important to note a number of different issues that still need to be addressed in evaluating ADLs for clinical purposes. Practitioners often see existing ADL scales as being too gross to be useful for describing current function, for pointing to possible interventions, or for sensing change. Clinically directed ADL assessment, then, requires the attention of measurement specialists.

As compared with health measurement in general and with ADL measurement in particular, Duncan and Studenski's chapter 4, on gait and balance, represents a much more restricted area. From the points of view of both physical mobility and the subjective confidence or security that accompanies everyday motor behavior, the functions of gait and balance are highly salient to everyday function and to quality of life in general. As the authors make clear, these functions typically have been studied in clinical fashion by professionals outside the mainstream of formal assessment in the psychometric sense. Duncan and Studenski clearly recognize the need to formalize. The further question as to whether gait and balance assessment can be incorporated into the pan-professional, generalized functional assessment battery remains an open question. Clinical judgments are still often required among the suggested measures, and issues of safety for the subject being evaluated are still acutely relevant. For these reasons, it is possible that gait and balance, more than many of the assessment domains reviewed here, will continue to fall in the specialty assessment area. Nonetheless, Duncan and Studenski have integrated an immense amount of hard-to-locate information on the technology and psychometrics of gait and balance assessment that will be helpful to both the generalist and the specialist.

From health, attention turns in chapter 5 to cognitive function. Albert's focus is on cognitive screening, rather than on the task of assessing cognition throughout its full range. Cognition is a function in which impairment often may be discerned through relatively simple testing that assumes that any positive sign is a signal for in-depth evaluation by neurological and neuropsychological methods. A number of options for such screening assessments are now available, including some that attempt to adjust scores in relation to educational experiences and another designed for telephone screening. Albert also reviews clinical ratings of dementia, a category that does not fit completely the criterion of nonprofessional use; nonetheless, professionally rated systems for designating degree of intactness or impairment have the great advantage of relative simplicity plus an ability to communicate clinical judgments among treatment staff.

Although behavioral pathology is not a category in Lawton's behavioral competence schema, in a sense, inappropriate behavior may occur in any of the health, cognitive, time-use, and social domains. "Incompetence" is a social normative judgment made regarding the adaptive quality of behavior in everyday situations. In chapter 6, Teri and Logsdon note the absence of a unitary defining structure for "behavioral disturbance." Yet clinicians have little difficulty comprehending the term, whether they are dealing with dementing illness, psychosis, or acting-out behavior. Nonetheless, in the absence of a firm theoretical structure, measurement technology for behavior pathology lags somewhat behind some of the areas more closely tied to social, psychological, or medical science. For example, very different manifestations of pathology might be expected to occur, depending on whether the underlying illness is dementia, depression, or schizophrenia. Yet, in practice, symptoms tend to co-occur, so that we have scales measuring "depression in dementia" and so on. Notably lacking in the literature, as well as in Teri and Logsdon's chapter, are attempts to measure behavioral disturbances that might be associated with personality disorders.

Their review describes current hurdles to successful behavioral measurement, for example, the tendency for investigators to construct their own measures, rather than to use standard ones. From a psychometric point of view, Teri and Logsdon assert that homemade measures tend to be incompletely analyzed and reported. Their overview makes clear to the reader the breadth of what is available, the very different purposes of each, and the psychometric beauties and blemishes of the array of measures.

The next two chapters' concerns move from issues that are particularly relevant to clinical assessment and the identification of pathology to realms that represent a much broader spectrum of the functioning of older people. Mannell and Dupuis' chapter 7 deals with measuring the activities and meaningful uses of time by older people in general. Although leisure has been a favorite topic throughout the history of gerontology, how one assesses the prevalence, amount, or quality of time use has been of relatively little concern to gerontological assessment. For one thing, pathology is not necessarily manifested in this domain. One also feels that because leisure activities have been discussed primarily in terms of their ability to enrich "normal" elders' life styles, they have been considered irrelevant to the lives of impaired or deprived elders. Mannell and Dupuis take on the very special task of reviewing a number of constructs that leisure researchers have found useful in research with people of younger ages. Their review illustrates how much remains to be done in applying this knowledge to understanding older people. Reviewing the meaning and measurement of leisure constructs used in the general adult literature will provide a major resource for researchers seeking to extend such research into gerontology.

In chapter 8, Rook discusses social relationships, another domain that is frequently absent from the typical assessment battery. In addition to reviewing the content of many measures of social relationships, the organization of her chapter provides a way of conceptualizing this very complex domain. Thus content and concepts mutually feed each other. She organizes the topic into broad areas of *social integration* (which includes the many structured and network features of social relationships), *functional content* (the substance of relationships, including such facets as social support, companionship, social control, and conflictual relationships), and *evaluations* (subjective judgments regarding the adequacy of the quantity and quality of social relationships and the satisfaction they produce). Although this chapter provides the last word on assessment of social relationships, it also contributes immensely to our understanding of the many ambiguities of both concepts and methods in this area. Characterizing Rook's focus as behavioral does it an injustice, of course, because subjective as well as countable phenomena are necessary to the assessment process.

Although there are exceptions, the focuses for assessment represented in the remaining chapters lie somewhat outside the typical realm of functional assessment. They also inevitably reflect the psychological bias of the editors. On the other hand, the primarily intraindividual domains reviewed in this section all represent domains easily accommodated to assessment by the generalist using instruments that do not require high-level clinical expertise.

The broadest topic is that of personality assessment, treated by Aldwin and Levenson in chapter 9. This topic does not fully meet one of the defining criteria for functional assessment, the susceptibility to evaluation along a desirable to undesirable continuum. Many personality traits, needs, or dispositions vary along stylistic, rather than evaluational, continua. Other personality dimensions, however, do possess the evaluative connotation and, therefore, this domain is included. A strong overlay of methodological concern is exhibited in this chapter. The authors feel that any attempt to measure personality among older people must confront the issue of aging specifically and must address age-related change versus stability. They use the latter question to delimit the scope of their chapter, that is, to discuss personality measures that have been used in longitudinal studies of some portion of the later life span. Thus in addition to their invaluable documentation of the measurement characteristics of a number of personality inventories, they provide a dispassionate integration of the evidence regarding change and stability. They find evidence for continued change through the life span, against a background of relative stability. They conclude that the need continues for methodological improvements before the balance sheet can be appropriately constructed.

The next two chapters share parts of their topics with the domain of personality. Unquestionably, some personality traits are defined in terms of the probability that prototypical affect states will occur in certain individuals. Nonetheless, Schulz, O'Brien, and Tompkins (chapter 10) provide a discussion of emotion measurement that makes clear both the conceptual overlap and the high points of measurement technology for characterizing the types of emotion experienced by older people.

They begin with a helpful introduction to the dimensions by which emotions may be characterized and the differentiation of emotion from related constructs. The reader is thus fully oriented to the position of emotion among a number of other psychological processes. The measures of affect are organized around several theoretical conceptions of emotions: basic emotions, a two-dimensional and hierarchically structured model, and a trait-oriented scheme. The strengths and weaknesses of a great many measures are critically discussed, to the great benefit of a researcher in search of the best measure for a specific purpose.

Chapter 11 by Pachana, Gallagher-Thompson, and Thompson moves toward the clinical area by reviewing depression as a focus for assessment. Some personality types appear especially susceptible to depression, and depression itself is one of the primary emotions. Depression warrants an entire chapter because it is one of the most common symptoms of psychological distress in older people, a fact that in turn explains the extensive use of various depression assessment tools among older people. There may be almost as much justification for the separate study of other emotions, such as anxiety, pleasure, or anger, in older people, but the requisite research for in-depth reviews of other affects is simply not yet in hand.

Pachana, Gallagher-Thompson, and Thompson cover assessment of depression both as a clinical diagnosis (primarily through structured diagnostic interviews) and as a negative affect (through both clinical interviews and structured, self-report instruments). Their chapter provides useful thoughts on special aspects of depression assessment: co-occurrence with physical illness; cognitive impairment; substance-abuse; differentiation from anxiety; and issues in assessing minority aged.

Caregiver stress and dynamics well may have been the favorite research topic of the past decade. To a greater extent than any other topic in this volume, caregiving assessment has relevance to gerontology when applied across the entire adult age span. That is, spouse caregivers and adult-child caregivers who are themselves over age 65 account directly for a substantial preponderance of caregiving. But more important, the well-being of caregivers of any age may have an impact on the well-being of the elder care receiver. Deimling's chapter 12 reviews the extensive literature on caregiving as a generic, rather than age-related role. Deimling begins with the excellent point that generalized indicators of well-being should be the starting point for assessing caregivers, and, furthermore, that there are excellent methodological reasons for making such assessments independent of any caregiving content. In a discussion specific to caregiving, Deimling provides considerable conceptual clarification as he addresses issues such as the frequently specious distinction between objective and subjective effects of caregiving and the role of attribution of well-being to caregiving activity. The bulk of the chapter is devoted to in-depth reviews of approaches to measuring caregiver burden, caregiver satisfaction, and other effects of caregiving on personal behavior and self-attitude, and to measuring the coping mechanisms used by caregivers. Throughout the chapter the relevance of assessment to service delivery is emphasized.

Pain, discussed in chapter 13 by Patricia Parmelee, constitutes another topic whose relevance for routine assessment has been inadequately recognized. As Lawton and Lawrence note in chapter 2, pain and subjective distress represent an essential component of illness. Despite general recognition of this fact, pain assessment has tended either to remain in the province of pain specialists or to be embedded in general or disease-specific indicators of health without differentiation from a number of other conceptually different aspects of health. By providing this first critical review of concepts and measures of pain, Parmelee's chapter serves as a potential beginning point for new research efforts that will result in an understanding of pain in relation to other aspects of well-being. Although we are regrettably short on brief measures of pain that have been tested on and deemed suitable for older persons, Parmelee provides a comprehensive review of the meaning of pain and its dimensions. With this conceptual overview, researchers of the future should be much better equipped to create and use age-specific measures while doing justice to the essential dimensions of pain.

Although the older person is also the focus of the next two chapters, the authors of both recognize the need to encompass the environmental context in what is measured. Carp provides an update and critical overview of approaches to measuring environments of particular interest to older people. Most assessment in this area has been driven by the need to design actual environments, such as those in housing, institutions, and, more recently, in ordinary community-based housing. Such pressure has resulted in a reduction of effort in theoretically relevant environmental research and a focus on market-oriented research. A historical review of the progression of this research results in the conclusion that there is much more potential for relating physically defined environmental measures to older persons' well-being than has yet been recognized. Continued use of theory in formulating research and the application of systematic quantitative and qualitative research methods are seen as necessary for environmental research to thrive.

Zautra, Affleck, and Tennen devote chapter 15 to the measurement of events in the lives of older people. The phenomenon that we refer to as "an event" almost always depends on both the person and the environment for its definition. Zautra and colleagues provide the conceptual basis for the meaning of events in discussions of the ambiguity of the location of an event (in the person? in the environment?) and the many possible dimensions by which events may be characterized. The central focus of the chapter lies in the authors' thesis that both major and minor events are relevant to the older person's life style and well-being. This chapter represents the first attempt to review new methodological approaches to the study of small events and to point out their potential for research with older people. As in other chapters on domains not well represented in research, this review should act as an effective stimulus for new research of this type.

The volume ends with George's chapter on multidimensional assessment instruments, a fitting final chapter because measures of many dimensions discussed in the separate chapters are included in the multidimensional packages. Because there are relatively few such instruments, George's discussions are detailed and scrupulously objective in discussing the strengths and weaknesses of each. She addresses the differences between the clinical assessment connoted by the term "comprehensive geriatric assessment" and the types of assessment best suited for research or for service screening outside the explicit medical context. She ends with a major challenge for multidimensional assessment: to generate evidence that justifies the expenditure of the extra time required for broad-spectrum, psychometrically acceptable assessment when performed in a service-relevant context. Short cuts are tempting and are often selected by busy service providers; empirical data regarding the merits of better methods are the only effective counteractant to this tendency.

WHAT ELSE IS THERE TO ASSESS?

Although the editors would have liked this volume to treat every topic worth assessing, no single volume could possibly do justice to such a task. We acknowledge such gaps and suggest, in this final section, topics where reviews of assessment technology would be welcome. The emphasis will be placed primarily on designating the omitted topics, without either offering reasons for the omissions or providing any extensive references to other treatments of the topic.

Health. Vision and audition assessment, mentioned in chapter 2, warrant more in-depth treatment. Gait and balance (chapter 4) are only two subdomains of many more that could be discussed in the category of motor function. Strength, dexterity, and range of motion each deserve consideration as possible elements of modules in a general-purpose assessment. Fine-grained, clinically oriented ADL assessment instrumentation could be developed with more input from the rehabilitation disciplines. Finally, a very complex area in which there is a large body of literature is the health decision-making area, where pathology and quality of life intersect—"health utility" research (see Kane and Kane, 1981; Kaplan and Bush, 1982). More remains to be done on the tradeoffs between length of life and quality of life and the conditions that mediate different tradeoffs.

Cognition. Functional assessment was never intended to subsume intellectual assessment of the type possible using the Wechsler Scales (Wechsler, 1981), or the research-oriented specialty assessments of memory, reasoning, and other forms of cognitive processing. Nonetheless, there is a range of such functions where rough screening may be of assistance for specific purposes. Situations where broad cognitive screening is appropriate include memory clinics, postretirement educational settings, or leisure counseling.

Other behavior. Psychopathology other than the varieties discussed in chapter 6 is deserving of treatment in age-specific terms. For example, schizophrenia, the various forms of personality disorders, and substance addiction do occur in older people. Although even basic clinical knowledge regarding these syndromes in old age is in short supply, a review of assessment-related issues would be helpful.

Coping behavior is a very important topic, alluded to in chapters 9 and 12, but clearly deserving of a separate critical review of the now substantial number of modes for assessing coping behavior.

Intrapersonal constructs. Although the subjective aspects of activities (chapter 7), social relationships (chapter 8), and residential environment (chapter 14) are good examples of specific domains of everyday life capable of being perceived and evaluated by the subject, they constitute only two of many other such domains that fall into the perceived quality of life sector posited as one of the four major categories of quality of life. Although the classic adult studies of quality of life (Andrew & Withey, 1976; Campbell et al., 1976) remain the source of most information regarding measurement in this sector, it is probably time for another broad search of the literature to find smaller studies that have advanced our ability to measure the perceived quality of different domains of older persons' lives, such as friendships, daily time use, or late-life marriage.

The set of domains often called life satisfaction or morale have been omitted from this volume. We felt that at this point in the development of gerontology, greater focus on more differentiated constructs representing psychological well-being would provide a better contribution and therefore commissioned the specific chapters on affect and depression.

Absence of material dealing with the self represents another gap. However, the editors are inclined to feel that this elusive construct is still not well-enough understood to afford any possibility of confident measurement, at least insofar as self can be clearly differentiated from other types of psychological well-being.

Attitudes may well require their own book. The same may be true of values. On the other hand, there is no compelling rationale for their inclusion in a standard functional assessment battery done either to provide a broad context within which to base a more focused research inquiry or to serve as an efficient clinical screening battery. Attitudes thus may constitute a stand-alone domain where research investigating problems dealing with attitudes are the focus.

In conclusion, although the editors deny the intent to be all-inclusive in representing all that is out there waiting to be assessed, that broad expanse is also finite. Our hope is that the largest part of that expanse has been included in this volume and that what is not included will be treated in timely fashion by others.

REFERENCES

Andrews, F. M., & Withey, S. B. (1976). *Social indicators of well-being*. New York: Plenum Press.

Bowling, A. (1991). *Measuring health: A review of quality of life measurement scales*. Philadelphia: Open University Press.

Burt, R. S., Wiley, J. A., Minor, M. J., & Murray, J. R. (1978). Structure of well-being. *Sociological Methods and Research, 6*, 365–406.

Campbell, A., Converse, P., & Rodgers, W. (1976). *Quality of life in America*. New York: Russell Sage.

Fisher, A. G. (1993). The assessment of IADL motor skills: An application of many-faceted Rasch analysis. *The American Journal of Occupational Therapy, 47*, 319–329.

Kane, R. A., & Kane, R. L. (1981). *Assessing the elderly*. Lexington, MA: Lexington Books.

Kane, R. L., & Kane, R. A. (1982). *Values in Long-term care*. Lexington, MA: Lexington Books.

Kaplan, R. M., & Bush, J. W. (1982). Health-related quality of life measurement for evaluation research and policy analysis. *Health Psychology, 1*, 61–80.

Lawton, M. P. (1970). Ecology and aging. In L. A. Pastalan & D. H. Carson (Eds.), *Spatial behavior of older people* (pp. 40–67). Ann Arbor: Institute of Gerontology, University of Michigan.

Lawton, M. P. (1983). Environmental and other determinants of well-being in older people. *The Gerontologist, 23*, 349–357.

Lawton, M. P. (1986). Functional assessment. In L. Teri & P. M. Lewinsohn (Eds.), *Clinical assessment and treatment of the older adult* (pp. 39–84). New York: Springer.

Lawton, M. P., & Storandt, M. (1984). Assessment of older people. In P. M. Reynolds & G.

J. Chelune (Eds.), *Advances in psychological assessment* (Vol. 6, pp. 236–276). San Francisco: Jossey-Bass.

Mangen, D. J., & Peterson, W. A. (Eds.). (1982). *Research instruments in social gerontology* (Vols. 1–3). Minneapolis: University of Minnesota Press.

McDowell, I., & Newell, C. (1987). *Measuring health: A guide to rating scales and questionnaires*. New York: Oxford University Press.

Stewart, A. L., & Ware, J. E. (Eds.). (1992). *Measuring functioning and well—being: The Medical Outcomes Study approach*. Durham, NC: Duke University Press.

Wechsler, D. (1981). *WAIS-R Manual: Wechsler Adult Intelligence Scale—Revised*. New York: Psychological Corporation.

CHAPTER 1

Overview of Methodological Issues in Gerontological and Geriatric Measurement

JEANNE A. TERESI
HEBREW HOME FOR THE AGED AT RIVERDALE
COLUMBIA UNIVERSITY CENTER FOR GERIATRICS AND GERONTOLOGY
NEW YORK STATE OFFICE OF MENTAL HEALTH

AND

DOUGLAS HOLMES
HEBREW HOME FOR THE AGED AT RIVERDALE

This chapter provides an overview of methodological issues raised by different authors with respect to constructs and measures presented in this volume. While some measurement problems (e.g., response bias) may apply to specific age cohorts, we argue that many measurement problems are not necessarily a function of the age cohort assessed, but of the varying distributions, rates, or ratios of the underlying attribute when measured across different samples of elderly, ranging from the normal well to the chronically impaired. Thus, although the focus of this review is on assessment of older persons, the concepts presented and the statistical problems and methods discussed are relevant to the entire age spectrum.

KEY MEASUREMENT ISSUES

Prerequisite to the tasks of classification and assignment is the availability of valid scales and/or procedures to be used in assessment. To the extent that scales tap domains extraneous to the desired classification, inappropriate assignments will follow.

Key measurement issues are (a) whether it is a state or a trait that is being assessed, (b) the extent to which the state or trait is observable, (c) the extent to which the state or trait is conceptualized as invariant across populations differing in such attributes as age and correlates of age, race/ethnicity, and education, (d) the extent to which the measures of states or traits are invariant, and (e) the prevalence of the state or trait in the study populations.

State Versus Trait

When Campbell and Fiske (Campbell & Fiske, 1959) published their landmark article on multitrait multimethod approaches to examining convergent and discriminant validity of measures, they were essentially referring to traits rather than to states. Two decades later, Fiske (1982), in summarizing the contemporary state of the art, conceded that the trait-method unit concept may have been too narrow. For example, traits referred primarily to "such attributes of persons as abilities and personality characteristics" (Fiske, 1982, p. 84). More recently, there has been concern about the trait-state distinction in measurement, particularly in the context of longitudinal assessment.

A *trait* is described as a stable entity, in its most narrow interpretation immutable and genetically predetermined (Hertzog & Nesselroade, 1987). Examples of such relatively stable traits are intelligence, aptitude, some personality constructs (e.g., extraversion), and some clinical conditions (e.g., low vision). On the other hand, constructs such as affect, disturbed behavior and caregiver burden are mutable, and, therefore, are viewed as *states*. However, the issue is somewhat more complicated than these simple examples suggest. It is possible for a construct to share elements of both states and traits. For example, attention deficit disorder is probably an inherited trait; the person always has this disorder, and thus has a high probability of exhibiting the indicators of the trait: rage reactions, inability to concentrate, impulsivity. Manifestation of any of these indicators, however, may be determined by hormonal fluctuations. Thus, the attention deficit disorder can be viewed as both a state and a trait. Rook (chapter 8 in this volume) suggests perceived social support as a construct which is viewed by some as a state, and by others as a personality trait because of traitlike stability in perceptions over time. Hertzog and Nesselroade (1987) give an example of extraversion as a stable trait; however, the indicator gregariousness can vary depending upon external situations. Aldwin and Levenson (chapter 9 in this volume) discuss extraversion and emotionality as examples of stable traits which may be heritable. However, they argue that longitudinal data supporting or refuting this interpretation is inadequate because intervals between measurement occasions are not of the length necessary to show change.

As these examples indicate, it is important first to provide a conceptual argument as to whether it is a state or a trait that is being assessed. Complicating this issue, while one may conceive of the latent underlying condition as a trait, the observed indicators may perform as state variables, that is, they may not be stable. This may be due to errors of measurement, or it may be because the paths of the observed indicators are such as to suggest that they cause, rather than are the effects of, the latent variable. If the latent variable is caused by the indicators, the estimated correlations among the indicators may be erroneously low. Chronic somatic disorder provides an example of the problem regarding the causal direction between a latent attribute and its indicators. The latent attribute is chronic illness; however, the attribute does not cause its indicators (arthritis, cardiovascular disease, circulatory disorder). Rather, the indicators are generative—they cause the latent variable. While the person is relatively stable in terms of having a disabling trait (chronic illness), the individual indicators themselves may change, depending upon medications, diet, etc. (see Cohen, Cohen, Teresi, Marchi, & Velez, 1990). For some structural equation modelling techniques, this can result in disattenuated (and spuriously higher or lower) estimates of longitudinal relationships between latent variables. These higher or lower longitudinal correlations or path coefficients will obscure the true nature of the latent variable, at times giving it the appearance of a state. This problem is relevant to the measurement and structural equation model presented by Lawton and Lawrence (chapter 2 in this volume). Are the indicators of health status causes of, or caused by, the latent variable? (this issue is discussed in more detail later in this chapter.)

Response format and the timing of the reporting period can determine whether the construct being measured is treated as a trait or a state. Schulz, O'Brien, and Tomkins (chapter 10 in this volume) refer to this in their chapter on measuring affect. They suggest that reporting on mood states over a period of 1 week, as contrasted with obtaining reports of current mood, may result in measurement of mood traits rather than states; this complicates attempts to measure, longitudinally, transient fluctuations related to environmental or other stressors.

Proper conceptual specification of constructs as states or traits has implications for study design and for the type of reliability analyses conducted. Specification is particularly germane to the selection of an analytic model, in terms of its relative degree of focus on either intraindividual or interindividual differences. As stated earlier, much of the literature focuses on traits, using nomothetic descriptors of interindividual differences (means and correlations). Hertzog and Nesselroade (1987) show that although examination of interindividual differences is useful for traits such as intelligence, intraindividual differences typically do not play a role because intelligence is not apt to change across measurement occasions. Yet, intraindividual differences are key to the measurement of states and to the determination of whether a construct is a trait or state (stable or not).

Hertzog and Nesselroade show that states can be measured reliably, and that fluctuations in states, although warranting careful interpretation, are not necessarily due to measurement error. However, they suggest that certain types of reliability estimates, for example, the test–retest procedure, are not appropriate for application to state measures. Two examples, presented in this volume, serve to illustrate this point. Some behavioral measures (see Teri & Logsdon, chapter 6) and some state aspects of environmental measures (see Carp, chapter 14) may not be best estimated using test–retest reliability. While certain aspects of agitated behavior (e.g., calling out) may act as trait variables, remaining relatively stable over time, other behavioral manifestations, such as physical aggression, may vary depending upon factors extraneous to the individual (presence of restraints, medications, environmental stimuli). Similarly, state components of the environment (e.g., odors) may change on an hourly basis, while trait components (size of a room) will not change at all.

Aldwin and Levenson (chapter 9, in this volume) grapple with the problem of interpreting longitudinal correlations as indicators of stability or change in personality measures. As they point out, "Given the lack of criteria for indicating change or stability, the same data set conceivably could yield opposite conclusions, depending upon the method of analysis and the predilections of the researchers" (p. 185). Statistics based on aggregated data (e.g., the correlation coefficient) leave the question of what constitutes significant change to subjective interpretation. Because correlations are not invariant with respect to prevalence, they will change as the sample characteristics change over time, making comparisons problematic. As Hertzog and Nesselroade (1987) state:

> A further complication is that attributions of stability seem to depend a great deal on the perspective of the interpreter. For example, a stability coefficient of +.60 over a period of 5 years can be interpreted as high or low, depending upon both psychometric concerns and one's theoretical orientation and expectations. (p. 94)

Kenny and Zautra (in press) provide an example of the difficulty in interpreting correlations between waves. Correlations of .53 or higher were observed between various 1-month waves of measures of life events. The authors conclude that these correlations might suggest an autoregressive factor indicative of stable individual differences associated with a trait. But the patterns might also be taken as evidence of a state variable with moderate correlations between waves. Because of this interpretive conundrum, Kenny and Zautra argue that one should examine both the trait component variance as well as the latent state variance.

In this context, simple autoregressive models (characterized by the regression of a variable on itself) may not be optimal models for examining states because there are several explanations for the magnitude of the autoregression (stability) coefficient (see Hertzog & Nesselroade, 1987). Longitudinal correlations of the same variable measured over several points in time will decrease with decreasing proximity of measurement times. The more proximal measures will correlate more highly (see Rogosa & Willet, 1985; Willet, 1985). This phenomenon of entropic stability over time may not be the ideal framework for modeling fluctuating constructs (see Hertzog & Nesselroade, 1987). However, recently, Kenny and Zautra (in press) present a model with autoregressive components as part of an overall examination of variance due to trait, state, and error (TSE) associated with a latent variable. Using structural equation modeling techniques to examine trait, state, and error variances for repeated measures of the small event, the authors view the stable individual differences in events as trait components and person-environment relationships as state components. While major life events are typically correctly viewed as states, Kenny and Zautra argue that it is realistic to view the small event as both a state and a trait. For example, they found an autoregressive statelike factor with respect to undesirable events suggesting a recurrence of small stressors; on the other hand, only 8% of the variance in desirable events were accounted for by state factors.

Aldwin and Levenson discuss the importance of ipsative studies of change, employing sequential designs and employing analytic methods such as growth curve analyses to disentangle both individual and group/cohort effects over time. A recent discussion of different approaches and the controversy surrounding the measurement of change can be found in an overview article by Teresi (1994) and in commentaries by Nesselroade (1994) and Rogosa (1994).

Observable or Not

Philosophy of Science Issues. A key issue in the measurement of traits and states is whether or not they are observable. Although some branches of science have well-developed theories and ultimate criteria against which measures can be validated, this is generally not the case in the behavioral and social sciences. Fallible signs or symptoms must serve to indicate the presence of a disorder, particularly when using self-reports rather than physiological indicators (see Teresi, Golden, Gurland, Wilder, & Bennett, 1984, p. 147).

Basic scientists often can sidestep the issue of validity. A lizard ear cell is precisely that—a lizard ear cell. At issue is not the question of recognition, but of the precision with which one counts these cells. The case is very different for the social, behavioral and medical sciences, where phenomena are less clearly observable, and valid and reliable systems for classification are not always available. One must rely on a series of laws relating observable measures to constructs, constructs to observable measures and constructs to constructs (Meehl, 1973) and this nomological network must be repeatable (Popper, 1959).

The focus of this book is on functional assessment. Most, if not all chapters in this volume are presentations of latent attributes, which must be measured by inference rather than by direct observation. The possible exception is offered by the chapter on gait and balance. Duncan and Studenski (chapter 4 in this volume) present some measures which are directly observable. Chapter 2 in this volume by Lawton and Lawrence focuses on functional health measures, which do not fit the category of directly observable phenomena, collectable via a blood assay. Similarly, chapter 13 by Parmelee presents pain measures which are largely subjective. Thus, validation is reliant on examination of the relational network among reputed measures of the same construct or among measures of different constructs. Although some of the chapters deal with clinical phenomena, which presumably could be validated against a "gold standard," such a measure is usually lacking or suspect. For example, chapter 11 by Pachana, Gallagher-Thompson, and Thompson, discusses screening and diagnostic measures of depression, and chapter 5 by Albert describes screening measures for dementia; both of these are constructs which can be validated using gold standards. However, the diagnostic gold standards themselves must also be validated. Cross-national gold standards themselves must also be validated. Cross-national studies of psychiatric disorder in the community provided evidence of differences in methods and patterns of diagnoses across sites and countries (Cooper et al., 1972; Sharpe et al., 1974). Specification of a conceptual model (nomological network) for measurement validation, therefore, is critical to the evaluation of the gerontological and geriatric constructs discussed in this volume. All authors have attempted to present such a model.

Adequate Definition. To the extent that the definition of the construct is murky, the measure will be inadequately applied. Some constructs, even if well-defined, are more difficult to assess because of their subjective nature (e.g., environmental constructs such as "warmth"; some affective states).

Measurement exists in the context of a theoretical causal structure; a construct is defined by its relationship to other constructs. As Teresi and colleagues note:

> Construct validation by definition assumes some theory of interrelationship; one predicts that given a certain condition, there is some likelihood that other conditions will also be present. If one fails to find the connection, then either the measure is lacking, the theory or parts of it is faulty, or both. If the expected association is present, then initial evidence, subject to cross-validation, is provided for the validity of the measure. (1984, p. 147)

Even a demographic data point such as gender is of interest only to the extent that there are individual differences in the variable that have some meaning (defined in relationships with other variables) beyond the mere existence of identification as male or female. The Eskimos' many words for snow differentiate beyond mere description: There are causal consequences associated with each definition of snow.

Affect and environment are two examples of domains which are particularly difficult to define and validate. Schulz and colleagues (chapter 10 in this volume) discuss the difficulty associated with operationally distinguishing affective disorders from life dissatisfaction, demoralization, and depression. They provide definitions and examples of how the constructs are different, but admit that the empirical differentiation is difficult. Similarly, Carp (chapter 14 in this volume) discusses the difficulty in validating environmental constructs. Generally, reliance is placed on examination of convergent and divergent posited relationships among environmental, other exogenous, and outcome variables. Finally, even a seemingly objective domain such as behavior disorder, if broadly enough defined can encompass many constructs which may or may not be conceptually and/or empirically distinct. Confusion, asocial activities, agitation, depression, and even self-care decrements can be viewed broadly as disturbed behaviors. Thus, a conceptual model is critical in differentiating among domains and constructs. Teri and Logsdon grapple with this problem in chapter 6 which deals with disturbed behavior.

While some phenomena, such as behavior disorder, are theoretically easier to measure because they are readily observable, there may be disagreement about the valence to attach to behaviors. Is pacing a maladaptive behavior in a demented person or an adaptive reaction to anxiety, more of a nuisance to the caregiver than to the patient? Additionally, as discussed here by Teri and Logsdon, if observational measures are used (short of extensive 24-hour observational periods), to what extent are they capturing a person's typical behavior? On the other hand, if informant reports are gathered, are perceptions consonant with reality? A similar problem is evident in the measurement of the small event. As Zautra, Affleck, and Tennen (chapter 15 in this volume) discuss, informant corroboration is better for some types of events than for others. Cutting across all domains discussed in this chapter is the ability of the older person to provide self-report data.

Returning to a point presented earlier, the type and validity of assessment may change as one moves from assessing a younger to an older population and within that from a well to a physically or cognitively impaired subpopulation. With a more cognitively impaired population, it may be necessary to converge upon valid assessment by collecting data from multiple sources (see Teresi, Lawton, Ory, & Holmes, 1994).

Invariance Issues in Assessing Scales

A central issue that is interwoven throughout the chapters in this volume is the extent to which age plays a role in measurement and assessment. Several issues emerge. First, to what extent are constructs invariant across age cohorts? Do the natures of the constructs change as one moves across age cohorts? Does the definition of the latent construct change?

A second issue is the extent to which the same measures can be applied across age cohorts. Are there response biases present which may alter the validity of the measure for certain age cohorts? Finally, at issue is how age is placed in conceptual models of relationships among constructs. Should age be considered as a moderator variable, as an interaction term, or as a main effect?

Invariance of States and Traits Across Populations. A basic assumption in comparing age cohorts is that the same construct is being measured across cohorts; however, there may be reason to question this assumption in some areas. For example, Mannel and Dupuis (chapter 7 in this volume) point out that the definition of leisure may be different across age groups. Similarly, Parmelee, in discussing the measurement of pain (chapter 13), considers the age by stimulus intensity interaction indicating that older people as contrasted with younger age cohorts are less likely to report low intensity stimuli as painful. The question can be raised as to whether pain is actually a different construct for older and younger cohorts. Is there a physiological difference at the biochemical level in reaction to a pain stimulus across age cohorts, implying a different definition of pain for older people, or do older people have the same sensory experience but report differential levels of pain due to bias—the "rosy response" described by Carp and Carp (1982), denial, or some other mechanism. A third hypothesis is that age interacts with physical illness so that those in chronic pain due to other disorders, when presented with the same stimulus, have the same physiological response, but evaluate their pain differently because it feels less intense than other chronic pain.

If the definition of leisure or of the physiological response of the organism to pain is different across age cohorts, the implication is that different measures should be constructed for different age cohorts and that comparisons across young and old age cohorts are not possible.

Invariance of Measuring Instrument Across Populations. A second issue regarding invariant measures is more difficult to address. Here, the definition of the state or trait is not different across age cohorts, but the measure is performing differently owing to response or other bias. At issue here is the adequacy of the measure in terms of precision, reliability, validity (including sensitivity, specificity, and positive and negative predictive values), breadth of coverage, range of values (floor or ceiling effects), and acceptability. Response bias may take the form of the rosy or the cautious response. Length of the measure and complexity may affect responses. Factors which are correlated with age (cognitive impairment, physical frailty, chronic illness, perceptual disorders, experience, and wisdom) may impact on measurement. It is necessary to assess how well a measure developed for younger people operates with an older group, and how well a measure developed for younger–old stands up when applied to the old–old. Duncan and Studenski (chapter 4) discuss this problem in reference to measures of balance; many well elderly individuals (as contrasted with younger age groups) cannot stand on one foot. One can speculate that there is a fundamental change in balance with age that is uncorrelated with a disease process.

In addition to changes in performance associated with age, there is the more common problem of changes due to factors correlated with age. For example, performance on many cognitive screening tests is affected by visual impairment, a correlate of age. Superimposed on possible age effects are effects due to the setting in which measurement occurs. As Duncan and Studenski point out, it is not unusual for the floor effects in the nursing home to become the ceiling effects in the community.

A major problem outlined by Albert (chapter 5) is the extent to which cognitive measures maintain their range. Floor effects are frequently observed among old–old cohorts, among whom the prevalence of severe dementia is higher. At issue is the extent to which we attempt to extend the sensitivity of the measures at the tails of the distribution or, alternately, abandon these measures and switch to severe impairment batteries, possibly measuring different constructs in the process (see Zandi, 1994).

Measures may be too long when applied to some elderly samples. For example, scales such as the Profile of Mood States (McNair, Lorr, & Droppleman, 1971) reviewed by Schulz, O'Brien, and Tompkins (chapter 10 in this volume) may be too long for frail elders. Similarly, the response format (self- vs. interviewer-administered) may play a role in valid comparisons across age cohorts. Pachana and colleagues (chapter 11 in this volume) point out that studies of different depression screening measures have found that frail elderly have a higher rate of nonresponse to self-administered rating scales. The authors also discuss the fact that complicated Likert-type or frequency response categories may be too difficult for some elderly with lower educational levels. Vocabulary level of the scale is an issue; if abstract terminology is used to describe mood states, this may result in cultural and educational bias. Education is also a major confound in cognitive assessment (see chapter 5 by Albert in this volume).

Carp (chapter 14) discusses age effects in a slightly different context. She calls for age-unbiased measures to be used across age cohorts, citing similar factor structures for environmental scales across six age cohorts from 18 to over 70 years old as evidence of lack of bias in a measure she developed (Carp & Carp, 1982). She points out that the "rosy" response bias (in assessing environments) which was frequently attributed to aging was actually present to some degree in younger cohorts as well. This points up a possible danger in studying only tails of the age distribution: In the absence of comparative data from younger groups, a distorted view about characteristics of older cohorts may result.

Such possible distortion is a major point of discussion in chapter 9 by Aldwin and Levenson. They point out that many personality measures are constructed using college-aged individuals; items may not be relevant to the experiences of older individuals. The authors note that even though age-neutral items are used, the factor structures may be different across age cohorts, indicating that items "may mean different things to an older population" (p. 184). Further, similarity of the factor structures across two age cohorts does not mean that they will be similar across populations differing in physical and mental frailty, both of which correlate with age). For example, Pachana, Gallagher-Thompson, and Thompson (chapter 11 in this volume) point out that although Hertzog, Van Alstine, Usala, and Hultsch (1990), using confirmatory factor analysis, found factor structure of the Center for Epidemiological Studies Depression Scale (CES–D) to be invariant across age cohorts, the scale response values (frequency ratings) have been found too difficult for some older cohorts. Just because a scale has an invariant factor structure does not mean that it is unbiased for all comparison subgroups. Lawton and Lawrence, in their chapter on health measures, point out that somatic symptoms, which may represent severe indicators of psychological health in a younger cohort, may have a different connotation with respect to older age cohorts, for whom they are also measures of physical health. Another way of viewing this phenomenon is that the items may be related in a mathematically different way to the underlying attribute measured for different subgroups. This point is discussed in more detail below.

In terms of the placement of age in causal models, Zautra and colleagues (chapter 15 in this volume) posit that life events such as illness or death of family members may interact with age because they are viewed by older cohorts as fateful events. The age by life event interaction may indirectly effect outcomes by influencing psychological well-being, whereas ill health of the older person will act directly on outcomes. Deimling (chapter 12) discusses caregiving in the context of comprehensive multidimensional models. The caregiving context (relationship, family structure, living arrangement), the caregiving effects (physical and mental health of the caregiver, positive and negative effects of caregiving) and the caregiver's coping resources are factors that can be placed in different conceptual models, the most prevalent of which is the stress model. Caregiver age may be a moderator variable. Because 35% of caregivers are elderly spouses and because a large proportion of adult–child caregivers are themselves elderly, different relationships among variables may be observed for these older caregivers in contrast with younger caregivers. Lawton and Lawrence in this volume discuss the causal role of health variables. In older cohorts, do somatic symptoms represent an outcome or an exogenous variable in structural equation causal analysis? Are they indicators of the latent physical health variable or the latent psychological health variable in a measurement model?

Prevalence

One factor complicating assessment is the low prevalence (base rate) of many states. Taking the case of the clinical traits or states [clinical depression, dementia, physical health, incapacity in activities of daily living (ADL)] discussed in this volume, the setting and prevalence influence the accuracy of assessment. It can be shown mathematically that a threshold score developed for one purpose (e.g., minimizing the variance of a prevalence estimate) may not be the best for another purpose (minimizing false negative misclassifications or maximizing overall correct classification rates) (see Hand, 1987). Many commonly used screening measures have been developed for prevalence estimation. This is relevant to the discussion by George (chapter 16 in this volume) of the transferability of comprehensive assessments across settings varying in modal response capability. She argues for the use of cutting scores, which are, indeed, important for comparison purposes; however, in screening cases for clinic referral, it may be necessary to adjust the score based on the characteristics of the population screened.

If a person presents with specific symptoms to a clinic and reports a history of disorder, it makes assessment easier; however, if the person is presenting for the first time or is observed in a community setting, assessment is much more difficult. The problem is even trickier when it is necessary to assess nonclinical constructs (e.g., personality or social supports) for which there may be few normative data and, thus, no expected distribution of the trait or state. As Gurland and colleagues (1977) discuss:

> The situation is very different with regard to persons who have been randomly selected from the community-based population. It cannot be assumed that their symp-

toms (if any) have clinical significance, nor if they do have significance, to which disciplinary domain they might pertain. For example, weight loss which may indicate depression in a hospitalized psychiatric patient may, in a community resident, just as well be normal (e.g., the person is on a reducing diet), due to a medical condition (e.g., a wasting disease), or due to a social condition (e.g., poverty, or lack of help in preparing food). (p. 18)

STATISTICAL/MEASUREMENT ISSUES IN GERONTOLOGICAL AND GERIATRIC ASSESSMENT

Problems Associated with Classical Test Theory

Problems of comparability in comparisons of psychometric properties across populations which vary in base rates plagues measurement research. As discussed in the previous sections, most chapters in this volume address constructs which are affected by the base rate.

There has been recent controversy regarding the use of statistics based on classical test theory to summarize the psychometric properties of measures (Hambleton, Swaminathan, & Rogers, 1991; Uebersax, 1988). For example, Rook (chapter 8 in this volume) discusses the fact that items measuring received support, as contrasted with perceived support, may not be expected to intercorrelate because they tap selected services used. Thus, conventional methods of estimating reliability (internal consistency) may not be appropriate.

There is further controversy regarding the use of coefficients that are estimated using marginal probabilities because they are not invariant. For example, the most widely used method of examining interrater agreement for nominal data is κ or weighted κ (Cohen, 1960; Fleiss & Cohen, 1973). These methods have been criticized because the values will vary across populations differing in base rate of disorder (Spitznagel & Helzer, 1985). However, such purported solutions as the use of Yule's *Y* also suffer from some of the same problems as does κ (Shrout, Spitzer, & Fleiss, 1987). Similar problems are associated with measures of internal consistency such as Cronbach's α. Reliant upon average interitem correlations and, thus, degree of heterogeneity in the sample, the coefficient will vary across populations varying in item prevalences, rendering comparisons across samples problematic. Similarly, reliability estimates derived from factor loadings developed by the measurement component of structural equation models (e.g., lambdas from LISREL), are influenced by the base rate. Although such maximum likelihood estimates are more efficient, because the basic inputs are correlations or covariances (variant parameters), the base rate problem remains.

An example of this invariance issue is drawn from data presented in the paper by George (chapter 16 in this volume) showing reliabilities of different comprehensive assessments across populations. George cites, for example, reliabilities for some short version Comprehensive Assessment and Referral Evaluation (SHORT–CARE) scales across two different studies, the cross-national New York and London probability samples, (Gurland, Golden, Teresi, & Challop-Luhr, 1984) and the sample of older single-room occupancy residents (Cohen & Rajkowski, 1982). To the extent that the prevalences of disorders vary across samples, so too will the average possible correlations among items and the internal consistency estimates. It is necessary to consider the maximum reliability coefficient obtainable, given the prevalence of the state or trait and its associated indicators in the sample. This principle is illustrated using two samples of older community-resident elderly of different age cohorts. The first samples were probability samples of elderly aged 65 and over residing in the cities of New York ($n = 445$) and London ($n = 396$) (Gurland & Wilder, 1984), while the second was a United States sample ($n = 551$) of people 60 and over participating in the systolic Hypertension in the Elderly Program (SHEP) trials (Gurland et al., 1988; Hulley et al., 1985). The latter (SHEP) group was also, by exclusionary criteria, free of clinically diagnosable dementia, stroke with residual effects, cancer, chronic obstructive pulmonary disease, or heart attack within the last 6 months. The effects of prevalence on maximum obtainable alphas can be shown using the SHORT–CARE depression, cognitive impairment and activity limitation scales. The observed alphas for each scale in the community sample were .87, .84, .95, while in the SHEP sample, the comparable alphas were .74, .51, .84. Because coefficient α is a function of the number of items and the average interitem correlation, given a constant number of items, the item base rates will affect the α. In the community study the estimated prevalence ratios for depression, cognitive impairment and activity limitation were .10, .05, .20, respectively. In the SHEP study the prevalences for these scales were .03, .02, and .07. The observed estimates of the average interitem correlations for the community samples were .19, .35, and .35. Given the prevalence ratios observed in the SHEP study, the maximum estimated average interitem correlations would be .09, .17, and .26. When the prevalence is less than .05, the average interitem correlation is about one—half of the original estimate, resulting in lower possible (maximum) observed alphas. This is not new information; in fact, Carmines & Zeller (1979) provide a table of Cronbach's α values observed under different assumptions about the number of items and the average interitem correlations. Their table shows that given an average interitem correlation of .2, a 4-item scale will have an α of .50 and a 10-item scale a value of .71. On the other hand, if the average interitem correlation is .4, the 4-item scale will have an α of .73, the 10-item scale .87.

The same situation obtains for interrater reliability coefficients such as κ. Dunn (1989) recommends that the maximum obtainable κ should be reported along with the observed values.

The reliance of reliability estimates on the base rate of the state or trait in the sample has long been known; however, it is sometimes forgotten or ignored in evaluation of the psychometric properties of measures. The lack of invariance is less of a problem when prevalences and correlations are higher (prevalences above .2 and correlations of .4 and higher), as is typically the case with more normally distributed variables, for example, some personality variables. However, the problem is particularly relevant to clinical constructs: depression, affect, caregiver burden, behavior disorder, cognitive impairment, and many chronic illnesses. As the preceding section indicated, age can be an important factor affecting invariance because of different prevalence ratios across age cohorts.

Classical test theory parameters are group dependent. As Hambleton, Swaminathan, and Rogers (1991) point out, scale and item characteristics vary according to context. Thus it is difficult to compare different groups or age cohorts using such statistics. For example, the classical item difficulty parameter is estimated using the proportion admitting to a symptom or the proportion answering incorrectly on a cognitive item. It is obvious that for many constructs (depression, affect, cognition, behavior disorder, function, gait, balance, physical health status, and pain), this proportion will change as one moves from a young–old to an old–old cohort with higher disability levels. Thus, comparison of items using this statistic is problematic. The classical test theory item discrimination parameter (the corrected item-total correlation) suffers from the same lack of invariance. This estimate will vary across samples varying in the base rate of the state or trait. (See Teresi, Cross, and Golden, 1989, for a discussion.) Finally, the reliability coefficient estimated using classical test theory is problematic because an assumption of equal errors of measurement are made across all individuals, regardless of their standing on the latent attribute, an unrealistic assumption (see Hambleton et al., 1991). Measurement is more precise at different disability levels. Modern psychometric theory, discussed below, allows individual performance on an item to be related to disability level for the underlying attribute measured.

Nor are we spared the base rate problem in validity assessment. There is no way to select items to ensure reliability, while at the same time maximizing measure validity (see Lord & Novick, 1968). (A discussion of the relationship between reliability and validity is complex and beyond the scope of this presentation; however, it is noted that in classical test theory there is a paradox in the mathematical relationship between reliability and validity.)

Even in the instance of the most rigorous form of validity testing against an accepted criterion variable, it can be shown that, holding reliability constant, the positive predictive value is attenuated by low prevalence (Shrout & Fleiss, 1981). Shrout and Fleiss show that even at reliabilities as high as .80, the maximum positive predictive value for prevalence ratios below .05 is less than .70.

Invariant parameter estimates, such as those derived from modern psychometric theory, are promising for use in scale development. Following is a brief discussion of modern psychometric theory and some of the applications to measurement in aging research.

Modern Psychometric Theory

It would be remiss to undertake a volume on gerontological and geriatric assessment without discussing applications of modern psychometric theory. Most scales currently in use for assessment of the elderly have been developed or evaluated using classical test theory. This volume describes the current state of the art with respect to scale development; 10 years from now a similar volume will contain many new scales developed or old scales reevaluated using modern psychometric theory. Although the senior author first applied these methods to geriatric assessment in 1977, and first reported the results in 1981 (Teresi, Cross, Gurland, & Golden, 1981), except for a few scattered efforts the methods were not applied outside of educational testing until the mid to late 1980s. These methods are now beginning to be applied to the disciplines of psychiatry, psychology, neuropsychology, rehabilitation and occupational therapy and, cutting across these disciplines, gerontology and geriatrics. We believe that these methods will become the standards for scale development in the 21st century.

This section describes several advantages of modern psychometric theory, briefly presents the model and provides extant examples of the technique as applied to measures used with older persons.

Advantages of Modern Psychometric Theory. As a preface to this section, it should be noted that no modern method will supplant the need for the theory-driven approach to scale construction. As obvious as this may seem to many readers, there is a disturbing trend toward abandoning theory for blind pragmatism (see Holmes, Teresi, & Ory, 1993). This translates into, "It it works, use it." Too often, what works is vaguely defined as having a high α and correlates weakly with some dubious criterion using a small *n* and a nonrepresentative sample.

There is too much emphasis on maximizing α and too little on definition. It is too easy to combine a set of items, compute an α, correlate the measure with an outcome and publish it as a "reliable" and "valid" measure which will then be used time and again without much further investigation of its psychometric properties or meaning. Zautra and colleagues comment in this volume on the unfortunate practice on the part of some investigators to attempt to artificially increase the reliability (i.e., the internal consistency) of life events scales by measuring the event several times by including different aspects of the event as separate items.

Modern psychometric tools, meant to add to the ability to examine theoretical models, often have been misapplied, becoming agents of atheoretical tinkering used to produce a good model fit, even if the result bears little relationship to the original intent and makes little theoretical sense (see Cohen et al., 1990). Turning for an example to the measurement components of structural equation modelling, which is frequently used in confirmatory factor analysis, we return to an issue raised briefly earlier in this article: whether or not indicators of latent variables are generative. Many structural equation modelling programs are based on the premise that the construct is defined in terms of the indicators on which it has an effect; the latent variable explains (is the cause of) the correlations among the observed indicators. Some constructs could be both causal and emergent, depending upon the types of indicators. This issue warrants consideration in model specification, and may be particularly relevant to the health measures presented by Lawton and Lawrence in this volume (see chapter 2). Cohen et al. (1990) discuss the mathematical results when a latent variable is inadequately specified so that it does not explain a large proportion of each indicator variable. (The indicators in this case are not highly intercorrelated.) In addition to possible identification problems as a result of misspecification of the causal nature of the latent variable measured, many structural equation models will perform a correction for attenuation for less reliably measured variables, frequently resulting in inflated or deflated causal estimates.

An alternative method of scale construction which avoids some of these pitfalls is based on latent trait models, derived from item response theory (IRT; Lord, 1980). These models produce invariant parameters which are not sample dependent and, therefore, are not affected by disorder or item prevalence ratio differences.

IRT models, developed out of educational testing, have been used for the last two decades to develop ability and aptitude tests and examine item bias in these scales. (See Mislevy & Bock, 1984; Wood, Wingersky, & Lord, 1976; and Wright & Mead, 1977 for descriptions of computer programs.) The three-parameter model is typically used for this purpose. The probability of passing or failing an item is modeled as a function of the individual's standing on the latent attribute and three item characteristics (pseudo-guessing, difficulty, and discrimination).

For most constructs assessed in reference to older persons, including nearly all those reviewed in this volume, either the one-parameter (Rasch) or two-parameter models are used. This is because, unlike educational tests, it is unlikely that guessing plays a role in item response. The two-parameter (item discrimination and item difficulty) model is favored for evaluation of most psychiatric, cognitive and psychological scales because there is an interest in examining how well items discriminate at various points along the latent continuum; items which discriminate at a particular point or at various points can be selected for inclusion in a measure, depending on its purpose. The Rasch (one-parameter) model has been applied to ADL scales; this model assumes that items discriminate equally at different points along the latent attribute, but that item difficulty varies, and is thus estimated. Some prefer the Rasch model for the measurement of ADL because respondents can be located easily on the latent attribute and because extensions of the model (the many-faceted models) can be used to model and control rater bias in ADL assessments. (See the chapter by Kovar and Lawton for a discussion of sources of bias-associated with ADL measures.)

Advantages of item response theory in evaluating screening measures include: (a) use of the information function, which provides information about how an item performs at various points along the latent attribute continuum, for better selection of items to tailor tests for a specific purpose (Duncan-Jones, Grayson, & Moran, 1986; Gibbons, Clark, VonAmmon-Cavanaugh, & Davis, 1985), (b) the ability to identify items which are sensitive to change and which measure disability or ability across the entire latent attribute spectrum (Ashford, Colm, Colliver, Bekian, & Hsu, 1989), (c) the invariance properties of IRT, which allow examination of item bias across gender, racial/ethnic, age, and education subgroups (Teresi, Cross, & Golden, 1989; Teresi & Golden, 1994).

A further advantage of IRT is that it frees us from the necessity of rigidly assessing all individuals using exactly the same set of items. IRT parameters are distribution free; that is, ability can be estimated independently of measure version and population assessed. Because items have characteristics (difficulty parameters) which are invariant with respect to the prevalence of the disorder in the population assessed, item pools of varying item difficulty can be constructed and related to the disability of the individual assessed. The principles behind adaptive testing (i.e., allowing an estimate of the individual's ability to dictate whether harder or easier items are administered) is very attractive for neuropsychological testing, particularly among populations representing a range of cognitive disability. Very severely impaired individuals will tire and may refuse to complete lengthy batteries comprised of many items beyond their capability; conversely, intact individuals often become irritated at being asked many easy items. Fisher (1993a) provides an example of this in relation to application of the Rasch IRT model to motor instrumental activities of daily living (IADL). The methods of IRT allow the person to choose tasks to complete from among sets of items of equal challenge (difficulty). This allows optimal assessment of capability because motivational factors, such as, being forced to perform activities which are undesirable, are minimized. Both items and persons can be located on a common latent attribute. For Rasch analyses, the item difficulty estimate is the location of the item on the underlying latent ADL attribute; similarly, the person ability estimate is the location of the person on the line defined by the item difficulty (see Wright & Stone, 1979). Because the task difficulties are calibrated on the same metric as the underlying motor ability attribute, person ability is adjusted for task difficulty.

Another advantage of the IRT model is its ability to take rater bias into account; for example, the many-faceted Rasch model allows rater bias to be evaluated and controlled. In rating IADL items, some raters are more severe in their ratings and this severity may vary within raters. Lunz and Stahl (1993) observe that ratings are a function of stringency and floor and ceiling effects. Ability of an individual should be evaluated after taking into account such factors as rater stringency and difficulty of the item set. In the model applied by Fisher (1993a), rater leniency, skill item ease, task simplicity, and person ability are estimated. Person ability estimates are corrected for rater bias.

A disadvantage of interval scales developed using classical test theory is that intervals are rarely equal; a difference of one point on a scale may represent varying actual difference in terms of the latent attribute. Thus the assumption of additive equal intervals is violated. Item response theory circumvents this problem.

Final advantages of IRT include the ability to examine the fit of individual subjects and raters and the ability to estimate the reliabilities (termed efficiency in the three-parameter model, and separation reliability in the Rasch model) in terms of standard errors computed for each facet of the model and for different points along the measure of the latent attribute.

Item response theory models are based on the premise that there exists an underlying continuous attribute, the same for all subgroups of interest, and measurable using a set of fallible indicators of the underlying attribute. Clearly if different constructs are measured across subgroups, comparisons using any method are problematic. For example, Deimling (chapter 12 in this volume) discusses the utility of global measures of caregiver physical and mental health, which can be compared across younger and older caregiver and noncaregiver groups. Measures of specific caregiver constructs (e.g., burden) will not allow such comparisons.

Assuming the same construct is measured, the models derived from modern psychometric theory produce invariant parameters (item difficulty, item discrimination) which are not sample dependent and, therefore, are not affected by disorder or item prevalence ratio differences. Because these models relate item characteristics to the underlying attribute, they take disability (ability) level into account. The most commonly used IRT model defines the conditional probability of passing an item, given standing on the latent attribute, using the cumulative logistic function. A detailed explication of the model is beyond the scope of this chapter. (See Hambleton et al., 1991, and Teresi et al., 1989, for reviews.)

Examples. Modern psychometric theory is beginning to be used in the development and evaluation of measures of behavioral, social, psychological, and gerontological constructs. Pachana, Thompson, and Gallager-Thompson comment in the current volume on the need for examining possible cultural differences and biases in the assessment of depression across minority groups. Item response theory is the preferred method for examining group invariance, and for estimating item difficulty and discrimination. Modern psychometric theory has demonstrable utility in the development and evaluation of mental health and depression measures. For example, Duncan-Jones, Grayson, and Moran (1986) used IRT to examine the 12-item General Health Questionnaire using a probability sample of 3,000 male and 3,000 female Australians. Two items (feeling constantly under strain and feeling unable to overcome difficulties) are more related to depression for females than they are for males.

Gibbons et al. (1985) discuss the applicability of item IRT to analyses of depression using the Beck Depression Inventory, comparing severity and discrimination parameters across two samples: medically ill inpatients and psychiatric patients. The authors identified items with poor discrimination parameters (vegetative symptoms such as sleep disorders, poor appetite, weight loss) as well as items which discriminate best for depression across both samples (sense of failure, dissatisfaction, suicidal thoughts, loss of social interest, indecision, and sense of punishment). The vegetative symptoms of weight loss and loss of sexual interest were particularly poor discriminators of depression severity among the medically ill sample. Two items (loss of satisfaction and loss of social interest) were found to best assess depression severity.

Grayson (1987) used IRT models to investigate the bimodality versus dimensionality of psychiatric constructs such as schizophrenia and depression. Item response theory was appropriate to this investigation because generated invariant parameters will identify where and how an item discriminates. If all items discriminate at one point on the latent attribute, this is suggestive of bimodality, which would indicate a taxonic (dichotomous) rather than a dimensional (continuous) construct). Grayson, however, points out that this result is frequently an artifact of a priori selection of items (such as suicide or hopelessness) for a scale where all items discriminate at a very severe level of impairment; or of selection bias associated with selecting artificially taxonic samples (inpatients vs. normals). He suggests use of community samples rather than clinic samples to develop measures of depression, concluding that IRT should be used to select items which discriminate best at varying points along the latent continuum in order to adequately represent all levels of depression.

In an examination using IRT of item bias associated with the SHORT–CARE Depression Scale as used in a study of a probability sample of Hispanic elderly in Los Angeles (Kemp, Staples, Lopez-Aqueres, 1987; Lopez-Aqueres, Kemp, Plopper, Staples, & Brummel-Smith, 1984), Teresi and Golden (1994) found that some of the somatic symptoms (i.e., headaches), crying, and lack of interest, were relatively less severe indicators of depression for minority group members. In concert, these studies show some of the merits of using item response theory to evaluate depression items.

One of the few published studies applying IRT analyses to cognitive screening items used with the elderly was conducted by Ashford et al. (1989), who examined Mini-Mental State Examination (MMSE) item difficulties (Folstein, Folstein, & McHugh, 1975), classifying items as early or late memory loss indicators. They found that items measuring recent memory (items recalled after distractors and serial sevens) constitute more difficult early loss items; middle loss items are orientation (time and place) and remote memory items (dates of past events) representing temporal-parietal brain function. Later loss items, measuring frontal lobe impairment, include simple commands. Late loss items are expressive language items such as naming objects, reading, and writing. Most recently, Teresi et al. (in press) identified several cognitive test items which were biased for educational and/or ethnic/race groups.

Finally, IRT has been used to evaluate or develop ADL scales. Teresi, Cross, and Golden (1989) used IRT to evaluate bias associated with setting (London vs. New

York nursing homes) using a measure of basic ADL. The results were used to correct epidemiological estimates of ADL impairment in nursing homes in the two cities.

Recently IRT has been applied to analysis of ADL and IADL measures used with elderly and nonelderly in rehabilitation settings (see Fisher, 1993b). Because the scales involve ratings made by rehabilitation specialists, the many-faceted Rasch model was used to estimate ability, controlling for rater severity and ADL task difficulty.

SUMMARY

This chapter has reviewed a number of methodological issues addressed by the authors contributing to this volume. Generally speaking, these are issues relevant to measurement across the age spectrum, and to any subgroup of any age cohort. For example, difficulties associated with the definition, recognition, and measurement of fallible indicators is characteristic of social science in connection with any population group. That is not to say that the relative emphasis placed on a particular issue will not differ across groups. Thus, while floor effects in cognitive assessment may require little attention among the general population, this becomes a matter of paramount concern when dealing with nursing home populations.

This observation reflects the intent and, hopefully, the function of this chapter: to sensitize the reader to issues which lie at the base of social gerontological measurement. Each of these issues is explored at some length in the body of this text. Throughout, the aim is to present material grounded in well-known principles of measurement that both alerts the reader to precepts often overlooked and, in some cases, "stretches the envelope" by presenting materials and concepts which have yet to receive widespread attention. Thus, the methods of modern psychometric theory are offered as possible solutions to some of the issues presented. These methods show promise for application to gerontological and geriatric assessment and will undoubtedly become widely used for scale construction and evaluation over the next decades.

REFERENCES

Ashford, W. J., Kolm, P., Colliver, J. A., Bekian, C., & Hsu, L. N. (1989). Alzheimer patient evaluation and the Mini-Mental State: Item characteristic curve analysis. *Journals of Gerontology: Psychological Sciences, 44*, P139–P146.

Campbell, D. T., & Fiske, D. W. (1959). Convergent and discriminant validation by the multitrait–multimethod matrix. *Psychological Bulletin, 56*, 81–105.

Carmines, E. G., & Zeller, R. A. (1979). *Reliability and validity assessment: Sage University paper on quantitative applications in the social sciences*. Beverly Hills: Sage.

Carp, F. M., & Carp, A. (1982). Perceived environmental quality of neighborhoods. Development of assessment scales and their relation to age and gender. *Journal of Environmental Psychology, 2*, 295–312.

Cohen, J. (1960). A coefficient of agreement for nominal scales. *Educational Psychological Measurement, 20*, 37–46.

Cohen, C., & Rajkowski, H. (1982). What's in a friend? Substantive and theoretical issues. *The Gerontologist, 22*, 261–266.

Cohen, P., Cohen, J., Teresi, J., Marchi, M., & Velez, N. (1990). Problems in the measurement of latent variables in structural equations causal models. *Applied Psychological Measurement, 14*, 183–196.

Cooper, J. E., Kendell, R. E., Gurland, B. J., Sharpe, L., Copeland, J. R. M., & Simon, R. J. (1972). Psychiatric diagnosis in New York and London: A comparative study of mental hospital admissions. Maudsley Monograph No. 20. London: Oxford University Press.

Duncan-Jones, P., Grayson, D. A., & Moran, P. A. P. (1986). The utility of latent trait models in psychiatric epidemiology. *Psychological Medicine, 16*, 391–405.

Dunn, G. (1989). *Design and analysis of reliability studies*. New York: Oxford University Press.

Fisher, A. G. (1993a). The assessment of IADL motor skills: An application of many-faceted Rasch analysis. *The American Journal of Occupational Therapy, 47*, 319–329.

Fisher, W. P. (1993b). Measurement-related problems in functional assessment. *The American Journal of Occupational Therapy, 47*, 331–338.

Fiske, D. W. (1982). Convergent-discriminant validation in measurements and research strategies. In D. Brinberg & L. Kidder (Eds.), *New directions for methodology of social and behavioral science: Forms of validity in research*. (pp. 77–92). San Francisco: Jossey-Bass.

Fleiss, J. L., & Cohen, J. (1973). The equivalence of weighted kappa and the intraclass correlation coefficient as measures of reliability. *Educational and Psychological Measurement, 33*, 613–619.

Folstein, M. F., Folstein, S. E., & McHugh, P. R. (1975). Mini-Mental State: A practical guide for grading the cognitive state of patients for the clinician. *Journal of Psychiatric Research, 12*, 189–198.

Gibbons, R. D., Clark, D. C., VonAmmon-Cavanaugh, S., & Davis, J. M. (1985). Application of modern psychometric theory in psychiatric research. *Journal of Psychiatric Research, 19*, 43–55.

Grayson, D. A. (1987). Can categorical and dimensional views of psychiatric illness be distinguished? *British Journal of Psychiatry, 151*, 355–361.

Gurland, B. J., Golden, R. R., Teresi, J. A., & Challop-Luhr, J. (1984). The SHORT–CARE: An efficient instrument for the assessment of depression, dementia and disability. *Journal of Gerontology, 39*, 166–169.

Gurland, B., Kuriansky, J., Sharpe, L., Simon, R., Stiller, P., & Birkett, P. (1977). The Comprehensive Assessment and Referral Evaluation (CARE)—rationale, development and reliability. *International Journal of Aging and Human Development, 8*, 9–42.

Gurland, B., Teresi, J., McFate-Smith, W., Black, D., Hughes, G., & Edlavitch, S. (1988). Effects of treatment for isolated systolic hypertension on cognitive status and depression in the elderly. *Journal of the American Geriatrics Society, 36*, 1015–1022.

Gurland, B. J., & Wilder, D. E. (1984). The CARE Interview Revisited: Development of an efficient, systematic clinical assessment. *Journal of Gerontology, 39*, 129–137.

Hambleton, R. K., Swaminathan, H., & Rogers, H. J. (1991). *Fundamentals of item response theory.* Newbury Park, California: Sage.

Hand, D. J. (1987). Screening vs. prevalence estimation. *Applied Statistics, 36,* 1–7.

Hertzog, C., & Nesselroade, J. R. (1987). Beyond autoregressive models: Some implications of the trait-state distinction for the structural modeling of developmental change. *Child Development, 58,* 93–109.

Hertzog, C., Van Alstine, J., Usala, P. D., & Hultsch, D. F. (1990). Measurement properties of the Center for Epidemiological Studies Depression Scale (CES–D) in older populations. *Psychological Assessment, 2,* 64–72.

Holmes, D., Teresi, J., & Ory, M. (1993). Serendipity and pseudoscience. *Evaluation and the Health Professionals, 16,* 363–378.

Hulley, S., Iurberg, C., & Gurland, B. J. (1985). The Systolic Hypertension in Elderly Program (SHEP): Antihypertensive efficacy of chlorthalidone. *American Journal of Cardiology, 56,* 913–920.

Kemp, B. J., Staples, F., & Lopez-Aqueres, W. (1987). Epidemiology of depression and dysphoria in our elderly Hispanic population—prevalence and correlates. *Journal of the American Geriatrics Society, 35,* 920–926.

Kenny, D. A., & Zautra, A. (in press). The Trait-state-error (TSE) model for multi-wave data. *Journal of Consulting and Clinical Psychology.*

Lopez-Agueres, W., Kemp, B., Plopper, M., Staples, F., & Brummel-Smith, K. (1984). Health needs of the Hispanic elderly. *Journal of the American Geriatrics Society, 32,* 191–198.

Lord, F. M. (1980). *Applications of item response theory to practical test problems.* Hillsdale, NJ: Erlbaum.

Lord, F. M., & Novick, M. R. (1968). *Statistical theories of mental test scores.* Reading, MA: Addison-Wesley.

Lunz, M. E., & Stahl, J. A. (1993). The effect of rater severity on person ability measure: A Rasch model analysis. *The American Journal of Occupational Therapy, 47,* 311–317.

McNair, D., Lorr, M., & Droppleman, L. (1971). *Manual for the Profile of Mood States.* San Diego: Educational and Industrial Testing Service.

Meehl, P. (1973). *Psychodiagnosis: Selected papers.* Minneapolis: University of Minnesota Press.

Mislevy, R. J., & Bock, R. D. (1984). BILOG: Maximum likelihood item analysis and test scoring with logistic models. Mooresville, IN: Scientific Software.

Nesselroade, J. R. (1994). Commentary: Longitudinal research with chronic care populations. *Alzheimer's Disease and Associated Disorders, 8,* Suppl. 1, S299–S301.

Popper, K. (1959). *The logic of scientific discovery.* New York: Basic Books.

Rogosa, D. (1994). Individual trajectories as the starting point for longitudinal data analysis. *Alzheimer's Disease and Associated Disorders, 8,* Suppl. 1, S302–S307.

Rogosa, D. R., & Willett, J. B. (1985). Understanding correlates of change by modeling individual differences in growth. *Psychometrika, 50,* 203–228.

Sharpe, L., Gurland, B. J., Fleiss, J. L., Kendell, R. E., Cooper, J. E., & Copeland, J. R. M. (1974). Comparisons of American, Canadian and British psychiatrists in their diagnostic concepts. *Canadian Psychiatric Association Journal, 19,* 235–245.

Shrout, P., Fleiss, J. (1981). Reliability and case detection. In J. K. Wing, P. Bebbington and L. N. Robins (Eds.). *What is a case?* (pp. 117–128). London: Grant Mcintyre.

Shrout, P., Spitzer, R., & Fleiss, J. (1987). Quantification of agreement in psychiatric diagnosis revisited. *Archives of General Psychiatry, 44*, 172–177.

Spitznagel, E. L., & Helzer, J. E. (1985). A proposed solution to the base rate problem in the kappa statistic. *Archives of General Psychiatry, 42*, 725–728.

Teresi, J. A. (1994). Methodological issues in the study of chronic care populations. *Alzheimer's Disease and Associated Disorders, 8*, Suppl. 1, S247–S273.

Teresi, J., Cross, P., Gurland, B., & Golden, R. (November, 1981). Measurement invariance: A method for detecting item bias in geriatric assessment scales. Paper presented at the 34th Annual Meeting of the Gerontological Society, Toronto, Canada.

Teresi, J. A., Cross, P. S., & Golden, R. R. (1989). Some applications of latent trait analysis to the measurement of ADL. *Journals of Gerontology: Social Sciences, 44*, S196–S204.

Teresi, J., & Golden, R. (1994). Latent structure methods for estimating item bias, item validity and prevalence using cognitive and other geriatric screening measures. *Journal of Alzheimer's Disease and Associated Disorders, 8*, Suppl. 1, 291–298.

Teresi, J. A., Golden, R. R., Cross, P. S., Gurland, B. J., Kleinman, M., & Wilder, D. E. (in press). Item bias in cognitive screening measures: Comparisons of elderly white, Afro-American, Hispanic and high and low education subgroups. *Journal of Clinical Epidemiology.*

Teresi, J. A., Golden, R. R., Gurland, B. J., Wilder, D. E., & Bennett, R. G. (1984). Construct validity of indicator-scales developed from the Comprehensive Assessment and Referral Evaluation Interview Schedule. *Journal of Gerontology, 39*, 147–157.

Teresi, J., Lawton, M. P., Ory, M., & Holmes, D. (1994). Measurement issues in chronic care populations: Dementia special care. *Alzheimer's Disease and Associated Disorder, 8*, Suppl. 1, S144–S183.

Uebersax, J. (1988). Validity inferences from interobserver agreement. *Psychological Bulletin, 104*, 405–416.

Willett, J. B. (1985). Questions and answers in the measurement of change. *Review of Research in Education, 15*, 345–422.

Wood, R. L., Wingersky, M. S., & Lord, F. M. (1976). *LOGIST: A computer program for estimating examinee ability and item characteristic curve parameters*. Princeton, NJ: Educational Testing Service.

Wright, B. D., & Stone, M. H. (1979). *Best test design*. Chicago, IL: MESA Press.

Wright, B. D., & Mead, R. J. (1977). *BICAL: Calibrating items and scales with the Rasch model* (Research Memorandum 23). Chicago: Statistical Laboratory, Department of Education, University of Chicago.

Zandi, T. (1994). Comments on measurement of severe dementia. *Alzheimer's Disease and Associated Disorder, 8*, Suppl. 1, S206–S208.

CHAPTER 2

Assessing Health

M. POWELL LAWTON

AND

RENÉE H. LAWRENCE

POLISHER RESEARCH INSTITUTE

PHILADELPHIA GERIATRIC CENTER

The conceptual meaning of the state of health has been in the process of development over most of this century. As long as the concepts defining health change, measures of health will also change. In terms of breadth of definition, health ranges from the absence of diagnosable conditions on the narrowest end to the World Health Organization's very broad definition: "A state of complete physical, mental, and social well-being" (WHO, 1948).

The present chapter chooses a moderate breadth, limiting the conceptual range of health to functions directly involving human biology and subjective and externally observable manifestations of physical pathology. Thus "positive health" in the WHO sense is excluded, as denoted in sectors of life outside the physical health realm, such as psychological health, social behavior, or goal achievement. These sectors are excluded to emphasize their qualitative differences from, despite their partial dependence on, health. Excluded also are functional health, gait and balance, and pain domains that would qualify for inclusion, but which are discussed in depth in chapter 3 by Kovar and Lawton, chapter 4 by Duncan and Studenski, and chapter 13 by Parmelee, respectively. Conceptual reviews of health and its measurement may also be found in Bowling (1991), McDowell and Newell (1987), Kane and Kane (1981), Patrick and Bergner (1990), Rubinstein et al. (1989), and Stahl (1984). The most complete review of the problems of health assessment and how this and other domains are measured by multiple-domain instruments is that of Fillenbaum (1984).

This work was partially supported by the National Institute on Aging (grants: AG07001 and AG-09344).

A MODEL OF HEALTH

Although the purpose of this chapter is to review instruments that measure health, the organization of the review is driven by a conceptual model of health. In addition to providing a coherent organizational framework for discussing the present state of the art in health measurement, a model also has the capacity to identify areas where measurement ability is lacking or where future instrumentation might develop. The model views the core concept, health, as a latent construct in statistical terms, that is, a construct that cannot be measured directly but one for which a variety of measurable indicators is available (see Liang, 1986, for an example of how such a model can be operationalized). In light of the complexities of such a construct, it is not clear whether one should even attempt to deal with health as a generic concept. For research purposes, however, it is essential to be able to develop measures that do their best to represent single or multiple aspects of the health of individuals. It is for such uses that this chapter is intended.

Some Possible Dimensions of Health

Inasmuch as health is very much in the "fuzzy set" category, defining health requires consideration of a number of differing facets. The facets are intercorrelated, but none is totally predictable from another. Further, assessment of some of the facets may not differentiate individuals across the full range of health.

A first conceptual partition of the health construct consists of three facets: life threat, pain and discomfort, and functional ability (Lawton, 1984). *Life threat* is a probabilistic statement regarding mortality. Some illnesses have relatively well-known risks (including zero risk) associated with them. *Pain and discomfort* is a subjective domain, but one that clinicians may be able to assess. (See chapter 13 by Parmelee on pain measurement.) *Functional ability* represents the competence with which the person is able to perform important roles in life. Although such functions may be required for complex roles, such as those of worker, citizen, spouse, parent, and so on, the roles most closely tied to physical health are the only ones included in this definition: physical self-care or activities of daily living (ADL) and instrumental activities of daily living (IADL) (see chapter 3 by Kovar & Lawton). Clearly, none of these three facets in itself defines health, but as a set of measurable indicators, they contribute most strongly, according to our hypothesis, to the operational definition of health. These facets are quite similar to the health dimensions proposed by Cameron, Leventhal, and Leventhal (1993): symptom seriousness, activity disruption, pain, and long-term consequences. In similar fashion, Travis, McAuley, and Taylor (1988) characterized poor health by including dimensions of seriousness and severity. Seriousness describes the degree of life threat, duration, and prognosis of the illness; severity is the amount of functional impairment and pain.

A second conceptual partition, or way of viewing health, is to make the basic distinction between *objective versus subjective* indicators of health. Objective indicators include those that can be read from an instrument (thermometer, laboratory titration, etc.), those whose presence is unmistakably evident from observation (tremor, pallor, amputation, hearing loss), and signs or behaviors on which statistical consensus, but not total agreement, is obtainable, such as many medical diagnoses. Subjective indicators are those based on a person's self-estimate of presence, severity, distress, or degree of functional impairment. Clearly there is overlap between the subjective and objective realms and, in fact, for many indicators there are objective and subjective aspects. For example, self-report inventories frequently ask the subject to report signs that could be confirmed or disconfirmed by others, or to place a check beside diagnoses that may have been made by physicians in the past and reported to the patient.

A third conceptual partition is the *source* of the health-relevant information, a classification that includes self-report and subdivisions of the objective realms. Thus, we might have histology, laboratory tests, psychophysiological measures, physician reports, medical records, family observations of functional competence, or gait, balance, and other performance tests in the objective realm, some of which are obtainable from archival sources.

The fourth conceptual partition is that of *scale*, from micro to macro aspects of health. Many objective indicators can be measured with great accuracy but represent very limited areas of functioning, such as cell count. Often, such microindicators have a wide range of possible variation. In the case of heart rate, for example, the range of normal function is very broad. Wide-range microindicators may be useful in assessing health only over a narrow, sub- or suprathreshold range. On the macro end of the scale dimension are global measures, such as the typical self-rated health measures or various attempts to turn the entire health domain into a single physician-rated scale ranging from normal to moribund.

A fifth conceptual partition is the *centrality* of the indicator's tie to biological health. Invasive laboratory tests and physical diagnoses are most central, encircled with successively more peripheral facets of subjective distress, functional competence, psychological well-being, and the many domains of quality of life not directly associated with health. At the periphery (less biologically central) health is more contingent on environmental opportunities and constraints than on biology. An example might be that a prosthetic environment enhances functional health, while its absence will be associated with poor functional health.

The dynamic interrelatedness of all facets of human life is underlined as this dimension of centrality is considered. Physical health is always present in the causal model of total well-being. There is no domain of quality of life that cannot be eroded by poor physical health. One of the strategies used to exclude other domains from the realm of health is the judgment that factors other than physical health are stronger determinants of quality of life in these domains. For example, temperament, preferences, motivation, past learning, and environmental opportu-

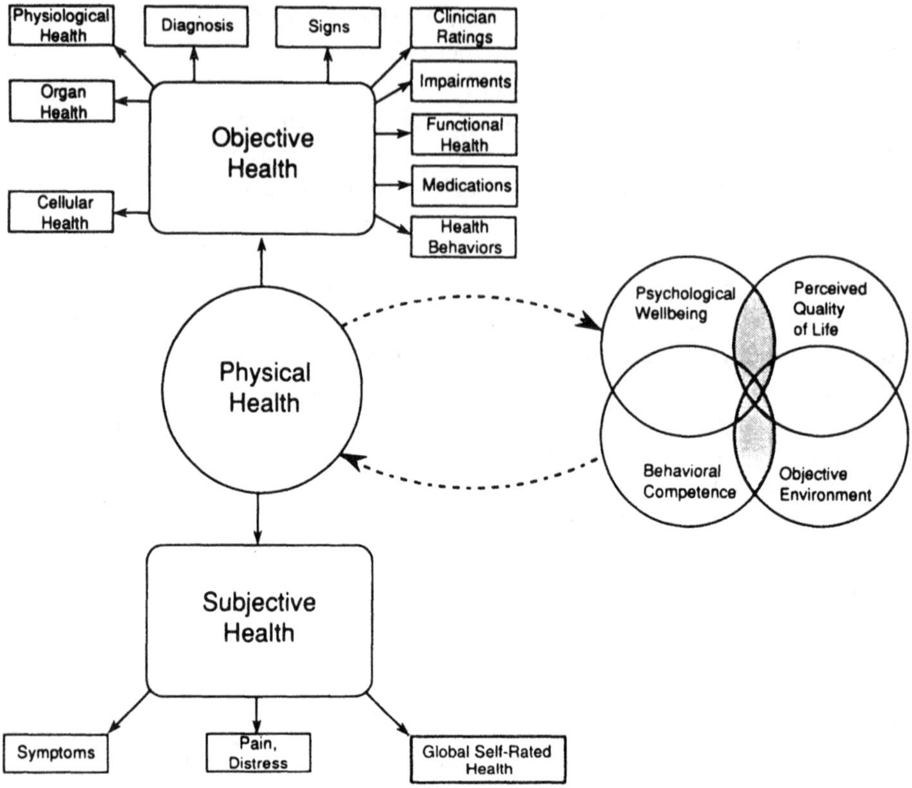

FIGURE 2.1 Model of physical health and its relationship to quality of life.

nity are probably more potent determinants of everyday social and goal-directed behavior than is physical health, except in a very narrow range of very poor health.

A final differentiation is that between *consequential* indicators and *essential* indicators. Essential indicators are intrinsic components of the state of good or poor health. Consequential indicators are the result (usually behavioral) of the basic health state, but may also be quite powerful indicators of health state. Consequential indicators, often used in health planning, include number of physician visits, nursing home and hospitalization rates, medication use, and other utilization data.

Figure 2.1 represents an attempt to depict, in simplified form, a structural model of health (left-hand portion) and its relationship to the broader aspects of life thought of as quality of life (Lawton, 1991), shown to the right. A different explicit model of health was built into the Comprehensive Assessment and Referral evaluation (CARE) (Gurland & Wilder, 1984). As a clinical, highly service-oriented assessment, the CARE model is very complex, incorporating a variety of social and service-context considerations. Another explicit model of health was presented by

Liang (1986), who conceptualized and specified linkages among five dimensions of physical health (chronic illness, sick days, ADL, IADL, and subjective ratings of health). In contrast are causal models of health that attempt to portray the dynamics of influence of one facet of health on another, such as that of Johnson and Wolinsky (1993). Health as depicted in Figure 2.1 is a second-order factor; objective and subjective health are first-order latent-variable factors, each with multiple measured indicators.

The partitions just outlined are overlapping and nonorthogonal; there is no neat way to nest all the elements. Life threat, for example, does not appear in the model, but its best single index is diagnosis, which, in turn, relates to cellular, organic, and physiological health, as well as to visible signs and subjective symptoms.

The nonhealth aspects of quality of life on the right of Figure 2.1 are all affected by the health model components. Further, all nonhealth components are causally associated with each other, and, in some circumstances, are reciprocal causal influences on health. With exception of functional health, pain, and gait and balance, which are considered in later chapters, measures of the proximal aspects of biological health are the topic of the discussion that follows. The more distal aspects of quality of life may be thought of as consequences, rather than indicators of biological health, despite their inclusion in conceptions of health offered by the WHO (1948), the RAND Medical Outcomes Study (Stewart & Ware, 1992), and many others.

One further area of ambiguity should be noted at this point. It is hazardous to separate health conceptually from psychological well-being and, especially, to exclude the latter from any definition of health. The relationship between soma and psyche introduces complexities far beyond the capacity of a single chapter to treat adequately. Suffice it to say that the two constructs in Figure 2.1 are separated for heuristic purposes only. Physical and psychological health have not been definitively separated either conceptually or empirically. The meta-analysis of Okun, Stock, Haring, and Witter (1984), for example, shows an average correlation of .31 between self-rated health and psychological well-being, across a wide variety of measures and research methods.

Aspects of Health Not Included in this Review

The measures to be reviewed all have in common an intention to evaluate health status by the classes of indicators shown on the left side of Figure 2.1. Many other health-related constructs can be measured but are excluded from consideration here because they do not array people in differential orders of good to poor health. A number of widely used health measures are composed wholly or partially of indicators such as health locus of control (Wallston, Wallston, Kaplan, & Maides, 1976), health beliefs (Rosenstock, 1974; Stewart & Ware, 1992), health utility (Bush, Fanshel, & Chen, 1972), risk avoidance and prevention (Langlie, 1977), perceived susceptibility to disease (Newcomb & Bentler, 1987), health efficacy (Grembowski et al., 1993), or attributions of functioning in nonhealth domains to state health (Bergner, Bobbith, Carter, & Gilson, 1981; Williamson & Schulz, 1992).

A very important exclusion is the illness-specific health measure. Examples are the Arthritis Impact Measurement Scales (Meenan, Gertman, & Mason, 1980) and the Dyspnea Index (Mahler, Weinberg, Wells, & Feinstein, 1984), which include symptoms or effects known to occur in these diseases. These are excluded because the psychometric development of disease-specific measures is just beginning and there have been few attempts as yet to use them with older subjects. Nonetheless, their aim—to rank the severity or bothersome qualities of symptoms and other manifestations of single diseases—is a complementary and necessary addition to the more general task of representing the overall latent construct of health, which is the topic of this chapter. A most informative conceptual treatment and measurement overview of illness-specific measurement is provided by Patrick and Deyo (1989). Clinical medical aspects of illness-specific health indicators are discussed in Smith (1988).

OVERVIEW OF SELECTED PHYSICAL HEALTH ASSESSMENT INSTRUMENTS

Fourteen instruments are reviewed in this section. They are summarized by conceptual domains in Table 2.1 and by psychometric information in Table 2.2. In Table 2.1 the instruments are listed in the first row, which also shows the primary reference. The rows correspond to the dimensions, as named in Figure 2.1, with objective health dimensions, listed first and subjective health dimensions listed last. Because of the significance of the global self-rated health item, there are two rows for self-rated health to distinguish between instruments which include global self-rated health and instruments which do not include the global rating. For completeness of presentation, rows for the dimensions covered in other chapters (functional health, gait and balance, and pain) are included in Table 2.1, but will not be discussed.

The goal of Table 2.1 is to provide an overview of the conceptual dimensions assessed by each instrument. An "X" signifies that an instrument includes items assessing a dimension and a scorable subscale of such items. A lower-case (x) signifies that items in a particular domain were included as part of a larger scale but were not evaluated as a separate subscale. Thus, Table 2.1 summarizes cases where a scale or subscale assesses more than one conceptual dimension. For example, the Cornell Medical Index (Brodman, Erdmann, Lorge, & Wolff, 1949) does not have separate subscales, but the summary score of physical health provided by this instrument includes items representing several of the conceptual dimensions (i.e., diagnoses and conditions, signs, impairments, symptoms, pain, and self-rated health).

Several criteria were used in selecting the instruments to include in the tables, with the overall goal of providing as broad a sampling of different approaches as possible. Here *breadth* includes both breadth of the conceptual dimensions portrayed in Figure 2.1, and breadth of sources of information (e.g., insurance claims, physicians). A major criterion was whether the instrument included a multi-item index, or at least a collection of items that could be indicators of a dimension of physical health as presented in Figure 2.1. A second criterion was that the instruments selected should have been frequently used, or likely to become frequently used with older subjects, as judged by the authors. Some scales have appeared in many variations or have been used in numerous research projects and applied contexts. Although such applications are important, we have included in Table 2.1 only the original article on instrument use and later articles with particularly high-quality samples or psychometric analyses. Where a variant on an earlier scale provides a unique application, we have tried to mention it in the discussion of the separate dimensions rather than include it in the tables.

A third criterion for inclusion in the tables was that the major focus of the instrument had to be on dimensions of health other than those which are covered in depth in other chapters. Thus several instruments which might otherwise qualify as measures of physical health are not included (for example, the Sickness Impact Profile, Gergner et al., 1981; the McMaster Health Index Questionnaire, Chambers, MacDonald, Tugwell, Buchanan, & Kraag, 1982; the Structured Assessment of Independent Living Skills [SAILS], Mahurin, DeBettignis, & Pirozzolo, 1991; Physical and Mental Impairment-of-Function Evaluation, Gurel, Linn, & Linn, 1972). Finally, instruments are included that measure more than one dimension of physical health or measure an otherwise underrepresented dimension. Although the ordering of instruments in Table 2.1 is rough, an attempt was made to list first those which assess a limited breadth of health, followed by those of increasing conceptual breadth.

An invaluable resource for psychometric research in health measurement are the national surveys, which offer representative and large samples. Among them are the Health Interview Surveys (National Center for Health Statistics [NCHS], 1985; Chyba & Washington, 1993), including the Longitudinal Study on Aging (NCHS, 1992), the Long-Term Care Surveys (Macken, 1986) and the National Health and Nutrition Examination Surveys (NHANES). All have relevant health data, most of which is not formally scaled. While recognizing the value of all of the surveys, we chose the NHANES III (NCHS, 1991) to represent this domain of assessment and instrumentation possibilities because it is the most recent, and therefore, likely to be the most complete in terms of self-report data, direct physical examination, and ages of subjects (no upper age limit). NHANES III appears in Table 2.1, where its conceptual breadth and fruitfulness for instrument development and evaluation are highlighted.

Additional information relevant to further evaluating the instruments is provided in Table 2.2. For each instrument, the primary psychometric reference or ref-

(continued on p. 34)

TABLE 2.1 Assessment Instruments by Conceptual Dimensions as Depicted in Figure 2.1

	Assessment Instrument		
	CIRS Cumulative Illness Rating Scale (Linn, Linn, and Gurel, 1968)	*SIRS Seriousness of Illness Rating Scale* (Wyler, Masuda, and Holmes, 1968)	*CMI Cornell Medical Index* (Brodman et al., 1949)
OBJECTIVE HEALTH			
Cellular, Organ, and/or Physiological	X		
Diagnoses & Conditions		(x)	(x)
Signs		(x)	(x)
ClinicianGlobal/ Summary Ratings			
Impairments		(x)	(x)
FUNCTIONAL HEALTH			
Gait and Balance[a]			
Functional Status[a]			
HEALTH BEHAVIORS			
Medications			
Physician Visits			
Disability Days			
Hospitalization			
SUBJECTIVE HEALTH			
Symptoms		(x)	(x)
Pain[a]	(x)		(x)
Self-Rated Health			
Items/Scale Includes Global[b] Rating			
Items Included (but without Global Rating)			(x)

Assessment Instrument			
SCL-90-R *Symptom Checklist* (Derogatis, 1992)	*DUHP* *Duke UNC* *Health Profile* (Parkerson et al., 1981)	*MOS-FWBP* *Medical Outcomes* *Study-Functioning and* *Well-Being Profile* (Stewart and Ware, (Ed.), 1992)	*MOS: SF-36* (Ware and Sherbourne, 1992)
	(x)		
	(x)		
	X	X	X
	X		
X	X	X	
		X	X
		X	X

(continued)

TABLE 2.1 (Continued)

	Assessment Instrument		
	Manitoba Longitudinal Study on Aging (Mossey et al., 1981)	*Alameda County Survey* (Belloc, Breslow, and Hochstim, 1971)	*SELF Self-Evaluation Life Function Scale* (Linn and Linn, 1984)
OBJECTIVE HEALTH			
Cellular, Organ, and/or Physiological			
Diagnoses & Conditions	(x)	X	(x)
Signs			
ClinicianGlobal/ Summary Rating			
Impairments		X	
FUNCTIONAL HEALTH			
Gait and Balance[(a)]			
Functional Status[(a)]	(x)	X	X
HEALTH BEHAVIORS			
Medications			(x)
Physician Visits	(x)		
Disability Days	(x)		(x)
Hospitalization	(x)		(x)
SUBJECTIVE HEALTH			
Symptoms		X	(x)
Pain[(a)]		(x)	(x)
Self-Rated Health			
Items/Scale Includes Global[(b)] Rating	X[(c)]		
Items Included (but without Global Rating)			(x)

Notes: (a) Although these dimensions are not covered in our chapter, we have provided an overview for completeness of the various physical health dimensions as presented in Figure 2.1.

(b) Global specifically refers to a variation of the item: "How would you rate your overall health at the present time: excellent, good, fair, or poor?"

X Indicates that a multi-item instrument or subscale, which assesses the dimension, is included.

Assessment Instrument			
OMFAQ *OARS Multidimensional Functional Assessment Questionnaire* (Duke University, 1978)	*MAI* *Multilevel Assessment Instrument* (Lawton et al., 1982)	*CORE-CARE* *CORE-Comprehensive Assessment and Referral Evaluation* (Golden, Teresi, and Gurland, 1984; Gurland and Wilder, 1984)	*NHANES III* *National Health and Nutrition Examination Survey* (NCHS, 1991)
			(x)
(x)	X	X	(x)
		(x)	(x)
			(x)
(x)	(x)	X	(x)
		(x)	(x)
X	X	X	(x)
(x)		(x)	(x)
(x)	(x)	(x)	(x)
(x)	(x)	(x)	
(x)	(x)	(x)	(x)
(x)	(x)	X	(x)
		(x)	(x)
(x)	X	(x)	(x)

Notes (continued)

(x) Indicates that items are included, but the items are part of a larger scale and do not form a separate multi-item scale as named in the column heading.

(c) Although the Manitoba Study does not have a multi-item subscale assessing Self-Rated Health, the single item is defined as a scale (i.e., X) and is an entry on Table 2.1.

erences were selected as main entries. When more than one reference is included, we have distinguished between them using lower case letters. The distinction is used, where appropriate, in each block of Table 2.2when summarizing information from the various reference articles.

Three major types of information are summarized. First, information relevant to administering the instrument is presented: who administers it, the number of items it includes, the amount of time it takes, and the availability of alternative forms. For several instruments there is a distinction between the number of total items in the instrument as a whole and the number of items assessing a particular subdimension of physical health.

Second, information about the sample used in the cited studies is summarized: size, age range, and sampling frame. In some instances the primary psychometric reference did not specifically evaluate older populations and/or there are additional references which are particularly relevant to gerontologists. We have provided this information in the column headed "Data on 65+ samples."

Third, information about psychometric properties (i.e., reliability and validity) is included. Often several types of reliability and validity were available in the original reports. It was not always feasible to report all types, particularly for validity. We have indicated when several types are available and, when possible, selected comparable types of information (e.g., convergent/conceptual validity and predictive validity).

As noted earlier, upper- and lowercase x's are used in Table 2.1 to denote the conceptual dimensions (as named in Figure 2.1) covered by each scale. For each instrument or subscale appearing in Table 2.1 (and referenced by an X), there is a corresponding entry in Table 2.2 summarizing the psychometric information, again excluding scales measuring functional health and pain. However, it is important to keep in mind that the conceptual framework depicted in Figure 2.1 was devised by the authors of the present chapter and was not the conceptual basis used in developing most of the assessment instruments. For five instruments the dimensions posited in Figure 2.1 correspond with the dimensions included in the instruments: Cumulative Illness Rating Scale (CIRS; Linn, Linn, & Gurel, 1968); the Symptom Checklist 90 (SCL–90–R; Derogatis, 1992); the Medical Outcomes Study (MOS–FWBP, Stewart & Ware, 1992); the MOS Short-Form 36 (SF–36, Ware & Sherbourne, 1992); and Alameda County Survey (Belloc, Breslow, & Hochstim, 1971). In those cases there is a one-to-one correspondence between the number of X's in Table 2.1 and the number of entries in Table 2.2 (i.e., there are uppercase X's and no relevant lowercase x's). Note that even in this subset, some instruments have a broader conceptual reference which needs to be kept in mind when selecting and evaluating the subscales (i.e., the total number of items exceeds the number of items discussed here). For another subset of three instruments there are only lowercase x's in Table 2.1 and one entry for the instrument in Table 2.2: Seriousness of Illness Rating Scale (SIRS; Wyler, Masuda, & Holmes, 1968); Cornell Medical Index (CMI; Brodman et al., 1949); and the Manitoba Longitudinal

(continued on p. 44)

Table 2.2 Summary of Instrument, Sample, and Psychometric Information for Assessment Tools and Relevant Subscales

CIRS (Cumulative Illness Rating Scale)

Primary Reference(s)

a) Linn, Linn, and Gurel, 1968
b) Linn, Linn, and Gurel, 1967
c) Conwell et al., 1993

Instrument Information

Administered by	*Number of Items*	*Amount of Time (Minutes)*	*Alternative Forms Available*
Clinician	13	varies	CIRS-G (Geriatric Version) Miller et al., 1992

Sample Information

Size	*Age Range*	*Sampling Frame*	*Data on 65+ Sample*
a) 20	NA	FL (Miami)-VA Hospital	Miller et al., 1992(a)
b) 172	55+	FL (Miami)-VA Hospital	Presented
c) 72	21+	NY (Monroe County) sample of suicides investigated by the Office of Medical Examiner	

Psychometric Information

Reliability: a) Interrater (6 raters) estimates (Kendall's W) ranged from .83–.91

Validity: b) Scores significantly correlated with death, previous illness, and vital organ involvement (values NA)

c) CIRS autopsy ratings predictive of ratings on historical data ($R^2 = .74$)

SIRS (Seriousness of Illness Rating Scale)

Primary Reference(s)

a) Wyler, Masuda, and Holmes, 1968
b) Rosenberg, Hayes, and Peterson, 1987
c) McAuley, Travis, and Taylor, 1987

Instrument Information

Administered by	*Number of Items*	*Amount of Time (Minutes)*	*Alternative Forms Available*
Clinician Interviewer	126		SIRS-R (Revised) Rosenberg, Hayes, & Peterson, 1987 McAuley, Travis, & Taylor, 1987

continued

TABLE 2.2 (Continued)

SIRS (Seriousness of Illness Rating Scale) (Continued)

Sample Information

	Size	Age Range	Sampling Frame	Data on 65+ Sample
a)	117	21–65	WA (medical sample)	
	141	20–65+	WA (nonmedical sample) Seattle University H	
b)	46	21–50+	IN (medical sample)	
c)	201	60+	VA (acute care patients Virginia)	Presented

Psychometric Information

Reliability: a) Interrater estimates (two methods) were .95 (Spearman's rho) and ranged from .60–.70 (Kendall's W)

b) Interrater estimate was .72 (Kendall's W)

Validity: c) Predictor of length of stay (b = .56), controlling for ADL

CMI (Cornell Medical Index)

Primary Reference(s) Brodman et al., 1949

Instrument Information

Administered by	Number of Items	Amount of Time (Minutes)	Alternative Forms Available
Self	195	10–20	

Sample Information

Size	Age Range	Sampling Frame	Data on 65+ Sample
179	NA	NY (new outpatients)	

Psychometric Information

Validity: Criterion based on comparing CMI responses with history recorded by attending physician: 95% answered identically

SCL-90-R (Symptom Checklist)

Primary Reference(s)
a) Derogatis,, 1992
b) Derogatis, Rickels, and Rock, 1976

Somatization (S)

Instrument Information

Administered by	Number of Items	Amount of Time (Minutes)	Alternative Forms Available
Self	90 12 (S)	12–15	BSI (Brief Symptom Inventory)

Sample Information

	Size	Age Range	Sampling Frame	Data on 65+ Sample
a)	94	NA	NA (psychiatric outpatients)	
b)	209	39.5 ($\overline{X}$)	PA (Philadelphia: 'symptomatic' volunteers)	

TABLE 2.2 (Continued)

SCL-90-R (Symptom Checklist) (Continued)

Psychometric Information

Reliability: Alpha; Test–Retest

a) Test–Retest = .86

b) Alpha = .86 (N = 565)

Validity: b) Several types available. Convergent (MMPI, Wiggins, and Tyron) reported here: r's ranged from .48–.66

DUHP (Duke UNC Health Profile)

Primary Reference(s) Parkerson et al., 1981

Disability Days (DD)
Symptom Status (SS)

Instrument Information	*Administered by*	*Number of Items*	*Amount of Time (Minutes)*	*Alternative Forms Available*
	Self	63	10	DUKE Health 17-Item
	Interviewer		30	
		2 (DD)		
		26 (SS)		

Sample Information	*Size*	*Age Range*	*Sampling Frame*	*Data on 65+ Sample*
	395	18–65+	NC (Durham) primary care setting	

Psychometric Information

Reliability: Test–Retest Correlations: (n = 55)
.35 (DD)
.68 (SS)

Validity: Several types evaluated. Convergent (n = 315) (SIP and Zung) reported: r's ranged from
.45 (DD) (SIP only)
.61–.66 (SS)

MOS-FWBP (Medical Outcomes Study-Functioning and Well-Being Profile)

Primary Reference(s) Stewart and Ware (Ed.), 1992

Physical/Psychophysiologic Symptoms (PPS)
Current Health Perceptions (CHP)

Instrument Information	*Administered by*	*Number of Items*	*Amount of Time (Minutes)*	*Alternative Forms Available*
	Self	149	23–28	(see below)
		8 (PPS)		
		7 (CPH)		

continued

MOS-FWBP (Medical Outcomes Study-Functioning and Well-Being Profile) (Continued)

Sample Information	*Size*	*Age Range*	*Sampling Frame*	*Data on 65+ Sample*
	3053	18+	MA (Boston) IL (Chicago) CA (Los Angeles)	

Psychometric Information

Reliability: Alpha:
.75 (PPS)
.88 (CHP)

Validity: Several types evaluated. Predictive (as measured by utilization: hospitalization, and medications) reported. Predictive (r's ranged from)
.038–.199 (PPS)
–.056 to –.211 (CHP)

MOS: SF-36

Primary Reference(s)
a) Ware and Sherbourne, 1992
b) McHorney, Ware, and Raczek, 1993

General Health Perceptions (GHP)

Instrument Information	*Administered by*	*Number of Items*	*Amount of Time (Minutes)*	*Alternative Forms Available*
	Self	36 5 (GHP)		

Sample Information	*Size*	*Age Range*	*Sampling Frame*	*Data on 65+ Sample*
	1014	18+	MA (Boston) IL (Chicago) CA (Los Angeles) Divided into 4 Groups of Conditions:	
	638		Minor chronic medical only	
	168		Serious chronic medical only	
	163		Psychiatric only	
	45		Serious medical and psychiatric	

Psychometric Information

Validity:
a) Convergent validity assessed using 22-item General Health Rating Index (Health Insurance Experiments): r = .96.
b) Criterion-group comparisons. GHP scale distinguished between groups as expected. Substantial relative validities reported for physical health conditions groups: .68 and .99.

Manitoba Longitudinal Study on Aging

Primary Reference(s)
a) Mossey and Roos, 1987
b) Mossey and Shapiro, 1982

Illness Scale (IS)
Self-Rated Health (SR)

Instrument Information

Administered by	Number of Items	Amount of Time (Minutes)	Alternative Forms Available
a) Self and Health Care Claim Files	NA	NA	
Insurance Claims	8 (IS)		
b) Self	1 (SR)	NA	

Sample Information

Size	Age Range	Sampling Frame	Data on 65+ Sample
a) 3,533	65+	Canada (Manitoba) Random sample of non-institutionalized population	Presented[(a)]
b) 3,128	65+		

Psychometric Information

Reliability: a) Various methods were used for each of the 8 years (1970–1977) estimates for the Illness Scale: Alpha: .82–.84; Stability: .35–.56

Validity: a) Several types were evaluated. Predictive validity (as measured by association with the probability of dying and hospitalization) reported below (range of odds ratios for 1973–1977):

	Death:	Hospitalization:
IS score > 10	1.85–4.30	2.36–3.00
IS score > 19	3.25–16.02	5.12–8.08

b) Predictive validity with poor self-rated health associated with increased risk of death (controlling for objective health reported by physician, age, sex life satisfaction, income, and urban/rural residence).

Adjusted Odds Ratio:
for Early Mortality (1–2 years) = 2.92
for Late Mortality (3–6 years) = 2.77

continued

Alameda County Survey

Primary Reference(s) Meltzer and Hochstim, 1970

Physical Health (PH)
Chronic Conditions (CC)
Impairments (I)
Symptoms (S)

Instrument Information

Administered by	*Number of Items*	*Amount of Time (Minutes)*	*Alternative Forms Available*
Self	35 (PH) 16 (CC) 3 (I) 11 (S)	NA	

Sample Information

Size	*Age Range*	*Sampling Frame*	*Data on 65+ Sample*
1,530	20+	CA (Alameda County) Probability sample of adults (persons 16–19 years old and ever married also included)	Seeman et al., 1989

Psychometric Information

Reliability: Cohen's Kappa:
.82 (PH)
.89 (CC)
.82 (I)
.79 (S)

Validity: Criterion validity (n = 739) (with medical observed agreement with medical records corrected for chance) (Index of Agreement):
.37 (PH)
.52 (CC)
.31 (I)
.28 (S)

SELF (Self-Evaluation of Function Scale)

Primary Reference(s) Linn and Linn, 1984

Symptoms of Aging (SA)

Instrument Information

Administered by	*Number of Items*	*Amount of Time (Minutes)*	*Alternative Forms Available*
Self	54 13 (SA)		

continued

SELF (Self-Evaluation of Function Scale) (Continued)

Sample Information

Size	Age Range	Sampling Frame	Data on 65+ Sample
	70.4 ($\overline{X}$)	FL (Miami)	
120		Institutional	Presented[(a)]
205		Outpatient	
115		Housing	
77		Counseling	

Psychometric Information

Reliability: Test-Retest (n = 105)
.93 (SA)

Validity: Criterion group comparisons (results as expected):
Predictive validity with SA significantly predicting future institutionalization, new disorders, physician visits, sick days, hospitalization and death; r's ranged from .16–.52 (SA)

OMFAQ (OARS Multidimensional Functional Assessment Questionnaire)

Primary Reference(s)
a) Fillenbaum and Smyer, 1981
b) Fillenbaum, 1988

Physical Health (PH)

Instrument Information

Administered by	Number of Items	Amount of Time (Minutes)	Alternative Forms Available
Interviewer	70 16	45	Discrete scales/subscales have been extracted

Sample Information

Size	Age Range	Sampling Frame	Data on 65+ Sample
		NC (Durham)	Presented[(a)]
997	65+	Community	Additional norms:
98	65+	Clinic	Cleveland, OH
102	65+	Institution	(Comptroller General, 1977) Virginia, McAuley et al., 1980)

Psychometric Information

Reliability: Test–Retest (n = 30)
7.3% of objective changed;
11.4% of subjective changed
r = .59 (PH-Subjective only)

Validity: Criterion-group comparisons of three samples (results as expected);
Criterion estimates (n = 31) based on physician ratings (tau and Spearman's r):
.75 & .82 (PH)

continued

TABLE 2.2 (Continued)

MAI (Multilevel Assessment Instrument)

Primary Reference(s) — Lawton et al., 1982

Physical Health (PH)
- Health Conditions (HC)
- Health Behavior (HB)
- Self-Rated Health (SR)

Instrument Information

Administered by	*Number of Items*	*Amount of Time (Minutes)*	*Alternative Forms Available*
Interviewer	135 31 (PH) 24 (HC) 3 (HB) 4 (SR)	50	Mid-length; Short; Best Item

Sample Information

Size	*Age Range*	*Sampling Frame*	*Data on 65+ Sample*
	($\bar{X}$)	PA (Philadelphia)	Presented[(a)]
253	76	Community	
173	74.1	Public Housing	
99	75.8–80	In-home services	
65	79.7–80.2	Institutional waiting list	

Psychometric Information

Reliability: Alpha; Test–Retest (n = 22)
.74; .95 (PH)
.61; .85 (HC)
.39; .99 (HB)
.76; .92 (SR)

Validity: Several types of validity evaluated. Only criterion-based estimates summarized here (criterion-group; clinical; administrative) r's ranged from
.41–.65 (PH)
.35–.58 (HC)
.29–.33 (HB)
.32–.65 (SR)

CORE-CARE (CORE Comprehensive Assessment and Referral Evaluation)

Primary Reference(s)
a) Golden, Teresi, and Gurland, 1984
b) Teresi et al., 1984
c) Teresi, Golden, and Gurland, 1984

Heart Disorder (HD)	Arthritis (A)	Hypertension (H)
Stroke Effects (SE)	Leg Problems (LP)	Service Utilization (SU)
Cancer (C)	Hearing Disorder (HD)	Somatic Symptoms (SS)
Respiratory Symptoms (RS)	Vision Disorder (VD)	

continued

TABLE 2.2 (Continued)

CORE-CARE (CORE Comprehensive Assessment and Referral Evaluation) (Continued)

Instrument Information	*Administered by*	*Number of Items*	*Amount of Time (Minutes)*	*Alternative Forms Available*
	Interviewer	314 15 (HD) 9 (SE) 6 (C) 6 (RS) 9 (A) 9 (LP) 14 (HD) 11 (VD) 4 (H) 15 (SU) 34 (SS)		Global CARE, Short-CARE, Merge-CARE, In-CARE

Sample Information	*Size*	*Age Range*	*Sampling Frame*	*Data on 65+ Sample*
	445	65+	NY (NY city)	Presented[(a)]
	396	65+	England (London) Random sample of older residents of New York City and comparable sample of older residents in London	

Psychometric Information

Reliability	Validity	
	Several validity coefficients (n = 162) are available. Convergent (with family-informant) and Predictive (for death) reported only (significant ones noted*).	
Alpha; Cohen's Kappa	Convergent (r)	Predictive (Odds Ratio)
.85; .83 (HD)	.54 (HD)	3.1*
.84; .86 (SE)	NA (SE)	1.4
.78; .87 (C)	NA (C)	2.3
.75; .86 (RS)	NA (RS)	2.0
.84; .62 (A)	.45 (A)	0.9
.84; .81 (LP)	NA (LP)	1.3
.91; .75 (HD)	.51 (HD)	0.7
.80; .81 (VD)	.59 (VD)	2.7
.85; .74 (H)	.45 (H)	0.4
.75; .75 (SU)	.48 (SU)	1.6
.85; .83 (SS)	.47 (SS)	2.9*

Note: [(a)]Indicates that an instrument was designed explicitly for use with elderly adults.

Study on Aging (Mossey, Havens, Roos, & Shapiro, 1981). This indicates that the instrument or subscale aggregates the various conceptual dimensions noted. Although the NHANES III fits into this subset, it is not included in Table 2.2 because psychometric information is not yet available.

The final set of five instruments is a mixture of lower- and uppercase x's: The Duke University North Carolina Health Profile (DUHP; Parkerson et al., 1981); the Self-Evaluation of Life Functioning Scale (SELF; Linn & Linn, 1984); the CORE–CARE (Golden, Teresi, & Gurland, 1984); the Older Americans Resources and Services (OARS) Multidimensional Functional Assessment Questionnaire (OMFAQ; Duke University Center for the Study of Aging [DUCFSA], 1978); and the Multilevel Assessment Instrument (MAI; Lawton, Moss, Fulcomer, & Kleban, 1982). All have one or more subscales embedded in a larger assessment tool. For the OMFAQ and SELF, only one subscale is listed and that subscale summarizes information across the various dimensions marked with an (x). For the remaining instruments—DUHP, CORE–CARE, and MAI—there are several subscales which tap various conceptual dimensions in Table 2.2. Three points should help clarify the relationships between Table 2.1 and Table 2.2 for these instruments: First, each instrument has a separate health behavior subscale. For the DUHP the subscale items only assess disability days, whereas for the CORE–CARE and the MAI, content of the health behavior subscales is indicated by the lower case x's in the relevant rows. Second, the DUHP's symptom scale also has items we have designated as signs. And, third, for the MAI and the CORE–CARE, the subscales assess several dimensions represented by X and (x). For example, signs and medications are assessed but as part of the subscale for health conditions (uppercase X). Further, for the CORE–CARE instrument several health conditions and impairments provide disease specific subscales.

OBJECTIVE HEALTH MEASURES

Cellular, Organ, and/or Physiological Indicators

A number of clinical indicators (e.g., blood pressure, laboratory studies, or exercise stress tests) have demonstrated utility as indicators of health status, but are infrequently encountered as research instruments with psychometric evaluation. In geriatric clinical assessment, numerous such tests and procedures are available (cf. Kane, Ouslander, & Abrass, 1984), but attempts to develop health status scales for research use, especially for use by less than fully trained professionals, are not generally reported or pursued. An example of possible indicators from this domain is the Cumulative Illness Rating Scale (Linn et al., 1968). This scale has been completed by physicians, nurse practitioners, and nurses on the basis of health records as well as by direct examination. The CIRS provides a composite index and individual ratings for thirteen different organ systems. Recent research that produced a manual for use with geriatric patients (Miller et al., 1992) and predictive validity estimates (Conwell, Forbes, Cox, & Caine, 1993) has affirmed the usefulness of this scale as a summary measure of body system health.

The larger surveys designed to assess health status as broadly as possible, such as the NHANES, include physical examination procedures, but they have not yet been subjected to psychometric treatment. There is no doubt that these indicators would be valuable additions to assessment instruments, but the trade-offs regarding cost, time, and the necessary professional expertise remain an obstacle to their full use.

Diagnoses and Conditions

One of the major modes of indexing health is to provide a list of illnesses and count the number reported. Such a conditions checklist is most often a collection of very general diagnoses (e.g., cancer, liver condition) phrased in laypersons' terms and sometimes including major signs or symptoms not necessarily specific to a single diagnosis (e.g., high blood pressure). Although more often than not reported by the subject, such conditions are classed as objective because the information has usually been reported to the subject by a physician. The conditions are also theoretically capable of being verified by an external observer or archive search.

Many conditions checklists were modeled on lists used by Shanas (1962) or the Alameda County community study (Belloc et al., 1971). Most are reasonably serviceable (see also Rosencranz & Pihlblad, 1970; Markides & Martin, 1979). Some like the CARE (Golden et al., 1984), the OMFAQ (DUCFSA, 1978), and the MAI (Lawton et al., 1982), have the advantage of including extensive data showing the relationships between the conditions checklist and other measures of health and nonhealth variables. The Seriousness of Illness Rating Scale (Wyler et al., 1968) does not count conditions, but sums numerical weights attached to each of 126 conditions. The weights were determined by a consensus of physicians and nonphysicians regarding the seriousness of the conditions. The utility of this scale for elders was demonstrated by McAuley, Travis, and Taylor (1987) and by Aldwin, Levenson, Ekerdt, and Bossé (1987). Both studies also provided a minor update in relevance to older people by including additional health problems (and weights). The weights may be applied to a list of diagnoses or material from health records (McAuley et al., 1987) or to the responses given to an open-ended question asking about health problems (Aldwin et al., 1987).

The CMI (Brodman et al., 1949) and the CARE provide item sets grouped by classes of illness. The CMI is the most extensive, but data on the illness-specific symptom groups or its psychometric characteristics when used with older people were not found in the literature. Because both the Boston Veterans Administration Normative Aging Study (Aldwin, Spiro, Levenson, & Bossé, 1989) and the Baltimore Longitudinal Study (Costa & McCrae, 1980) used the CMI, its usability with elders is at least confirmed. Further development of subscales for the CMI would be a welcome addition to the health measurement repertory. The CARE yields 11 system scores, which have been psychometrically treated, with some estimates of concurrent and predictive validities. These scores could be considered to represent either conditions or symptoms, illustrating how uncertain the line is between the two categories. The OMFAQ and the MAI checklists also have extensive standardization data. The NHANES conditions list is one of the longest (31 items), but no psychometric treatment of indices constructed from this list or from that of the Supplement on Aging of the Health Interview Survey (18 conditions) have been reported (NCHS, 1992).

Signs

Signs (externally observable indicators of illness) appear in many of the measures designated as conditions checklists. No composites composed only of signs were found.

Clinician Global Ratings

Physician ratings appeared in only one instrument reviewed in Table 2.1, NHANES III. This, in part, reflects the self-report focus of most of the instruments reviewed. Nevertheless, the research of Hooker and Siegler (1992), using the Duke Second Longitudinal Study, and that of Hall, Epstein, and McNeil (1989), evaluating the multidimensionality of health status, are examples of the effective use of global ratings made by physicians. Both studies underscore the unique frames of reference of physicians and patients when providing overall health assessments and affirm the validity of physician ratings. This source of data does not fit the criterion of usability by many types of raters, but when a physician is involved in some of the data collection, it may add only a small cost to obtain such summary ratings.

Although not included for review, the Quality of Life Index (QL–Index, Spitzer et al., 1981) is worth mentioning because it has been so frequently cited. The QL–Index was developed for use by physicians to obtain global summary ratings for five domains of quality of life. Three are directly related to health: Two are within the functional health domain, and one is a physician's global rating. Nonetheless its form as a single index that includes two nonhealth indicators make it impossible to use as a health index by our definition.

Impairments

Many of the instruments include measures of sensory and motor impairments, but only the Alameda County Study and the CORE–CARE have separate indices for these functions. The Alameda index uses three general impairment questions (one for hearing, one for vision, and one for loss of extremities), which are common to many of the instruments reviewed. The CORE–CARE, as well as the NHANES III, permit a finer grained analysis of visual and auditory impairments because they include questions sensitive to specific situations. For example, for vision they assess ability to read labels, see traffic signs, or see steps; for hearing they ask about ability to hear normal, group, and telephone conversation).

Although many of the instruments did not evaluate a separate impairment scale, Laforge, Spector, and Sternberg (1992) provided an example of the effective use of the general impairment questions. They used the two impairment items assessing hearing and vision to create an impairment index and found significant relationships between impairment and both functional decline and 1-year mortality. These relationships were particularly strong for those with vision only or both vision and hearing impairment.

Increasing appreciation of the need to measure sensory impairments as a separate facet of health and to include finer grained assessment is reflected in several other impairment-specific indices not listed in Table 2.1. Rosenhall, Pedersen, and Møller (1987) used eight items assessing hearing problems, and included items sensitive to different situations (e.g., TV, phone, and conversation). In addition, several other self-reported hearing problems scales developed for use with older persons are available: the Your Hearing Questionnaire (Slawinski, Hartel, & Kline, 1993); the Self-Assessment of Communication (Schow & Nerbonne, 1982); and the Hearing Screening Inventory (Coren & Hakistian, 1992). All of these are sensitive to different situations and have proven to be useful. However, to date, the Your Hearing Questionnaire provides the most comprehensive assessment of hearing disability in the natural environment, assessing seven areas of auditory functioning (e.g., temporal resolution, distorted speech, and background noise). Overall, the seven subscales were found to have good reliability (alphas ranged from .70 to .94) and good validity based on criterion-group comparisons (Slawinski et al., 1993). Horowitz, Teresi, and Cassels (1991) reported a vision scale (15 items), derived in part from the CORE–CARE vision indicator scale, which, like the hearing problems scale, attends to different situations for vision problems (e.g., difficulty reading labels, recognizing faces across a room, needing to sit close to the television). The scale has good reliability (α of .84) and validity (80% correct classification with cut-score of 9). Finally, although multi-item scales were not developed, the analysis of three hearing and five vision indicators from the Longitudinal Study of Aging (NCHS, 1992) has the advantage of working with a large, nationally representative longitudinal sample (Rudberg, Furner, Dunn, & Cassel, 1993).

Health Behaviors

Several instruments include measures of health behavior. In one instance, the Duke–UNC Health Profile (DUHP; Parkerson et al., 1981), the measure reflects only one type of health behavior listed in Table 2.1, disability days. More often, when a subscale exists, it represents a health behavior index assessing various types of health behavior, including the three core ones identified in Table 2.1: physician visits, disability days, and hospitalization. As can be seen in Table 2.2, the MAI has a Health Behavior subscale, the the CORE–CARE has a Service Utilization subscale. However, the conceptual scope of the Service Utilization subscale in the CORE–CARE is much broader, including receiving assistance with daily activities of living. This subscale therefore does not serve as a pure measure of health behavior as defined here. The OMFAQ, the SELF, and the Alameda County survey have items measuring health behaviors as summarized in Table 2.1, but they do not include separate subscales for these items. Rather, the items are part of the conceptual definition of the physical health instrument which is presented in Table 2.2 for the OMFAQ and the Alameda County survey. In the case of the SELF, the items are part of a larger subscale, which is not directly related to the dimensions of health on which this review is focused (i.e., the items are part of the physical disability or ADL subscales).

As can be seen in Table 2.2, where psychometric information is available, health behavior subscales have acceptable validity and reliability. Test-retest reliability was less than ideal for the disability days subscale in the DUHP, but may be considered reasonable given the nature of these items (i.e., disability days would not necessarily be stable across time).

Medications

Some attempt to determine number of medications was found in a number of the instruments noted in Table 2.2. For example, Whitelaw and Liang (1991) used a simple count of the OMFAQ medications list as an analytic index. A weighted coding system for the typical medications used for 17 major classes of chronic diseases was devised for enrollees of a major health maintenance organization (Von Korff, Wagner, & Saunders, 1992). This overall index showed many favorable psychometric characteristics and was shown to be a useful indicator of health in a large sample (Wagner, LaCroix, Grothaus, & Hecht, 1993). One should note, however, the ambiguity inherent in the use of medication and other consequential indicators of health: Their consequences, for example, the outcomes of service use and medication, may themselves be therapeutic. At one and the same time, their use is an indicator of pathology, but their consequence may be improvement. Therefore, the possible double meaning of some consequential indicators must always be acknowledged in discussion of results based on their use.

SUBJECTIVE HEALTH MEASURES

Symptoms

Symptom checklists typically mix symptoms of various physical illnesses with symptoms traditionally considered to be indicators of somatization and other psychiatric syndromes. Because of the high prevalence in the elderly of physical illnesses that can include similar symptoms, there is built-in ambiguity as to whether "somatization" symptoms should be viewed as belonging in the somatic or psychological arena.

The 28-item Symptom Status scale of the DUHP (Parkerson et al., 1981) includes both types. The Physical and Psycho-physiological Symptom Scale from the RAND Medical Outcomes Study (Stewart & Ware, 1992) consists of eight items deliberately selected to provide a mix of symptoms that are likely to be due to physical conditions and to psychological conditions, but these two types are combined into a single index. The Alameda County study used an 11-item Symptom Scale that included more frankly physical than somatizing symptoms. The SCL–90 (Derogatis, 1992) includes a 12-item Somatization Scale which is more heavily weighted toward traditional psychosomatic symptoms. A similar 34-item Somatization scale constitutes one of the 11 CARE conditions subscales. Many of the symptoms classed as subjective indicators of health do or could appear in the conditions checklist.

Self-Rated Health

All of the self-rated health measures shown in Table 2.1 have in common the request that the subject give a global assessment of health, rather than a report of any particular condition, sign, symptom, or illness-specific rating.

The last two rows of Table 2.1 summarize information about self-rated health measures. As mentioned earlier, we included two rows to distinguish between instruments which include (next-to-last row in Table 2.1) and which do not include (last row) the global self-rated health item: "How would you rate your health?" Because of the usefulness and uniqueness of this single item we discuss it as a separate topic and then discuss multi-item indices of self-rated health.

Single-Item Global Self-Rated Health. The self-rated health item ("How would you rate your health? Excellent, good, fair, poor?") has appeared in dozens of studies, including early ones by Shanas et al. (1968), the First Duke Longitudinal Study (Palmore, 1974) and those listed in the next-to-last row of Table 2.1. The utility of this item was nicely demonstrated in its superiority over objective medical indicators in predicting mortality (Mossey & Shapiro, 1982). Their finding has been replicated many times since (see Idler & Kasl, 1991). This latter study and the MAI provide a number of concurrent validity estimates of this question.

Multi-Item Indices of Self-Rated Health. Several composite scales include the single-item rating reviewed above. Multi-item composites of general health are provided by the four-item self-rated health subindex of the MAI, the seven-item Current Health Index of the MOS, and the five-item General Health Perceptions Index of the SF-36. The OMFAQ self-rated health items were used as indicators of a latent construct of self-reported health by Whitelaw and Liang (1991), although psychometric characteristics were not fully reported in a way that would make this item composite completely usable by others. Self-rated health appears only as items embedded in more general health indices in the remainder of the scales (in the last row of Table 2.1).

GUIDELINES FOR CHOOSING A HEALTH MEASURE

The choice of an instrument will naturally be a function of the purpose of the research or the type of evaluation being performed. Below we summarize five guidelines which are useful to keep in mind in different research situations.

Health as a single measure. There are many research situations where it is desirable to represent health, but to do so using a single or small number of variables. For those situations where time and cost permit use of only a single indicator of health (most usually research with a focus that is not on physical health per se) the global self-rated health item provides a good option. When a more complete assessment of physical health is possible, but analytically a single variable is necessary, the MAI, OMFAQ, and the Alameda County instruments provide a single overall score which represents a broad sampling of health status information. The CMI, CIRS, and SIRS also provide a summary score, but sample fewer of the dimensions of health identified in Table 2.1. The CIRS is being used very widely. Its total score summed across all body systems represents one of the most comprehensive indicators. A disadvantage is that all systems are weighted equally, and thus an extremely severe illness in one body system may not be adequately weighted in the overall index.

New ad hoc dimensional scales. Although some instruments lend themselves to creating subscales (e.g., OMFAQ, CMI) separate subscales were not originally planned or evaluated. The relative costs and benefits of extracting subscales should be considered. It would seem, for example, that the OMFAQ and the CMI items deserve considerable psychometric exploration. The ease with which subscales or items may be extracted from a larger assessment instrument depends on the conceptual framework of the instrument. If having both a summary score and dimension-specific subscales is desirable, it may be preferable to select an instrument designed for that option, such as the MAI, CORE–CARE or the Alameda County scales.

Confounding of independent and dependent variables. As noted in the introduction, there is a hazard in attempting to separate physical and emotional health. The form this hazard takes is a function of the research question. If one is looking for a predictor of psychological outcomes, the most objective indicator of physical health as possible (e.g., health condition scales) is preferable to self-rated health, because this latter construct shares considerable variance with psychological well-being and therefore risks confounding the independent and dependent variables.

Conceptual dimensions of health. Perhaps the most important determinant of instrument choice is the concept of health under investigation. The dimensions shown in Figure 2.1 and Table 2.1 have differential significance depending on what is being studied. We did not include all the possible conceptual groupings of items. As noted earlier, one important approach is disease-specific measures. If a single disease is of interest, disease-specific scales or subscales should be considered. Of the instruments we reviewed, only the CORE–CARE has disease-specific subscales. Even within disease-specific research, it may be advisable to assess a broader spectrum of physical health. Again, including a global rating of health by a professional provides a good alternative when cost and time are of concern.

Returning to the initial alternative ways of examining health, there are many traditional measures representing life threat, pain and discomfort, and functional ability. Although pain is treated in chapter 13, there is room for further attempts to measure disease-specific pain and distress. The ideal end point would be a set of modules for the major illness classes that could represent separately the objective and subjective aspects of each illness.

Sources of data. Although the concordance among representations of health by data from different sources continues to be of both theoretical and applied interest, one cannot make a case for the superiority of any one of the major sources (physician examination, laboratory data, professional judgment, observable behavior, archives, or self-report) for all situations. Although some will be clearly preferable in certain situations, the ideal measure for each situation is not always available. It may, therefore, be necessary to use an imperfect indicator sometimes, and to recognize and discuss possible sources of error.

In broadest summary, preference clearly must go to measures derived from large sample population surveys, which only the Manitoba study and the NHANES (and its cousins such as the Health Interview Survey (HIS) fulfill. However, the Alameda study, the CARE and the OMFAQ originated in large local samples and thus have the advantage of providing normative comparison data for new studies. Large, but not representative, samples, were used by other investigators (DUHP, MOS–FWBP, MAI). For breadth and choice among a number of health dimensions, the CARE and the MAI stand out, with the NHANES providing potential data for the development of such indices.

In summary, health is complex, multifaceted, and easy or difficult to measure, depending on the researcher's needs and perspective. Knowing what one should measure depends heavily on being able to locate one's problem and the aspect of health under study within a conceptual framework. The framework offered here also points out some elements that are poorly covered by present assessment technology: easy-to-use direct indicators of organ health, scaled summary indictors of medication use, and both objective and subjective measures of disease-specific health.

REFERENCES

Aldwin, C. M., Levenson, M. R., Ekerdt, D. J., & Bossé, R. (1987). Mental health differences among retirees and workers: Findings from the normative aging study. *Psychology and Aging, 2*, 383–389.

Aldwin, C. M., Spiro, A. S., Levenson, M. R., & Bossé, R. (1989). Longitudinal findings from the Normative Aging Study: I. Does mental health change with age? *Psychology and Aging, 4*, 295–306.

Belloc, N. B., Breslow, L., & Hochstim, J. R. (1971). Measurement of physical health in a general population survey. *American Journal of Epidemiology, 93*, 328–336.

Bergner, M. B., Bobbitt, R. A., Carter, W. B., & Gilson, B. S. (1981). The sickness Impact Profile: Development and final version of a health status measure. *Medical Care, 19*, 787–798.

Bowling, A. (1991). *Measuring health: A review of quality of life measurement scales.* Philadelphia: Open University Press.

Brodman, K., Erdmann, A. J., Lorge, I., & Wolff, H. G. (1949). The Cornell Medical Index: An adjunct to a medical interview. *Journal of the American Medical Association, 140*, 530–534.

Bush, J. W., Fanshel, S., & Chen, M. M. (1972). Analysis of a tuberculin testing program using a health status index. *Social and Economic Planning Science, 6*, 49–68.

Cameron, L., Leventhal, E. A., & Leventhal, H. (1993). Symptom representations and affect as determinants of care seeking in a community-dwelling, adult sample population. *Health Psychology, 12*, 171–179.

Chambers, L. W., MacDonald, L. A., Tugwell, P., Buchanan, W. W., & Kraag, G. (1982). The McMaster Health Index Questionnaire as a measure of quality of life for patients with rheumatoid disease. *Journal of Rheumatology, 9*, 780–784.

Chyba, M., & Washington, L. (1993). Questionnaires from the National Health Interview Survey, 1985–1989 (National Center for Health Statistics Series 1, No. 31) (PHS 93–1307). Hyattsville, MD: Public Health Service.

Comptroller General. (1977). *The well-being of older people in Cleveland, Ohio.* Washington, DC: U.S. General Accounting Office.

Conwell, Y., Forbes, N. T., Cox, C., & Caine, E. D. (1993). Validation of a measure of physical illness burden at autopsy: The Cumulative Illness Rating Scale. *Journal of the American Geriatrics Society, 41*, 38–41.

Coren, S., & Hakistian, R. A. (1992). The development and cross-validation of a self-report inventory to assess pure-tone threshold hearing sensitivity. *Journal of Speech and Hearing Research, 35*, 921–928.

Costa, P. T., & McCrae, R. R. (1980). Somatic complaints in males as a function of age and neuroticism. *Journal of Behavioral Medicine, 3*, 245–257.

Derogatis, L. L. (1992). *SCL–90–R revised manual.* Towson, MD: Clinical Psychometric Research Inc.

Derogatis, L. R., Rickels, K., & Rock, A. F. (1976). The SCL–90 and the MMPI: A step in the validation of a new self-report scale. *British Journal of Psychiatry, 128*, 280–289.

Duke University Center for the Study of Aging. (1978). *Multidimensional functional assessment: The OARS methodology* (2nd ed.). Durham, NC: Duke University.

Fillenbaum, G. G. (1984). *The well-being of the elderly.* Geneva: World Health Organization.

Fillenbaum, G. (1988). *Multidimensional functional assessment of older adults.* Hillsdale, NJ: Erlbaum.

Fillenbaum, G. G., & Smyer, M. A. (1981). The development, validity, and reliability of the

OARS Multidimensional Functional Assessment Questionnaire. *Journal of Gerontology, 36*, 428–434.

Golden, R. R., Teresi, J. A., & Gurland, B. J. (1984). Development of indicator scales for the Comprehensive Assessment and Referral Evaluation (CARE) interview schedule. *Journal of Gerontology, 39*, 138–146.

Grembowski, D., Patrick, D., Diehr, P., Durham, M., Beresford, S., Kay, E., & Hecht, J. (1993). Self-efficacy and health behavior among older adults. *Journal of Health and Social Behavior, 34*, 89–104.

Gurel, L., Linn, M. W., & Linn, B. S. (1972). Physical and Mental Impairment-of-Function Evaluation in the aged: The PAMIE Scale. *Journal of Gerontology, 27*, 83–90.

Gurland, B. J., & Wilder, D. E. (1984). The CARE interview revisited: Development of an efficient, systematic clinical assessment. *Journal of Gerontology, 39*, 129–137.

Hall, J. A., Epstein, A. M., & McNeil, B. J. (1989). Multidimensionality of health status in an elderly population. *Medical Care, 27*, S168–S177.

Hooker, K., & Siegler, I. C. (1992). Separating apples from oranges in health ratings: Perceived health includes psychological well-being. *Behavior, Health, and Aging, 2*, 81–92.

Horowitz, A., Teresi, J. A., & Cassels, L. A. (1991). Development of a vision screening questionnaire for older people. *Journal of Gerontological Social Work, 17*, 37–56.

Idler, E. L., & Kasl, S. (1991). Health perceptions and survival: Do global evaluations of health status really predict mortality? *Journals of Gerontology: Social Sciences, 46*, S55–S65.

Johnson, R. J., & Wolinsky, F. D. (1993). The structure of health status among older adults: Disease, disability, functional limitation, and perceived health. *Journal of Health and Social Behavior, 34*, 105–121.

Kane, R. A., & Kane, R. L. (1981). *Assessing the elderly.* Lexington, MA: Lexington Books.

Kane, R. A., Ouslander, J. G., & Abrass, I. (1984). *Essentials of clinical geriatrics.* New York: McGraw-Hill.

Laforge, R. G., Spector, W. D., & Sternberg, J. (1992). The relationship of vision and hearing to one-year mortality and functional decline. *Journal of Aging and Health, 4*, 126–148.

Langlie, J. K. (1977). Social networks, health beliefs, and preventive health behavior. *Journal of Health and Social Behavior, 18*, 244–260.

Lawton, M. P. (1984). Investigating health and subjective well-being: Substantive challenges. *International Journal of Aging and Human Development, 19*, 211–227.

Lawton, M. P. (1991). A multidimensional view of quality of life in frail elders. In J. E. Birren, J. E. Lubben, J. C. Rowe, & D. E. Deutchman (Eds.), *The concept and measurement of quality of life* (pp. 3–27). New York: Academic Press.

Lawton, M. P., Moss, M., Fulcomer, M., & Kleban, M. H. (1982). A research and service-oriented Multilevel Assessment Instrument. *Journal of Gerontology, 37*, 91–99.

Liang, J. (1986). Self-reported physical health among aged adults. *Journal of Gerontology, 41*, 248–260.

Linn, M. W., & Linn, B. S. (1984). Self-Evaluation of Life (SELF) Scale: A short comprehensive self-report of health for the elderly. *Journal of Gerontology, 39*, 603–612.

Linn, M. W., Linn, B. S., & Gurel, L. (1967). Physical resistance in the aged. *Geriatrics, 22*, 134–138.

Linn, B. S., Linn, M. W., & Gurel, L. (1968). The Cumulative Illness Rating Scale. *Journal of the American Geriatrics Society, 16*, 622–626.

Mahler, D. A., Weinberg, D. H., Wells, C. K., & Feinstein, A. R. (1984). The measurement of dyspnea. *Chest, 85*, 751–760.

Mahurin, R. K., DeBettignies, B. H., & Pirozzolo, F. J. (1991). Structured Assessment of Independent Daily Living Skills: Preliminary report of a performance measure of functional abilities in dementia. *Journals of Gerontology: Psychological Sciences, 46*, P58–P66.

Markides, K. S., & Martin, H. W. (1979). Predicting self-rated health among the aged. *Research on Aging, 1*, 97–112.

McAuley, W. J., Arling, G., Nutty, C. L., & Bowling, C. A. (1980). *Final report of the Statewide Survey of Older Virginians*. Richmond, VA: Virginia Center on Aging.

McAuley, J., Travis, S., & Taylor, C. A. (1987). Long-term patients in acute care facilities. *Journal of Applied Gerontology, 6*, 67–81.

McDowell, I., & Newell, C. (1987). *Measuring health: A guide to rating scales and questionnaires*. New York: Oxford University Press.

McHorney, C. A., Ware, J. E., & Raczek, A. E. (1993). The MOS 36-Item Short-Form Health Survey (SF–36): II. Psychometric and clinical tests of validity in measuring physical and mental health constructs. *Medical Care, 31*, 247–263.

Meenan, R. F., Gertman, P. M., & Mason, J. M. (1980). Measuring health status in arthritis: The Arthritis Impact Measurement Scale. *Arthritis and Rheumatism, 23*, 146–152.

Meltzer, J. W., & Hochstim, J. R. (1970). Reliability and validity of survey data on physical health. *Public Health Reports, 85*, 1075–1086.

Miller, M. D., Paradis, C. F., Houck, P. R., Mazumdar, S., Stack, J. A., Rifai, A. H., Muisant, B., & Reynolds, C. F. (1992). Rating chronic medical illness burden in geropsychiatric practice and research: Application of the Cumulative Illness Rating Scale. *Psychiatry Research, 41*, 237–248.

Mossey, J. M., Havens, B., Roos, N. P., & Shapiro, E. (1981). The Manitoba longitudinal study on aging: Description and methods. *The Gerontologist, 21*, 551–558.

Mossey, J. M., & Roos, L. L. (1987). Using insurance claims to measure health status: The Illness Scale. *Journal of Chronic Diseases, 40*, 41S–50S.

Mossey, J., & Shapiro, E. (1982). Self-rated health: A predictor of mortality among the elderly. *American Journal of Public Health, 72*, 800–808.

National Center for Health Statistics. (1985). The national health interview survey design, 1973–84, and procedures, 1975–1983. *Vital and Health Statistics*, Series 10, No. 18 (PHS 85–1320). Hyattsville, MD: Public Health Service.

National Center for Health Statistics. (1991). *National health and nutrition examination survey III data collection forms*. Hyattsville, MD: Public Health Service.

National Center for Health Statistics. (1992). The longitudinal study of aging: 1984–90. *Vital and Health Statistics*, Series 1, No. 28 (PHS 91–1304). Hyattsville, MD: Public Health Service.

Newcomb, M. E., & Bentler, P. M. (1987). Self-report methods of assessing health status and health service utilization: A hierarchical confirmatory analysis. *Multivariate Behavior Research, 22*, 415–436.

Okun, M. A., Stock, W. A., Haring, M. J., & Witter, R. (1984). Health and subjective well-being: A meta-analysis. *International Journal of Aging and Human Development, 19*, 111–132.

Palmore, E. (Ed.). (1974). *Normal aging II*. Durham, NC: Duke University Press.

Parkerson, G. R., Gehlbach, S. H., Wagner, E. H., James, S. A., Clapp, N. E., & Muhlbaier, L. H. (1981). The Duke–UNC Health Profile: An adult health status instrument for primary care. *Medical Care, 19*, 806–829.

Patrick, D. L., & Bergner, M. (1990). Measurement of health status in the 1990s. *Annual Review of Public Health, 11*, 165–183.

Patrick, D. L., & Deyo, R. A. (1989). Generic and disease-specific measures in assessing health status and quality of life. *Medical Care, 27*(Suppl. 3), S217–S232.

Rosenberg, S. J., Hayes, J. R., & Peterson, R. A. (1987). Revising the Seriousness of Illness Rating Scale: Modernization and re-standardization. *International Journal of Psychiatry in Medicine, 17*, 85–92.

Rosencranz, H. A., Pihlblad, C. T. (1970). Measuring the health of the elderly. *Journal of Gerontology, 25*, 129–133.

Rosenhall, U., Pedersen, K., & Møller, M. B. (1987). Self-assessment of hearing problems in an elderly population: A longitudinal study. *Scandinavian Audiology, 16*, 211–217.

Rosenstock, I. M. (1974). The health belief model and preventive health behavior. *Health Education Monographs, 2*, 354–386.

Rubinstein, L., Calkins, E. R., Greenfield, S., Jette, A. M., Meenan, R. F., Nevins, M. A., Rubenstein, L. Z., Wasson, J. H., & Williams, M. E. (1989). Health status assessment for elderly patients. *Journal of the American Geriatrics Society, 37*, 562–569.

Rudberg, M. A., Furner, S. E., Dunn, J. T., & Cassell, C. K. (1993). The relationship of visual and hearing impairments to disability: An analysis using the Longitudinal Study of Aging. *Journals of Gerontology: Medical Sciences, 48*, M261–M265.

Schow, R. L., & Nerbonne, M. A. (1982). Communication screening profile: Use with elderly clients. *Ear and Hearing, 3*, 135–147.

Seeman, T. E., Guralnik, J. M., Kaplan, G. A., Knudsen, L., & Cohen, R. (1989). The health consequences of multiple morbidity in the elderly. *Journal of Aging and Health, 1*, 50–66.

Shanas, E. (1962). *The health of older people*. Cambridge, MA: Harvard University Press.

Shanas, E., Townsend, P., Wedderburn, D., Friis, H., Milhøj, P., & Stehouwer, J. (1968). *Old people in three industrial societies*. New York: Atherton.

Slawinski, E. B., Hartel, D. M., & Kline, D. W. (1993). Self-reported hearing problems in daily life throughout adulthood. *Psychology and Aging, 8*, 552–561.

Smith, G. T. (1988). *Measuring health: A practical approach*. New York: Wiley.

Spitzer, W. O., Dobson, A. J., Hall, J., Chesterman, E., Levi, J., Shepherd, R., Battista, R. N., & Catchlove, B. R. (1981). Measuring the quality of life of cancer patients: A concise QL index. *Journal of Chronic Diseases, 34*, 585–597.

Stahl, S. M. (1984). Health. In D. J. Mangen & W. A. Peterson (Eds.), *Health, program evaluation and demography* (pp. 85–116). Minneapolis: University of Minnesota Press.

Stewart, A. L., & Ware, J. E. (Eds.) (1992). *Measuring functioning and well-being: The Medical Outcomes Study approach*. Durham, NC: Duke University Press.

Teresi, J. A., Golden, R. R., & Gurland, B. J. (1984). Concurrent and predictive validity of indicator scales developed for the Comprehensive Assessment and Referral Evaluation interview schedule. *Journal of Gerontology, 39*, 158–165.

Teresi, J. A., Golden, R. R., Gurland, B. J., Wilder, D. E., & Bennett, R. G. (1984). Construct validity of indicator-scales developed from the Comprehensive Assessment and Referral Evaluation interview schedule. *Journal of Gerontology, 39*, 147–157.

Travis, S. S., McAuley, W. J., & Taylor, C. A. (1988, November). Experience with a Seriousness of Illness Rating Scale in long-term care research. Paper presented at the annual meeting of the Gerontological Society of America, San Francisco.

Von Korff, M., Wagner, E. H., & Saunders, K. (1992). A chronic disease score from automated pharmacy data. *Journal of Clinical Epidemiology, 45*, 197–203.

Wagner, E. H., LaCroix, A. Z., Grothaus, L. C., & Hecht, J. A. (1993). Responsiveness of health status measures to change among older adults. *Journal of the American Geriatrics Society, 41*, 241–248.

Wallston, B. S., Wallston, K. A., Kaplan, G. D., & Maides, S. A. (1976). Development and validation of the Health Locus of Control Scale. *Journal of Consulting and Clinical Psychology, 44*, 580–585.

Ware, J. E., & Sherbourne, C. D. (1992). The MOS 36-item short-form health survey (SF–36). *Medical Care, 30*, 473–483.

Whitelaw, N. A., & Liang, J. (1991). The structure of the OARS physical health measures. *Medical Care, 29*, 332–347.

Williamson, G. M., & Schulz, R. (1992). Physical illness and symptoms of depression among elderly outpatients. *Psychology and Aging, 7*, 343–351.

Woodruff, S. I., & Conway, T. L. (1992). Impact of health and fitness-related behavior on quality of life. *Social Indicators Research, 26*, 39–405.

World Health Organization. (1948). *Constitution of the World Health Organization*. Geneva, Switzerland: WHO Basic Documents.

Wyler, A. R., Masuda, M., & Holmes, T. H. (1968). Seriousness of Illness Rating Scale. *Journal of Psychosomatic Research, 11*, 363–374.

CHAPTER 3

Functional Disability: Activities and Instrumental Activities of Daily Living

MARY GRACE KOVAR
NATIONAL OPINION RESEARCH CENTER
WASHINGTON, D.C.

AND

M. POWELL LAWTON
POLISHER RESEARCH INSTITUTE
PHILADELPHIA GERIATRIC CENTER

THE CONCEPT OF FUNCTIONAL DISABILITY

It is valuable to have a conceptual framework for any measure. Probably the most widely known concept for assessing the impact of injury and disease on the individual is that of the World Health Organization (WHO). Although the International Classification of Impairments, Disabilities, and Handicaps (ICIDH), which was published for trial purposes in 1976 (WHO, 1976), is not yet widely used in the United States, it is currently being revised with active participation from the United States.

The authors of the ICIDH pointed out that the medical model of disease was, and continues to be, useful for acute infectious and life-threatening chronic diseases. However, diseases that are self-limiting or amenable to cure account for only part of the spectrum of morbidity. In fact, the success of various medical and public health measures for the control of such diseases has resulted in the increasingly recognized importance of the residue of conditions, including the effects of trauma, impairments of special sense organs, mental retardation and mental illness, and the chronic diseases.

The ICIDH authors went on to say that the medical model, which they described as

Etiology ⟶ Pathology ⟶ Manifestation

fails to describe the full range of problems. Therefore, they proposed a broader model to measure the consequences of disease. They defined three consequences:

1. An *impairment* is any loss or abnormality of psychological, physiological, or anatomical structure or function.
2. A *disability* is any restriction or lack (resulting from an impairment) of ability to perform an activity in the manner or within the range considered normal for a human being.
3. A *handicap* is a disadvantage for a given individual, resulting from an impairment or disability, that limits or prevents the fulfillment of a role that is normal (depending on age, sex, and social or cultural factors) for that individual.

Disease → Impairment (exteriorized) → Disability (objectified) → Handicap (socialized)

Despite some major limitations in the categories of the ICIDH, especially the categories of handicaps, the ICIDH has been used extensively in other parts of the world, except in the United States. Perhaps its first wide visibility in the United States was in the Institute of Medicine report, "The Second Fifty Years: Promoting Health and Preventing Disability" (Institute of Medicine [IOM], 1990). After consideration of the difficulties in classifying disability, the committee decided to advocate the WHO model. They discussed many reasons for their decision but ended their discussion by writing:

> Much of the appeal of the WHO classification system lies in the new health care goals made explicit in its subcategories. It is in this context that the Committee on Health Promotion and Disability Prevention for the Second Fifty Years encourages physicians to shift their attention—and with it their frame of reference—toward providing comprehensive help for their elderly patients (IOM, 1990, p. 30).

That paragraph is important because it shows two major reasons why the committee chose this model for disability among older people. They felt that it was useful to measure progress toward health care goals and that its use would encourage physicians caring for elderly patients to shift their attention toward providing comprehensive help for their elderly disabled patients.

Unfortunately, the ICIDH was written as if medical records were the only source of health data and the only purpose of the classification was evaluating health services, which may account for some of the limitations. There are many other reasons for measuring the consequences of disease and many ways of gathering information.

This chapter on the activities of daily living (ADL) and the instrumental activities of daily living (IADL) is designed to evaluate one way of measuring disability and, sometimes, handicap and particularly their use in population-based surveys, with occasional discussion of contrasts between survey and clinical issues. The ADL and IADL fit the ICIDH model well when they include a measure of severity. Difficulty with an activity of daily living would be a disability in the ICIDH framework (Verbrugge, 1990); inability to perform an activity is a handicap. The IADL also fits well for both disability and handicap when the qualifying phrase on social and cultural factors is included. Earlier useful critical reviews of this area of assessment may be found in Ernst and Ernst (1984), Feinstein, Josephy, and Wells (1986), Kane and Kane (1981), and McDowell and Newell (1987).

MEASURING ACTIVITIES OF DAILY LIVING

The ADL was originally developed for assessing the potential of institutionalized people to regain functioning; by the early 1980s it had become the preferred method of assessing the health of older community-dwelling populations.

Katz and his colleagues (Katz, Ford, Moskowitz, Jackson, & Jaffee, 1963) developed the activities of daily living as a means of assessing rehabilitation, and the potential for rehabilitation, for chronically ill older people. Katz continued to work on and improve the scale (Katz, Downs, Cash, & Gratz, 1970) and in 1976 published a theoretical basis for using the items that he had selected (Katz & Akpom, 1976).

The theoretical framework is based on the concept that recovering patients pass through three stages:

1. Return of independence in feeding and continence,
2. Recovery in transferring and going to the toilet, and
3. Recovery of independence in dressing and bathing.

These stages have an interesting parallel with early childhood development. Katz observed that elderly patients lose functioning in these areas in approximately the reverse order in which children acquire them. Patients then follow the same order as children in recovering function. All of these functions are defined in terms of independence, or lack of assistance, with assistance defined as active physical assistance, directive assistance, or supervision. Katz and his colleagues used the evaluation of functional independence (or dependence) to develop an Index of Independence in Activities of Daily Living with seven defined categories. That index is structured as a hierarchical scale and has been extensively validated. A good review that includes the questions, the index, and a review of validation studies can be found in Ernst and Ernst (1984).

MEASURING INSTRUMENTAL ACTIVITIES OF DAILY LIVING

At about the same time, Lawton and Brody (1969) developed a scale for the instrumental activities of daily living (IADL), which they used for community dwelling applicants for long-term care as well as for institutional residents. The IADLs were designed to tap a more complex range of functioning, in that they require more skill, judgment, and independence than the ADLs. They measure an individual's functioning in the social world and the world outside the home; difficulty with one or more IADLs is far more prevalent than difficulty with an ADL.

USE OF ADLS AND IADLS ON LARGE SURVEYS

Although ADL-like questions were included in the three-nation study by Shanas et al. (1968), the first use of the full set of ADLs in a population-based survey was for the Massachusetts Health Care Panel Study in 1974 (Katz et al., 1983). The questions on the 1979–1980 Home Care Supplement to the National Health Interview were influenced by the Katz work but were not really an ADL set. However, by the early 1980s questions on the ADLs had been included on many smaller surveys, and by the middle 1980s on at least three large national longitudinal studies: the Long-Term Care Survey (Macken, 1986), the National Health and Nutrition Examination Survey Epidemiological Follow-up Study (Cohen et al., 1987), and the Longitudinal Study of Aging (Kovar, Fitti, & Chyba, 1992), which was based on the Supplement on Aging to the 1984 National Health Interview Survey (Fitti & Kovar, 1987). The Supplement on Aging and the Longitudinal Study of Aging also included the IADLs. Wiener, Hanley, Clark, and Van Nostrand (1990) review in greater detail how these ADL measures were used in 11 different nationally representative surveys.

These large longitudinal surveys provide strong evidence for the power of the ADL and IADL measures. The best evidence is from the longitudinal analysis of the Long-Term Care Survey across two years (1982–1984) (Manton, 1988) and seven years (1982, 1984, 1989) (Manton, Corder, & Stallard, 1993a). A clearly measurable increased risk of growing morbidity and increase in mortality was noted as the baseline categories progressed from nondisabled to IADL-only disability to disabilities marked by one or two ADL disabilities, three, four, five, or six disabilities, institutional residence, and death (Manton et al., 1993, Table 2). For example, of those nondisabled in 1984, 86.5% were still nondisabled in 1989, 1.3% were in institutions, and 5.7% had died. Compare these low-risk figures with transitions observed for one of the moderately impaired categories, that is, those with one or two ADL impairments in 1984: Only 3.4% had improved to a nondisabled state, whereas 8.0% had become institutionalized, and 19.5% had died. For the most severely impaired in 1984 (those with five to six ADL impairments),

7.6% were institutionalized, and 39.2% had died. Evidence from the first follow-up on the Longitudinal Study of Aging shows the same thing. Of those receiving help with an ADL at baseline, only 65% were alive 2 years later; in contrast, 78% of those receiving help only for IADLs were still alive, whereas 86% of those who had no difficulty with either an ADL or an IADL were still living (Kovar, 1987). The comparable figures for predicting living in an institution from the three levels of disability were 10.5%, 4.7%, and 1.3%. The predictive power of such data in making transition estimates is of major usefulness in planning future health services.

ISSUES IN MEASURING ADLS AND IADLS

The literature is filled with demonstrations of the power of ADL and IADL measurements in making predictions. Yet, as they have become widely used, many issues of both conceptual and methodological import have arisen, forcing us to recognize that there are sources of error in both epidemiological and clinical applications of ADL and IADL measurements. The 10 issues discussed in this chapter are (1) which activities should be included in the set of ADLs or IADLs, (2) the differing goals of assessment for clinical and survey use, (3) the expected prevalence of disabilities, (4) the context within which disability is assessed, (5) frames of reference for defining disability, (6) social roles and cultural context, (7) self-reporting versus proxy reporting, (8) cognitive factors in reporting, (9) subjective estimation versus performance as the measurement object, and (10) technical measurement and methodological issues.

Which Activities Should be Included?

There is no universally accepted list of activities to include on surveys. The original Katz Index of Independence in Activities of Daily Living included six activities; in current practice, toileting and continence are not always distinguished, and a question on mobility is frequently added. The original Instrumental Activities of Daily Living scale included an eight-item scale for women and a five- or six-item scale for men. Self-rated versions of the IADL were developed later. They include a five-item (Fillenbaum, 1985), a seven-item (Duke University, 1978), and a nine-item (Lawton, Moss, Fulcomer, & Kleban, 1982) scale for both men and women; none of the large population-based surveys conducted during the 1980s included all nine of the original Lawton and Brody items. Wiener et al. (1990) review these differences in the actual items included in different national surveys. Such differences are important determinants of the varying sizes of the national estimates of disability obtained from the surveys.

The issue of which items and how many of them to include is especially important for the ADL because much legislation is based on a criterion for dependence defined by national estimates of the number of people evidencing a specified num-

TABLE 3.1 Percentages of 65+ Population with Activity Limitations[a]

	Receive help with activity	*Difficulty performing activity*
Self-care activities		
Eating	1.1	1.8
Using toilet	2.2	4.3
Dressing	4.3	6.2
Transferring	2.8	8.0
Getting outside	5.3	9.6
Bathing	6.0	9.8
Walking	4.7	18.7
One or more activities	9.6	22.7
Home management activities		
Using telephone	3.0	4.8
Managing money	4.8	5.1
Preparing meals	6.0	7.1
Doing light housework	6.2	7.1
Shopping	10.5	11.1
Doing heavy housework	19.3	23.8
One or more activities	22.2	26.9

[a]From Dawson, Hendershot, & Fulton (1987).

ber of ADL disabilities (usually two); the chance of being dependent in two functions obviously rises as the number of ADLs on the list increases. If there are two questions on toileting, one on ability to get to the toilet and one on continence, a person who needed help with both would be dependent in two ADLs; if they are combined into one question, the same person would be dependent in only one. A specific example of the actual items that appear on one of the major surveys illustrates the typical range of such functions and their prevalence, as measured in survey situations (Table 3.1).

A related question concerning the choice of which activities to include in an ADL or IADL set is that of the breadth of representation needed to cover the important facets of everyday task performance. There appears to be a natural limitation of ADL tasks to a relatively small number of candidates, but the number of possible IADL tasks seems almost limitless. For example, cutting's one's own toenails was used in the cross-national survey (Shanas et al., 1968) but is not included among scales now in use. In contrast to the relatively short IADL scales in most general use, a recent scale attempted to broaden the scope of knowledge about a person yielded by an IADL assessment. Myers (1992) reported on the psychometric testing of a 50-item IADL instrument. When a clinical evaluation is required, the advantages of such a broad range of skills is obvious. In fact, to rehabilitation-oriented staff, the usual ADL and IADL instruments appear to be inappropriately gross (see Duncan and Studenski's chapter on gait and balance for one way to probe more deeply into the fine-grained measurement of clinically relevant functioning). For survey purposes, however, a short, five- to eight-item scale is appropriate.

Finally, one also must be concerned about the "difficulty" of all items in a set, that is, variations in the proportion of the population who are unable to perform the task. Obviously, the presence of more difficult items will result in a higher estimate of disability than will a set with fewer difficult items. Such considerations will affect both national policy and individual eligibility decisions for services (see Jackson, Burwell, Clark, & Hanrahan, 1992, for a discussion of the functional criteria for service eligibility).

Clinical Versus Survey Use of Functional Assessment

It is important to distinguish between performing functional assessments for an individual, as is usually done in a clinical setting, and a survey designed to estimate the prevalence of disability. The individual assessment needs to minimize false positives and negatives, even at the expense of ease and economy of administration, and usually requires a highly trained professional to perform the assessment. In contrast, group assessment sacrifices the accurate assessment of individuals in favor of high levels of interrater reliability and ease of administration (Guralnik & LaCroix, 1992). On population surveys, the questionnaires are usually administered by an interviewer who is trained in survey techniques, which includes accepting the respondent's answers without interpretation. That is quite different from the setting in which the person who is asking the question is also evaluating the respondent.

The ADLs and IADLs have been used both ways. They were originally developed for clinical use, especially in institutional settings, but both have now been used extensively on both local and national surveys.

Prevalence of Disability

Both the ADLs and IADLs were developed to be used by trained observers in specified situations, usually clinical situations where few people would be free of any disability along one of the dimensions. Because the ADLs were designed to measure the functional status of chronically ill people, they only measure the extremely disabled end of the scale. In a community-dwelling population, the prevalence of ADL disability is low, and the scales' ability to discriminate above very low levels of disability is poor. The same is true of the IADLs, although disabilities in this realm are more prevalent. The data in the first column of Table 3.1 show the prevalence of dependence in ADLs and IADLs among community-dwelling people age 65 and over.

Even the most prevalent disability, difficulty doing heavy housework, affects less than one-quarter of community-dwelling elders. The ADL and IADL scales thus are best at identifying the most-disabled minority. There has, therefore, been a search for more complex tasks on which to base assessments that would distinguish among high-functioning people. Because such tasks inevitably have major social and cognitive components and vary with preference and environmental opportunity, they fall outside the realm of the ADLs.

The Context of Disability Assessment

The effect of contextual factors on ADL and IADL scores is substantial. Proper interpretation requires an account to be taken of the manner in which the ADL questions are framed and how such wording interacts with the residential care context. For example, in the National Medical Expenditure Survey (NMES) of 1987, ADL disabilities were determined by asking whether personal assistance was needed to perform the task (Lair & Lefkowitz, 1993). Although this question is meaningful for some ADLs in some institutions, in many nursing homes residents are required to receive assistance in such tasks as bathing. Many of the IADLs are routinely performed for the resident. Therefore, the estimates of functioning on these scales reflect an unknown mix of personal disability and contextual constraint when used on institutional residents. Even in more independent residential situations, such as life care or congregate housing, some IADL tasks may be part of the bundle of services provided for everyone, whether needed or not.

Context is also important on the micro level of the individual home environment. Performing an interview in the person's home means that there is no standardization of the context of the person's life, and the questions on large surveys cannot be worded to provide that standardization. It should be noted that the Supplement on Aging did include questions regarding three home-supportive design features at two levels: first, whether the feature exists, and, second, whether the respondent "needs" it.

Whether an individual has difficulty getting to and using the toilet may depend a great deal on whether there is a toilet easily accessible and whether there are grab rails to aid rising and sitting. Whether that person has difficulty dressing may depend on the type of clothes he or she wears; dresses that fasten in the front and shoes that do not lace simplify dressing. Difficulty preparing meals may depend not only on the equipment in the kitchen but the type of meal the person considers normal; a microwave makes preparation of prepackaged food easy in comparison with, say, peeling and cooking potatoes. Some people may have difficulty bathing because they have only a deep tub, whereas others with a walk-in shower may have no trouble. With the growing prevalence of special home modifications to support self-maintaining behaviors, it may be necessary to begin reporting ADL disability rates stratified for the presence of such supports (Manton, Corder, & Stallard, 1993b). For example, they found that the most prevalent and fastest-growing group of disabled (those with one to two ADL impairments in 1982) also showed a greater rate of increase by 1989 in the use of equipment relative to other help than did those with more ADL impairments. The home context would thus seem to affect ADL measurement especially strongly at mild, rather than low or severe, levels of impairment.

Frames of Reference for Defining Disability

It is unfortunate that the concepts, wording, and items to be included in measuring ADL are not more consistent across large national surveys because data from those surveys are used to formulate public policies that affect large numbers of older people. The difference between "requiring" and "receiving" help is conceptually important. However, both are used, and many people assume "need" without reading how the question was asked. It may not even matter to respondents; there has been no research to indicate whether respondents notice the difference between such wordings. The difference between hands-on help given by a person who is physically present with the older person and help provided by another person who furnishes equipment to make it possible for the older person to do something alone is also important; research has shown that some respondents do not make that distinction (Keller, Kovar, Jobe, & Branch, 1993). It seems strange that research on questions whose answers affect so many older people has received so little attention. Much more such research needs to be done.

At least four different frames of reference for assessing ADLs have been used: task description, assistance from others, latent ability to perform, and difficulty experienced.

The *task-descriptive* approach defines each scale point in terms of specific behaviors, rather than using a single dimension, such as help received. It has been used primarily in small-sample and clinical, but not survey, situations. The prototype was the Langley-Porter Physical Self-Maintenance Scale for ADLs (Lowenthal, 1964) (e.g., grooming, with scale points ranging from 1 = "always neatly dressed" to 5 = "actively negates all efforts of others" in dressing); the amount of help received was a component of many scale points but not the central concept. A similar approach was used in the original IADL (Lawton & Brody, 1969); for example, the telephone use item's scale points where 1 = "operates telephone on own," 2 = "dials a few well-known numbers," 3 = "answers but does not dial," and 4 = "does not use at all." The Functional Independence Measure (FIM; Granger, 1987) has become the standard in rehabilitation settings. The FIM requires 7-point ratings on 24 functions, 16 of which are basic ADLs. Each scale point is phrased as a hybrid of task description and help required. This task-oriented approach requires a trained observer to make such ratings. The validity of self-ratings on such direct measures of competence may be more problematic than when attention is focused on either whether the task is performed or whether assistance is received. In addition, the focus on task performance resulted in the inability to use the same scales for men and women in the original Lawton and Brody IADL. The problems in obtaining valid and role-relevant observations have led to a neglect of the task-descriptive approach in most ADL research. For clinical and small-scale research, there is room for considerable development of task descriptive measures. For example, the application of ergonomic task-analytic methods has shown promise in the work of Czaja, Weber, and Nair (1993) on several ADLs and in the study of meal preparation behavior (Falleti, 1984).

Assistance from others, or ADL dependence, is the most used approach to defining disability. Assistance is defined as active physical assistance. This concept of assistance for judging independence in the ADLs has not always been defined in the same way. This frame of reference is intrinsically more global and subjective than the task-descriptive perspective. A single dimension of "how much help" constitutes the criterion, and most such approaches use a three-point ordinal scale, such as none—some—not performed except with help. There are subtle differences in how the inquiry is phrased that may affect population estimates. Some surveys ask whether personal assistance is "needed," and others ask if it is "received;" only the Long Term Care Survey appears to have asked the question both ways in the full survey (Wiener et al., 1990). Unfortunately, no data are on hand to suggest whether one frame of reference or another elicits more valid information or whether the differences are meaningful.

It should also be noted that receiving "assistance" may not always be assigned the same significance in different perspectives. For example, the approach often taken by advocates for the rights of disabled persons is that the outcome, that is, the final performance of the task, is a more important indicator than the manner by which the outcome was obtained. Thus, the use of assistive devices and even a personal helper would be seen as affording independence (Simon-Rusinowitz & Hofland, 1993).

Latent ability to perform a task is a frame of reference introduced by the Older Americans Resources & Services Multidimensional Functional Assessment Questionnaire (OARS; Duke University, 1978) to correct for the possibility that factors other than impairment could account for a functional disability (e.g., an environmental barrier, a gender role, a preference). Therefore the OARS IADL items are phrased as, "Can you . . .?" rather than "Do you . . .?" with the subject's response being accepted as given. The Multilevel Assessment Instrument (MAI; Lawton et al., 1982) extended the inquiry in stepwise fashion to obtain maximum knowledge, which was coded finally by the interviewer: First, "Do you?" perform the task. If not, "Why not?" If a non–impairment-related response is given to explain nonperformance, the latent-ability question is asked. "Could you . . . if . . . (the explanatory factor were not in existence)?" In light of the fact that self-ratings are often more favorable than those produced by professionals, and the optimism tends to become greater as objective impairment increases (Rubenstein, Schairer, Wieland, & Kane, 1984; Weinberger et al., 1992), the "Could-you" approach to IADL measurement is not a completely satisfactory alternative to the "Do-you" version.

Difficulty in performing everyday tasks has been introduced as an alternative to task performance, that is, "Do you have no difficulty, some difficulty, a lot of difficulty, or are you unable to . . .?" The Comprehensive Assessment and Referral Evaluation (CARE) activity limitation scale items are of this format, "Do you have difficulty . . .?" (Gurland et al., 1977–78). Verbrugge (1990) has argued that difficulty should be the focal frame of reference for defining disability because it is clearly a characteristic of the person. By contrast, "do with assistance" Verbrugge sees as more of a "handicap" in the WHO sense and, therefore, only a indicator of personal impairment. Doing with assistance dilutes the disability measure by adding the social support element. A further argument offered by Verbrugge in favor of difficulty ratings is that they are easy to elicit.

A first question concerns what one measures when obtaining difficulty ratings. Self-ratings of difficulty would seem to have better face validity than ratings by an observer of such a subjective phenomenon, which has substantial built-in error. One major survey, the Supplement on Aging, and its longitudinal follow-ups (Kovar et al., 1992) inquired about both receiving help and difficulty (both dichotomously). Table 3.1 shows the comparison between percentages based on these two frames of reference. Without exception, the disability rates are higher for difficulty. If we could be certain that the difficulty rate is the sum of the receive-help, need-help, or latent-ability rate plus the percentage who actually perform the task, but with difficulty, there would be every reason to include both the help and the difficulty frames of reference routinely. One's confidence in making such an assumption is moderated somewhat, however, by evidence documenting a third influence on difficulty ratings whose strength and bias when used for ADL ratings is unknown, what Carp and Carp (1981) called the "self-defensive" response set. In a test of the effect of descriptive versus competence-oriented survey question wordings, they found that a set of judgments by older people of several objects (e.g., housing) showed a lower prevalence of negative evaluations when the evaluation was framed in terms of "problem to you" than when judged in more descriptive terms. That is, people admitted less ideal housing when the emphasis was on objective quality of the housing, rather than on whether it was a problem to the respondent. It is likely that ego defensiveness or its opposite, a self-deprecating tendency, may enter into judgments of difficulty. Such tendencies may be unequally distributed among subgroups of elders as they rate their ADLs and IADLs. One way of disentangling such effects might be to explore whether personality factors or response styles might contribute to the error in these estimates.

The Longitudinal Study of Aging contains the requisite data to test the predictive ability of the ADL difficulty items for transitions similar to those reported by Manton et al. (1993a) from the Long-Term Care Study data. Such an analysis, compared to the predictive ability of the help-received version, would instruct us better on the properties of these alternative response formats.

To summarize this section on frames of reference for ADLs, both help received and help needed (the task dependence framework) have been widely used, with little evidence to suggest whether one is superior to the other. The task-oriented approach is less well suited to the survey but deserves considerably more attention for clinical use. The latent-ability or "could-do" approach is recommended for IADL use, with recognition of the many limitations of this use, especially for self-ratings. Difficulty ratings clearly offer an additional perspective of potential value but should not be substituted for the task dependence approach.

Social Roles and Cultural Context

Many of the factors discussed earlier under contextual factors apply specifically to the use of ADL and IADL measures with people of varying social statuses and cultural backgrounds. Socially or culturally assigned roles are obvious conditioners of IADL task performance and, conceivably, capability. The widower who is truly incapable of cooking a meal is well known in service settings.

Such measures have rarely been used cross-culturally in such a way as to explore essential differences in the actual structure and meaning of ADL competence or disability. Smaller scale studies of subgroups defined by language, income, race, or other characteristics will be needed before any attempt to accommodate subgroup diversity in epidemiological surveys can be made. In the section on measurement that follows, one possible approach to increased representation of such structural diversity will be offered.

Self-Reporting Versus Proxy Reporting

If any two people are asked about the ability of a third person to perform certain activities they are liable to give different answers. Davies (1991) reported that in a study by Factor and colleagues in Israel, elderly persons on waiting lists for admission to long-term care institutions were assessed at the time of application and were later reassessed. Forty-three percent of the elderly who were moderately disabled in performing ADLs said that they could remain in the community. The informal caregivers thought that only 37 percent could remain. However, the multidisciplinary assessment team felt that 82 percent could remain in the community. In general, proxy respondents are more likely to report disability, and to report more disability, than self-respondents (Rubenstein et al., 1984). That has led to suggestions that caretakers overreport disability and individuals underreport it. Neither is necessarily true nor supported by research. In the Supplement of Aging, great care was taken to have every person respond for himself or herself, and 91.5 percent of the sample participants did so (Fitti & Kovar, 1987). People who reportedly received help with one or more ADLs or IADLs were far less likely to respond for themselves than those who did not receive help. People age 85 and older were also more likely to have proxy respondents than younger people (27% vs. 6%). Given such substantial age and probable health differences, it does not seem surprising that proxy respondents would be more likely to report disability.

At the present time, there has been too little research on the effect of proxy reporting, and conclusions on what has been completed are conflicting (see reviews by Herzog & Rodgers, 1992, pp. 68–69; Magaziner, 1992). It does seem clear that large surveys must continue to mix self-reporting and proxy reports. It is also clear that surveys, such as those that include the oldest-old, will have more proxy reports. The need for research on proxy reporting where large samples of subjects of differing statuses (socioeconomic, age, or health) are assessed in both ways is obvious.

Cognitive Factors in Reporting

The cognitive demand on the respondent is an important issue to understand, especially in the ADL area, where the target population of self-respondents may be frail, poorly educated, or of uncertain intellectual competence. For example, an ADL or an IADL problem is usually defined as not being able to perform "by yourself and without the help of another person." That concept is not always easy for a respondent. Keller et al. (1993) conducted a small study of older people using cognitive probes and found that the older people did not always interpret the concept "help of another person" (which was read to them as part of the question) in the same way. In particular, they did not always interpret help from another person as meaning that the person had to be present. Some thought that they had help if someone had brought them a telephone with large numbers or installed a seat in the shower. The study identified similar problems that were related to memory for the occurrence of instances of disability, comprehension of the terms used in the question, and to the error introduced by either ignoring or improperly involving conditional definitions (e.g., difficulty experienced only in certain contexts). Their "think aloud and probe" technique should be applied much more extensively in order to improve question wording and coding rules.

It should also be noted that respondents are not always consistent in the same interview. Brief questions on needing help with a list of ADLs and IADLs were asked on the core National Health Interview Survey questionnaire before the detailed questions in the Supplement on Aging. A few respondents who reported a need for help with some item on the ADL list reported later during the same interview that they had no difficulty with any of the same items.

Subjective Estimates Versus Performance Estimates

The error inherent in estimates by either the subject, a professional, or other proxy of such global concepts as need, amount of assistance, or difficulty have been commented on. Such concerns have led to a number of attempts to develop performance tests of ADLs, where a standard task in a controlled setting is presented to a subject, with behavioral criteria for quality of performance. One of the first was the Performance Activities of Daily Living (Kuriansky & Gurland, 1976). A prototypical item is to ask a subject to put on and take off a sweater, with separate components of the larger tasks being scored separately. A newer measure receiving considerable use is the Structured Assessment of Independent Living Skills (SAILS; Mahurin, DeBettignies, & Pirozzolo, 1991). The SAILS is longer and tests for a broader range of competence, from simple cognitive-motor skills like picking up coins to following a simple cooking recipe. All performance measures take several times longer and have other major problems that counteract their virtue of objectivity.

Guralnick, Branch, Cummings, and Curb (1989) review a number of other performance tests and their generic advantages and disadvantages. Two systematic comparisons of a traditional and a performance approach may be noted. The Performance ADL when compared with the traditional ADL showed higher external validity for the performance test (Kuriansky, Gurland, Fleiss, & Cowan, 1976). Myers, Holliday, Harvey, and Hutchinson (1993) designed a 14-task physical performance test whose cognitively intact subjects also completed Myers's (1992) 50-item IADL. They could not document any improved subject acceptance, ease of administration, or better psychometric qualities in the performance tests. Such utility should also be tested among cognitively impaired subjects. Despite the lack of compelling evidence for performance test superiority, it seems likely that the major use of performance tests will be to test in greater depth a variety of component skills, rather than to evaluate the more complex chain of acts that compose a single ADL. Continued exploration of human-factors approaches for this purpose is highly desirable. For example, Czaja et al. (1993) analyzed three ADL and three IADL tasks in terms of "problems" experienced in their performance (being, lifting, fatigue, etc.). Such analyses will ultimately be of assistance in identifying component skills of relevance to both rehabilitation activity and environmental design.

Technical Measurement and Methodological Issues

Feinstein et al. (1986), Ernst and Ernst (1984), and other review articles provide overviews of traditional psychometric treatments of various ADL measures. Although many instruments have been deficient in such analyses, whenever reliability and validity data have been reported, most instruments perform reasonably well. By comparison with many assessment domains, the ADL appears to be better developed in a psychometric sense.

One measurement issue not yet resolved is the question of whether hierarchically scaled ADL measures should be used in preference to aggregated composites derived through traditional test-theory analysis. The Lawton and Brody (1969) ADL and IADL in their original forms were scaled according to Guttman criteria. The OARS version of the Lawton and Brody IADL was subjected first to factor analysis, which suggested reducing the number of items from seven to five, and then to scalogram analysis (Fillenbaum, 1985). The Katz ADL was similarly scaled (Katz & Akpom, 1976), as was a scale using six ADL and IADL tasks (Spector, Katz, Murphy, & Fulton, 1987). Such hierarchically ordered scales have the advantage of producing a score that describes much more precisely which ADL tasks a person does and does not perform, in contrast with the aggregated composite, whose total score could be obtained by many different combinations of higher and lower scores across the different skills. Intuitively, a hierarchical scale would seem to describe an individual better and, therefore, communicate better among professionals in a clinical situation. The aggregated composite clearly makes more complete use of multiple-scale-point data, however, and is, therefore, better as a predictive variable.

Some psychometric techniques discussed by Teresi and Holmes in Chapter 1 may assist in dealing with several issues discussed or implied in this chapter. Specifically, context dependence and subgroup variation in the meaning and structure of a domain are possible to document using traditional methods, but simply documenting their existence does not offer a satisfactory method for producing measurement identity across contexts or subgroups. Item response theory, as discussed by Teresi and Holmes, offers an alternative approach. As a very concrete example, this approach would allow a highly diverse group of IADL indicators to be assembled in order to represent central daily activity functions for several cultures. Rather than constraining the instrument to generate scores for each subject on every item, even those foreign to their culture (as the classical test would require), the item-response theoretic approach would allow the single domain, IADL competence, to be represented by item clusters relevant to each culture. Item bias due to variability in item difficulty is thus removed without compromising the ability to compare across subject groups or cultures. Rater bias (i.e., the tendency of some raters to be more stringent than others) may also be removed from the disability estimates through the use of multifaceted item-response models. An extended illustration of this technique showed how gender and cross-national differences could be accounted for in the ADL realm (Teresi, Cross, & Golden, 1989).

CHOICE OF ADL OR IADL MEASURES

Earlier reference has been made to the relatively good psychometric performance and predictive power of many ADL and IADL measures. In fact, the authors are willing to suggest that for prediction purposes, which includes most research uses, one can hardly go wrong, regardless of which reasonably tested measure of ADL, IADL, or their combination, one chooses. For this reason, it does not seem profitable to provide an inventory of a large number of measures and to compare their psychometric characteristics. The Katz ADL, the Lawton and Brody ADL and IADL, and their transformation as embedded in multidimensional batteries such as

CARE (Gurland et al., 1977), the OARS (Duke University, 1978), or MAI (Lawton et al., 1982) are equally usable and have the advantage of having been used widely, with large-sample descriptive data (see Chapter 16 by George on these multidimensional measures). Other assessment compendia (Ernst & Ernst, 1984; Kane & Kane, 1981; McDowell & Newell, 1987) provide further concrete information on these and many other ADL and IADL instruments.

CONCLUSION

The scales formed by the ADLs and IADLs together, whether they are used in original or revised form, measure an important range of the consequences of injury or disease along the dimensions recommended by the WHO. They are especially useful for populations of older people where the prevalence of disability is high.

It is clear, however, that this domain of assessment is full of unanswered questions and sources of error in measurement. Even for prediction purposes, ridding ADL measurement of some of its sources of error would sharpen its predictive utility. For the other two major uses, population estimates and clinical use, no such sanguine view is possible at the present time.

The diversity of methods used in national studies to make population estimates is very sobering. It does seem, however, that with the variations in question wording now in hand and the prospect for more outcome data to be generated by longitudinal studies now in process, there will be the opportunity for a meta-analysis of the correlates of differences in question wording. The experimental modules on the Health and Retirement Survey should also help, even though the prevalence of disability will be low among the middle-aged participants in that survey. The cognitive processes involved in comprehending and responding to particular content and modes of inquiry deserve in-depth study.

Continued exploration of new methodologies, including item-response theory methods, could contribute to this sorting-out process. Within a few years, enough data ought to be in hand to allow selection of one best way (until the next one comes along) to ask such questions, thereby reducing both measurement error and conflicts among epidemiological estimates.

Such development should also improve clinical measurement. Fine-detail task analysis and other clinical approaches will produce some creative approaches to measurement that may be adapted to large-scale use. Measurement in physical therapy, occupational therapy, and other rehabilitation disciplines has been slow to develop. Part of the explanation for the lag probably lies in the unsuitability of the standard ADL measures for individual use. The ADL and IADL measures in the form used for large-scale surveys are insufficiently sensitive to reflect change on an individual level. There has thus been a tendency to conclude that standardization is incompatible with the individual-therapeutic approach. The success of the FIM belies this conclusion, however, and the creative use of ergonomics should further bridge the gap between research and practice. Continuation of the development of performance testing should also be of assistance in this regard, particularly if its purpose be seen not as that of replacing global ADL assessment with a more precise measure but as a technology much better suited to individual clinical use than the relatively gross ADL and IADL judgments.

REFERENCES

Carp, F., & Carp, A. (1981). It may not be the answer, it may be the question. *Research on Aging, 3*, 85–100.

Cohen, B. B., Barbano, H. E., Cox, C. S., Feldman, J. J., Finucane, F. F., Kleinman, J. C., & Madams, J. H. (1987). Plan and operation of the NHANES I Epidemiological Followup Study, 1982–84. *Vital and Health Statistics, 1*(22). Washington, DC: U.S. Government Printing Office.

Czaja, S. J., Weber, R. A., & Nair, S. N. (1993). A human-factors analysis of ADL activities: A capability-demand approach. *Journal of Gerontology, 48* (special issue), 44–48.

Davies, A. M. (1991). Function in old age: Measurement, comparability, and service planning. In M. Feinleib (Ed.), *Proceedings of 1988 International Symposium on Data on Aging. Vital and Health Statistics, 5*(6). Washington, DC: U.S. Government Printing Office.

Dawson, O., Hendershot, G., & Fulton, J. (1987). National Center for Health Statistics: Functional limitations of individuals age 65 years and over. *Advance Data, Vital and Health Statistics, 133*. Hyattsville, MD: U.S. Public Health Service.

Duke University Center for the Study of Aging. (1978). *Multidimensional functional assessment: The OARS methodology* (2nd ed.). Durham, NC: Duke University.

Ernst, M., & Ernst, N. S. (1984). Functional capacity. In D. J. Mangen & W. A. Peterson (Eds.), *Research instruments in gerontology* (Vol. 3, pp. 9–84). Minneapolis: University of Minnesota Press.

Faletti, M. V. (1984). Human factors research and functional environments for the aged. In I. Altman, M. P. Lawton, & J. F. Wohlwill (Eds.), *Elderly people and the environment: Human behavior and environment* (Vol. 7, pp. 191–237). New York: Plenum Press.

Feinstein, A. R., Josephy, B. R., & Wells, C. K. (1986). Scientific and clinical problems in indices of functional disability. *Annals of Internal Medicine, 105*, 413–420.

Fillenbaum, G. G. (1985). Screening the elderly: A brief instrumental activities of daily living measure. *Journal of the American Geriatrics Society, 33*, 698–706.

Fitti, J. E., & Kovar, M. G. (1987). The Supplement on Aging to the 1984 National Health Interview Survey. *Vital and Health Statistics, 1*(21). Washington, DC: U.S. Government Printing Office.

Granger, C. (1987). The functional independence measure. Buffalo: Research Foundation of the State University of New York.

Guralnik, J. M., Branch, L. G., Cummings, S. R., & Curb, D. (1985). Physical performance measures in aging research. *Journal of Gerontology: Medical Sciences, 44*, M141–M146.

Guralnik, J. M., & LaCroix, A. Z. (1992). Assessing physical function in old populations. In R. B. Wallace & R. F. Woolson (Eds.), *The epidemiologic study of the elderly* (pp. 159–181). New York: Oxford University Press.

Gurland, B., Kuriansky, J., Sharpe, L., Simon, R., Stiller, P., & Birkett, P. (1977–78). The Comprehensive Assessment and Referral Evaluation (CARE) rationale development and reliability. *International Journal of Aging and Human Development, 8*, 9–42.

Gurland, B. J., & Wilder, D. E. (1984). The CARE interview revisited: Development of an efficient, systematic clinical assessment. *Journal of Gerontology, 39*, 129–137.

Herzog, A. R., & Rodgers, W. L. (1992). The use of survey methods in research on older Americans. In R. B. Wallace & R. F. Woolson (Eds.), *The epidemiologic study of the elderly* (pp. 60–90). New York: Oxford University Press.

Institute of Medicine. (1990). *The second fifty years: Promoting health and preventing disability.* Washington, DC: National Academy of Science Press.

Jackson, M., Burwell, B., Clark, R., & Hanrahan, M. (1992). Eligibility for publicly-financed home care. *American Journal of Public Health, 82*, 853–856.

Kane, R. A., & Kane, R. L. (1981). *Assessing the elderly.* Lexington, MA: Lexington Books.

Katz, S. C., & Akpom, C. A. (1976). A measure of primary sociobiological functions. *International Journal of Health Services, 6*, 493–508.

Katz, S. C., Branch, L. G., Branson, M. H., Papsidero, J. A., Beck, J. C., & Greer, D. S. (1983). Active life expectancy. *New England Journal of Medicine, 309*, 1218–1224.

Katz, S. C., Downs, T. D., Cash, H. R., & Gratz, R. C. (1970). Progress in development of the index of ADL. *Gerontologist, 10*, 20–30.

Katz, S. C., Ford, A. B., Moskowitz, R. W., Jackson, B. A., & Jaffee, M. W. (1963). Studies of illness in the aged. The Index of ADL: A standardized measure of biological and psychosocial function. *Journal of the American Medical Association, 185*, 914–919.

Keller, D. M., Kovar, M. G., Jobe, J. B., & Branch, L. G. (1993). Problems eliciting elders' reports of functional status. *Journal of Aging and Health, 5*, 306–318.

Kovar, M. G. (1987). The Longitudinal Study of Aging: Some estimates of change among older Americans. *Proceedings of the Public Health Conference on Records and Statistics.* Hyattsville, MD: National Center for Health Statistics.

Kovar, M. G., Fitti, J. E., & Chyba, M. M. (1992). The Longitudinal Study of Aging: 1984–90. *Vital and Health Statistics, 1*(28). Washington, DC: U.S. Government Printing Office.

Kuriansky, J. B., & Gurland, B. J. (1976). The performance test of activities of daily living. *International Journal of Aging and Human Development, 7*, 343–352.

Kuriansky, J. B., Gurland, B. J., Fleiss, J. L., & Cowan, D. (1976). The assessment of self-care capacity in geriatric psychiatric patients by objective and subjective methods. *Journal of Clinical Psychology, 32*, 95–102.

Lair, T. J., & Lefkowitz, D. C. (1993). Mental health and functional status of residents of nursing and personal care homes. *Research Findings.* Rockville, MD: Agency for Health Care Policy and Research.

Lawton, M. P., & Brody, E. M. (1969). Assessment of older people: Self-maintaining and instrumental activities of daily living. *The Gerontologist, 9*, 179–185.

Lawton, M. P., Moss, M., Fulcomer, M., & Kleban, M. H. (1982). A research and service-oriented multilevel assessment instrument. *Journal of Gerontology, 37*, 91–99.

Lowenthal, M. (1964). *Lives in distress.* New York: Basic Books.

Macken, C. L. (1986). A profile of functionally impaired elderly persons living in the community. *Health Care Financing Review, 7*, 33–49.

Magaziner, J. (1992). The use of proxy respondents in health surveys of the aged. In R. B. Wallace & R. F. Woolson (Eds.), *The epidemiologic study of the elderly* (pp. 120–129). New York: Oxford University Press.

Manton, K. G. (1988). A longitudinal study of functional change and mortality in the United States. *Journal of Gerontology: Social Sciences, 43*, S153–S161.

Manton, K. G., Corder, L. S., & Stallard, E. (1993a). Estimates of change in chronic disability and institutional incidence and prevalence rates in the U.S. elderly population from the 1982, 1984, and 1989 National Long Term Care Survey. *Journal of Gerontology: Social Services, 48*, S153–S166.

Manton, K. G., Corder, L., & Stallard, E. (1993b). Changes in the use of personal assistance and special equipment from 1982 to 1989. *The Gerontologist, 33*, 168–176.

Mahurin, R. K., DeBettignies, B. H., & Pirozzolo, F. J. (1991). Structured assessment of independent living skills: Preliminary functional abilities in dementia. *Journal of Gerontology: Psychological Sciences, 46*, P58–P66.

McDowell, I., & Newell, C. (1987). *Measuring health: A guide to rating scales and questionnaires.* New York: Oxford University Press.

Myers, A. M. (1992). The clinical Swiss army knife: Empirical evidence on the validity of IADL functional status measures. *Medical Care, 30*(Suppl.), 96–111.

Myers, A. M., Holliday, P. J., Harvey, K. A., & Hutchinson, K. S. (1993). Functional performance measures: Are they superior to self-assessments? *Journal of Gerontology: Medical Sciences, 48*, M196–M206.

Rubenstein, L. Z., Schairer, C., Wieland, G., & Kane, R. (1984). Systematic biases in functional status assessment of elderly adults: Effects of different data sources. *Journal of Gerontology, 39*, 686–691.

Shanas, E., Townsend, P., Wedderburn, D., Friis, H., Milhøj, P., & Stehouwer, J. (1968). *Old people in three industrial societies*. New York: Atherton Books.

Simon-Rusinowitz, L., & Hoflund, B. F. (1993). Adopting a disability approach to home care services for older adults. *The Gerontologist, 33*, 159–167.

Spector, W. D., Katz, S., Murphy, J. B., & Fulton, J. P. (1987). The hierarchical relationship between activities of daily living and instrumental activities of daily living. *Journal of Chronic Diseases, 40*, 481–490.

Teresi, J. A., Cross, P. S., & Golden, R. R. (1989). Some applications of latent trait analysis to the measurement of ADL. *Journal of Gerontology: Social Services, 44*, S196–S204.

Verbrugge, L. (1990). The iceberg of disability. In S. M. Stahl (Ed.), *The legacy of longevity: Health and health care in later life*. Newbury Park, CA: Sage Publications.

Weinberger, M., Samsa, G. P., Schmader, K., Greenberg, S. M., Carr, D. B., & Wildman, D. S. (1992). Comparing proxy and patients' perceptions of patients' functional status. *Journal of the American Geriatrics Society, 40*, 585–588.

Wiener, J. M., Hanley, R. J., Clark, R., & Van Nostrand, J. F. (1990). Measuring the activities of daily living: Comparisons across national surveys. *Journal of Gerontology, 45*, S229–S237.

World Health Organization. (1976). *The International Classification of Impairments, Disabilities, and Handicaps*. Geneva, Switzerland: WHO.

CHAPTER 4

Balance and Gait Measures

PAMELA W. DUNCAN
CENTER FOR POLICY RESEARCH EDUCATION
DUKE UNIVERSITY

AND

STEPHANIE STUDENSKI
CENTER ON AGING
UNIVERSITY OF KANSAS MEDICAL CENTER

Balance and gait are complex neuromuscular tasks which require integration of sensory, motor, and neural processes. With aging there is often a progressive decline in balance and gait (Blanke & Hatgeman, 1989; Horak, Shupert, & Mirka, 1989; Oberg, Karsznia, & Oberg, 1993; Stelmach & Worringham, 1985; Winter, 1991; Woollacott, 1990). Deterioration of the ability to perform these tasks is usually a manifestation of losses in such physiological functions as sensory, motor, and neural processing, and endurance. Aging, disease, or a combination of both contribute to these changes. There is little doubt that declines in balance and gait are major contributing factors to falls in the elderly (Campbell, Borrie, & Spears, 1989; Campbell, Reinken, Allen, & Martinez, 1981; Gryfe, Amies, & Ashley, 1977; Nevitt, Cummings, Kidd, & Black, 1989; Overstall, Smith, Imms, and Johnson, 1974; Robbins, et al., 1989; Tinetti, Speechley, & Ginter, 1988; Tinetti, Williams, & Mayewski, 1986). Impaired balance and gait also contribute to the fear of falling syndrome which itself leads to restrictions in mobility, and further declines in functional independence. Moreover, decreased balance has been associated with increased mortality in the elderly (Wild, Mayak, & Issacs, 1981). The cycle of impaired balance and gait, decreased mobility, and falls presents a major health issue whose magnitude will continue to increase with the aging of the population.

Assessment of balance and gait includes physical performance measures that reflect functional limitations. Objective measurements of balance and gait detect declines in function that impose a threat to safety and can lead to restriction in activities of daily living (ADL). By relating balance and gait to physiological impairments we may clarify the contributions of these impairments to restricted mobility, instability, and falls. Ideally, we hope to identify impairments and functional limitations that may be responsive to interventions. Assessments may also identify individuals who are in need of assistive devices or other support services. Finally, reliable and valid measures of gait and balance are necessary to evaluate the effectiveness of therapeutic interventions or to monitor patients over time in longitudinal studies of aging.

Balance and gait have been assessed by a number of different tests. Sophisticated laboratory methods of gait and balance assessment have been employed as well-as practical and easy clinical measures. The measures discussed in this chapter are limited to well characterized clinical measures that are easily used and can be administered by professional or nonprofessional staff.

SELECTING BALANCE AND GAIT MEASURES

The quality of a measure is reflected by its sensibility, reliability, validity, and sensitivity to change (Applegate, Blass, & Williams, 1990; Feinstein, 1987; Guyatt, Walter, & Normal, 1987; Kirshner & Guyatt, 1985). Assessment of the sensibility of a measure asks the questions: Based on current knowledge, does utilization of this measure make sense? What is its intended purpose? In what setting could the measure be applied? How easily can the measure be used? A measure that is sensible must be accompanied by clear instructions and replicable procedures (Feinstein, 1987).

Reliability should be assessed both between observers (interrater) and over time (test–retest) (Applegate et al., 1990; Feinstein, 1987; Kirshner & Guyatt, 1985). Individual characteristics of the observers and the characteristics of the elderly population of interest may affect reliability assessment. For example, interrater reliability may depend on the consistent interpretation of procedures and scoring. Test–retest reliability is influenced both by variability in the scoring of the test and by true variability in a subject who is tested on two different occasions. Certain types of patients who have conditions that fluctuate, such as Parkinson's disease or rheumatoid arthritis, may score quite differently on successive tests. The result is an apparently low test–retest reliability. To assure that measurements are reliable, reliability assessment should be an ongoing process to be applied each time the test is used in a new setting or a new subject population.

Validity represents the ability of the measure to reflect the unknowable "truth." Face validity describes the overall sense that the measure is capturing the problem (Applegate et al., 1990; Feinstein, 1987; Kirshner & Guyatt, 1985). Face validity tends to be high for balance and gait measures. A valid measure should tend to agree with other measures of the same function. The validity of balance and gait measures is often assessed against self- or proxy reports of function and against other existing gait and balance measures.

Sensitivity to change implies the ability to detect differences in an individual over time (Guyatt et al., 1987). Precise measures that use continuous or fine scaling tend to be more sensitive than coarse scales with only a few levels. For example, measuring the amount of time an individual can balance on one foot is a more precise measure than rating one–foot standing balance as good, fair, or poor. High sensitivity to change improves power in a research study; the more sensitive the measure, the smaller the number of subjects required. However, very sensitive measures have disadvantages. They may detect such small changes that the difference is not clinically meaningful. For example, a change in walking velocity from 1.1 to 1.2 meters per second might be statistically significant, but no one knows if this difference is of any benefit to the individual.

The range of a measure reflects its ability to capture both very low and very high levels of performance. A measure with extensive range allows a broad spectrum of people to be tested with a common instrument. A wide range can maximize sensitivity to change. If there is always room for improvement or deterioration, there will be no "floor" and "ceiling" problems. Some balance measures are prone to floor problems. For example, one-foot standing is often employed in studies of the elderly, yet many elderly cannot perform this task.

Other factors that should be considered in selecting gait and balance measures include safety, portability, convenience, expense, performance time, and the training and expertise required of the examiner. Respondent burden—how much trouble we cause the subjects—should always be considered. Burden includes fatigue, frustration, discomfort, and danger imposed by the test. Safety of measures is enhanced when the tasks are hierarchically organized, and progression is based on successful completion of lower level tasks. All testing personnel must be well trained in the measures. The training must include instructions for guarding of patients and guidelines for test progression.

Balance or gait performance cannot be assessed by one single measure. In selecting the measures to be used, there is often a process of trade–offs and compromise. The tests that best meet the needs of a project in terms of feasibility and low respondent burden may not be as sensitive or reliable as other tests that consume more resources. Evaluators need to be open to using more than one test and to using different tests as settings and populations change. Finally, balance and gait are very complex physical constructs that cannot usually be characterized by one single test.

BALANCE

Balance can be defined in biomechanical terms as the ability to maintain the center of gravity over the base of support. Most traditional measures of balance capture stability. Also called static balance, stability is the ability to remain upright over a fixed base of support. However, living organisms also need to remain upright while moving. This type of balance, which requires the ability to continuously adjust the center of gravity over a moving base of support (e.g., walking), is called dynamic balance. Balance assessment should capture both static and dynamic balance.

There are two mechanisms of balance control. The first mechanism, which is called *feedback*, occurs as the individual attempts to maintain a position or respond to external perturbations (Stelmach & Worringham, 1985). A second mechanism, which is called *feedforward*, occurs when a standing subject lifts the upper extremity rapidly. Prior to initiation of the upper extremity movement, there are anticipatory postural adjustments that stabilize the body (Belenkii, Gurfinkel, & Paltsev, 1967; Bouisset & Zattara, 1986; Bouisset & Zattara, 1987). In order to characterize balance, both feedback and feedforward mechanisms of balance control should be assessed.

Clinical Balance Measures

The Romberg Test. For over 100 years clinicians have attempted to assess balance by progressively narrowing the base of support and altering sensory inputs. In 1853 Romberg introduced a balance test to assess the effects of posterior column disease on standing balance (Romberg, 1853). This test qualitatively assesses postural sway as individuals: a) stand with feet together and eyes open and then with eyes closed (standard Romberg) and b) stand with their feet tandem (heel to toe) with eyes open and then with eyes closed (sharpened Romberg). Although its characteristics had never been adequately assessed, the Romberg test was used for years as part of the standard neurological exam.

In 1982 Black and colleagues used force platform recording of the Romberg test to assess its measurement characteristics (Black, Wall, Rockette, & Kitch, 1982). They concluded that the Romberg performance in individuals under age 20 and over age 50 was too variable to develop a systematic normal data base. They warned that "unless further studies can identify, control, and resolve sources of these variances, clinical application and interpretation of results of the Romberg test in the younger (less than 20) and older (more than 50) age groups should be performed with caution" (p. 314). Even when they restricted their analyses of Romberg performance measures to individuals between 20 and 49 years of age, the analysis of test-retest reliability demonstrated large variability upon repetition of the Romberg test over five consecutive days. Assessment of trial–to–trial reliability demonstrated that performance for the eyes–closed task improved considerably with repeated trials. Black's study is very significant in that it demonstrates how clinicians may accept a measure for interpretation of pathology without adequately testing the measurement properties.

One-Leg Stance Measures. The time an individual can balance on one leg with eyes open or closed is a frequently recommended measure of balance in the elderly. One–leg stance measures have the advantage of being easily performed in any location and requiring no complex equipment. However, several investigators have recently questioned this method of clinical balance assessment in the elderly (Bohannon & Larkin, 1984; Heitman, Gossman, & Shaddeau, 1989; Potvin, Syndulko, Tourtellotte, Lemmon, & Potvin, 1980). The ability to stand on one foot declines with age. Potvin et al. (1980) reported in an assessment of 138 neurologic tests that one-leg stance with the eyes closed was more sensitive to age than any other item. In their sample, the ability to do this task declined 100% with increasing age. The decline in one-leg stance with the eyes open was 32% with increasing age. Bohannon and Larkin confirmed that subjects over age 60 were impaired in their ability to perform one leg stance with eyes closed (Bohannon & Larkin, 1984). Heitmann et al reported that one-leg stance and sharpened Romberg test did not discriminate fallers from non-fallers.

The one–leg standing test may be further limited in its ability to discriminate function in the elderly because of the wide range in performance ability within this group. Many frail elderly cannot perform the test at all (floor effect). Conversely, in the very fit elderly, everyone may be able to perform this task (ceiling effect). In addition, the static nature of the one–leg stance measures is not reflective of the conditions in which most people fall since falls occur during movement (e.g., walking, reaching, or changing position).

The Sternal Shove. In order to assess an individual's ability to balance in response to postural perturbations, several clinicians have designed tests to stress standing balance. The simplest clinical measure was developed by Wild, Mayak, and Issacs (1981). In this test, the clinician subjectively evaluates balance responses by pushing subjects on the sternum ("the sternal shove"). The response is considered normal if the patient sways slightly and abnormal if the patient steps back, falls, or demonstrates a startle response. The force of the sternal shove was not quantified. In 1984, Weiner, Nora, and Glantz (1984) attempted to define more precisely the scoring of the responses to the sternal shove. However, the reliability and validity of this crude measure has not been established.

The Postural Stress Test. Wolfson, Whipple, Amerman, and Kleinberg (1986) developed a quantifiable measure of balance, the postural stress test (PST), in response to postural perturbations of varying force. In this test, motor responses to different degrees of perturbations are measured for a standing subject. The PST measures an individual's ability to withstand a series of destablizing forces applied at waist level. Scoring of the postural responses is based on a 9–point ordinal scale. Wolfson et al. established reliability of interobserver scoring for the PST and Hill, Vandervoort, and Kramer (1990) established test–retest reliability of the measure. Wolfson et al. (1986) demonstrated in a nursing home population that performance on the PST could discriminate fallers from nonfallers. They also reported that the nonfalling nursing home subjects did not perform as well as individuals residing in the community. A subsequent study by Chandler, Duncan, and Studenski (1990) demonstrated that community dwelling elderly perform as well on the PST as younger community dwelling individuals. They also confirmed in a community sample that performance on the PST discriminated fallers from nonfallers.

In summary, the PST is a reliable measure; poor performance on the PST is associated with falls. The equipment required to perform this test is inexpensive and clinically accessible. However, the equipment is not portable and could not be used easily in the community.

The Functional Reach Test. A recently developed measure of balance is the functional reach test (Duncan, Weiner, Chandler, & Studenski, 1990). Functional reach is defined as the maximal distance one can reach forward beyond arm's length while maintaining a fixed base of support in the standing position. Functional reach is measured using a simple apparatus consisting of a leveled yardstick attached to the wall at the height of the right acromion. Subjects are asked to assume a position of comfortable stance and to stand so that the shoulder is perpendicular to the yardstick. They are then asked to make a fist and extend their arm forward. While the subject is in this position the placement of the end of the third metacarpal along the yardstick is recorded (Position 1). Subjects are then asked to reach as far forward as they can without losing their balance or taking a step, and the placement of the end of the third metacarpal is again recorded (Position 2). Functional reach is defined as the difference between Position 1 and Position 2. Five measures of functional reach are recorded. The first two trials are considered practice trials and the last three are averaged to establish the functional reach measure.

Functional reach represents a feedforward mechanism of balance control (stabilization during voluntary movements). Reaching produces sudden shifts of the center of gravity which may not be compensated for if the subject has impaired balance. An individual's functional reach might deteriorate with balance impairments so as to minimize disturbance of the center of gravity.

Functional reach has been compared to laboratory measures of center of pressure excursion and has been tested for reliability, precision, and validity in 128 community volunteers aged 21–87 (Duncan et al., 1990). The influence of age and anthropometrics on functional reach has also been established. In a sample of 45 community-dwelling persons aged 66–104, functional reach was established as an estimator of physical frailty (Weiner, Duncan, Chandler, & Studenski, 1992). It was correlated with physical and instrumental activities of daily living, 10-foot walk time, one–foot standing balance, tandem walking, and social mobility.

In a prospective study of falls which included a sample of 217 community dwelling elderly male veterans, functional reach was demonstrated to be predictive of falls (Duncan, Studenski, Chandler, & Prescott, 1992). Subjects who were able to stand but unable to reach were 8 times more likely to fall than subjects who could reach 10 inches or farther. Subjects who reached less than or equal to 6 inches were 4 times more likely to fall than those who reached 10 inches or farther and those who reached farther than 6 but less than 10 inches were 2 times more likely to fall than those who reached 10 inches or farther (Duncan et al., 1992). More recently, Weiner, Bongiorni, Studenski, Duncan, and Kochersberger (1993) demonstrated in a nursing home population receiving therapy to improve balance that functional reach is sensitive to changes in balance.

Functional reach is a simple balance measure that is easily incorporated into clinical practice and can be performed in any setting. Functional reach, however, is not universally applicable. It may be difficult to perform in patients with severe dementia, extreme spinal deformities, severely restricted upper extremity function and in frail individuals who are unable to stand unsupported for at least 30 seconds.

Functional Tests to Assess Mobility and Balance

Several investigators have developed functional tests to assess an individual's mobility and balance. The purpose of these tests is to evaluate stability during a series of tasks that require both static and dynamic balance. These tests include the Get Up and Go Test (Mathias, Mayak, & Issacs, 1986), the Tinetti Performance–Oriented Mobility Assessment (Tinetti, 1986), the Berg Balance Scale (Berg, Wood–Dauphinee, Williams, & Gayton, 1989) the Duke Progressive Mobility Skills Test (Hogue, Studenski, & Duncan, 1990), the Physical Performance Mobility Examination (Winograd, et al., 1994), and the Established Population for Epidemiologic Studies of the Elderly (EPESE) Mobility Assessment (Guralnik et al., in press).

The Get Up and Go Test. Mathias, Mayak, and Isaacs (1986) developed the Get Up and Go Test to identify balance impairment in the elderly. This test requires that subjects stand up from a chair, walk a short distance, turn around, return and sit down. Performance on these functional tasks is graded on a 5–point ordinal scale. The authors reported that poor performance on these items may be due to impairment of balance. Interrater reliability was established for this test, and test function was correlated with sway and other clinical measures of balance. The test–retest reliability, sensitivity to change, and predictive validity of the Get Up and Go Test have not been established.

Podsiadlo and Richardson (1991) modified the Get Up and Go Test by timing performance rather than by assessing quality of performance (Table 4.1). The timed test was evaluated in 60 patients with a mean age of 79.5, referred to a geriatric day hospital. Both interobserver and test–retest reliability were reported to be excellent. The timed test correlated well with the Berg Balance Scale, gait speed, and ADL and it was predictive of those who could independently ambulate outside. The measure is simple, and can be performed in any setting by nonprofessional staff. It takes approximately five minutes to administer.

The Tinetti Performance-Oriented Assessment of Mobility. This test is a performance–based measure of balance and gait. Tinetti's (1986) original balance assessment included 15 performance activities which were rated dichotomously as normal or abnormal. Interobserver reliability assessment revealed that there was more than 90% agreement between a nurse and a physician on scoring individual items in 10 subjects. A prospective study of falls in 79 nursing home residents 60 years and older demonstrated that the mobility score was predictive of subjects who fell (Tinetti, 1987). In a subsequent prospective community–based study of falls, Tinetti, Speechley, and Ginter, (1988) reduced the number of items involved in the assessment. With the restricted measures, impaired balance and gait were identified as moderate but significant risk factors for falls in community dwelling individuals. Tinetti suggested that simplification of the scale may have been at the expense of sensitivity. In addition, with such gross scoring, this measure may not respond adequately to change, and the test is very likely to demonstrate ceiling effects in many community-dwelling elderly.

The Tinetti measure has recently been expanded to include the items listed in Table 4.1 (Mary Tinetti, personal communication, 1993). These activities are scored on a 3–point ordinal scale. The newest edition of the Tinetti scale is being used in community-dwelling persons 70 years and older and takes an average of 20 minutes to perform. The Tinetti measure is reliable, valid and predictive of falls, fall injuries, and nursing home placements. The sensitivity of the measure to change is currently being investigated. Performance on the Tinetti measure has been correlated with performance on more sophisticated laboratory measures as well as the Reuben physical performance measure (Lichenstein, Burger, Shields, & Shiavi, 1990; Reuben & Siu, 1990). The measure is simple, brief, and may be administered by nonprofessional staff. The measure may demonstrate ceiling effects in more fit individuals and floor effects in more dependent subjects.

The Berg Balance Scale. Berg et al. (1989) developed a balance measure to assess function in elderly subjects. It includes 14 items (Table 4.1) and is scored using a 5-point ordinal scale. The reliability and validity of the measure has been assessed in several different populations. It has been compared with laboratory measures of postural sway and other clinical measures of balance and mobility in 31 elderly subjects (Berg, Maki, Williams, Holliday, & Wood–Dauphinee, 1992). It correlates with other balance measures (Tinetti, Barthel Mobility Index, and the Timed Get Up and Go Test) as well as with motor function. Both intertester and test–retest reliability have been established. In two longitudinal studies of 114 elderly subjects and 70 acute stroke patients the Berg Balance assessment was predictive of falls and could discriminate subjects by their use of assistive devices; it was also sensitive to changes in functional status (Berg, 1992). The measure is simple, can be performed in any setting, and takes an average of 10 to 15 minutes to administer. Although the measure has only been administered by professional staff, it could be performed by nonprofessional staff with minimal training. The test probably has a ceiling effect in fit elderly subjects.

The Duke Progressive Mobility Skills Test. Thirteen mobility items that capture static and dynamic balance comprise this test(Table 4.1) (Hogue et al., 1990). The items are scored on a 3–point ordinal scale and are hierarchically organized with

TABLE 4.1 Items Assessed on Mobility Measures

Timed Get Up and Go (Mathias et al., 1986)	*Tinnetti Performance-Oriented Assessment* (Tinetti, 1986)	*Berg Balance Assessment* (Berg et al., 1989)
Get up from chair	Chair	Sitting to standing
	sitting balance	Standing unsupported
Walk 3 meters	sit to stand	Sitting unsupported
	stand to sit	Standing to sitting
Turn	Bed	Transfer
	stand to sit	Standing—eyes closed
Walk back 3 meters	sit to lie	Standing—feet together
	lie to sit	Reaching forward
Sit down	sit to stand	Retrieving object from floor
	Standing	Turning to look behind
	tandem (eyes open)	Turning 360 degrees
	semitandem	Placing alternate foot on stool
	pull at waist	Standing, one foot in front
	lean backward	Standing on one foot
	toe standing	
	one leg stand	
	Gait—flat surface	
	initiation	
	path deviation	
	turning	
	missed steps	
	step over obstacle	
	Gait—uneven surface	
	initiation	
	path deviation	
	turning	
	missed steps	
	step over obstacle	

the following Guttman characteristics: coefficient of reproducibility is .9, minimum marginal reproducibility is .7–.8 ; coefficient of scalability is .6. The instrument has been tested in four populations: (a) 45 community-dwelling elderly, mean age 79, (b) 40 nursing home residents, mean age 66.5, (c) 184 community-dwelling elderly men, mean age 75, and (d) 12 elderly individuals from the community or a nursing home. The interrater and test–retest reliability of the measure is high (intraclass correlation coefficient was .97). The Mobility Skills correlates

Duke Mobility Skills (Hogue et al., 1990)	*Physical Performance Mobility Assessment* (Winograd et al., 1993)	*Established Populations for Epidemiologic Studies of the Elderly* (Guralnik et al., in press)
Sitting balance	Bed mobility	Timed side-by-side stand
Sitting reach	Transfer skills	Semitandem stand
Transfer	Multiple chair stands	Tandem stands
Rising from a chair	Standing balance	Timed 8-foot walks
Standing balance	Step-up	Timed chair rise
Pick up object from floor	Ambulation	
Walking		
Turning		
Abrupt stop		
Obstacle		
Standing reach		
Stairs		

well with walk time, functional reach, and physical activities of daily living (Weiner et al., 1992). In nursing home subjects the correlation with the Functional Independence Measure (FIM) (Granger, 1990) of mobility was .74 and with FIM gait was .81. The sensitivity to change index for the mobility skills protocol was assessed in a Veterans' Administration nursing home by comparing the results in a population undergoing rehabilitation to results in residents not undergoing rehabilitation (Weiner et al., 1993). The responsive index, a measure of sensitivity to change calculated as the average change score in treatment subjects divided by the square root of 2 times the mean square error of the control group, was 4.63, indicating good sensitivity (Guyatt et al., 1987). The Mobility Skills Test is predictive of falls in elderly male veterans (Studenski et al., in press). The measure is simple, requires approximately 10 minutes to administer and may be administered in any environment. It may be administered by nonprofessional staff, but training is required. The Mobility Skills may not be able to discriminate function among fit older adults.

The Physical Performance and Mobility Examination (PPME). The PPME (Winograd et al., 1994) tests bed mobility, transfer skill, multiple stands from a chair, standing balance, step–up, and ambulation. The scoring is either pass–fail or a 3–level ordinal scoring. This mobility measure was developed to assess hospitalized older adults. The measure has been evaluated in a sample of over 500 hospitalized patients 65 years and older. Interrater and test–retest reliability have been established. The PPME correlates with physical activities of daily living and physical performance on the Medical Outcomes Scale (Stewart & Ware, 1992). The sensitivity of this measure to change has not been assessed. This brief assessment is portable and can be administered by nonprofessional staff.

The EPESE Mobility Assessment. Guralnik et al., (in press) have evaluated the use of a mobility assessment that has been employed in the Established Populations for Epidemiologic Studies of the Elderly (EPESE). This assessment includes timed side–by–side , semitandem, and tandem stands, timed 8-foot walk, and time to rise from chair 5 times. The measure has been employed in over 5,000 community–dwelling individuals over the age of 71. The measure may be scored as continuous (timed) or as categorical variables, using nonperformance as poorest category and quartiles of performance as four additional categories. The reliability of the measure is high and it has demonstrated construct validity. The categorical scoring of tasks is predictive for nursing home admission and death. The instrument takes approximately 10 minutes to administer. It can be administered by nonprofessional staff in any environment. The sensitivity of the measure to change has not been assessed.

Self–Report Measures of Balance

Tinetti, Richman, and Powell (1990) have developed an instrument to measure fear of falling. This is a self–report instrument in which individuals are asked to assess confidence in their ability to avoid a fall during 10 routine ADLs. The reliability and validity of the Falls Efficacy Scale (FES) have been assessed in two small samples: (a) 18 cognitively intact, ambulatory persons over age 65 residing in the community or in intermediate care facilities, and (b) 56 cognitively intact subjects 65 years or older recruited from senior centers or an elderly housing project. The predictors for Falls Efficacy scores include walking speed, anxiety, and depression. This instrument is continuing to be evaluated in other studies. Preliminary results demonstrate that it is a good measure of the patient's own assessment of his stability and will be a useful supplement to performance–based measures of balance.

GAIT

The Tinetti Performance Oriented Mobility Assessment (Tinetti, 1986) and the Duke Progressive Mobility Skills Test (Hogue et al., 1990) incorporate gait into their mobility assessments. In these assessments, gait is rated on ordinal scales. However, gait can be described in more specific and quantitative ways. The kinematics and kinesiology of gait can be characterized by sophisticated and highly technical laboratory assessments. In addition, there are several gait measures that can characterize velocity, stride length, step strength, and cadence with minimal equipment or technical training.

The simplest measure of gait is velocity. This is easily assessed by marking designated distances and capturing the time to negotiate the distance. The most commonly used distances for gait velocity measurements are 10–foot or 10–meter paths. There are age-referenced norms that can be used for comparisons (Blanke & Hatgeman, 1989; Oberg et al., 1993; Winter, 1991). Gait velocity does slow with age but excessive slowness is a marker of frailty, predictive of falls and nursing home placement. Velocity of gait is a continuous measure that may be very sensitive to change and may detect early decline in more fit populations.

The 6–minute walk is a measure that was originally developed to assess cardiopulmonary function (Guyatt, Sullivan, & Thompson, 1985). In this test, individuals are allowed 6 minutes to walk as far as they can at a pace normal to them. Individuals pace themselves and rest as needed. The distance they cover is measured and recorded. A low performance in this test is associated with limited cardiovascular endurance as well as sensorimotor impairments. The 6–minute walk is also a continuous measure that will be sensitive to change and may be useful in identifying early decline.

Stride length and step length can be measured with very simple equipment: stopwatch, felt–tip marking pen, and paper walkway. Felt–tip pens are taped to the back of the patient's shoes so that the tip reaches the floor when standing (Cerny, 1983; Robinson & Smidt, 1981). The patient is instructed to walk at his or her usual walking speed from one end of the walkway to the other. Measurements are made of distances from one heel contact to the next heel contact on the same side (stride length) and of distances between alternate sides (step length).

Wolfson et al. have developed a more detailed analysis of gait, the Gait Assessment Rating Score (Wolfson, Whipple, Amerman, & Tobin, 1990). This assessment requires that an individual's gait be videotaped. Then sixteen parameters of the gait are assessed via video analysis and the parameters are scored on a 4–point ordinal scale. In addition to the resulting 16 parameters of gait, stride length and walking speed are measured. This instrument has been tested in 71 nursing home residents. The interrater reliability of the gait assessment was reported to be high. In addition, decreased stride length and the summary score of the gait assessment scale were correlated with each other and were found to be impaired in fallers compared to nonfallers. Further reliability tests and validation of the gait assessment scale is needed. At this time, the reliability of the measure has only been tested as administered by professional staff.

SUMMARY

In the last few years, physical performance measures of balance, mobility, and gait are proliferating in response to the needs of health professionals working with older adults. The expected advantages of these physical performance measures over self–reports or professional observations include increased precision, reliability, the potential to detect subtle dysfunction, and increased sensitivity to change. Precision may be increased because many physical performance measures use continuous metrics such as time or distance as opposed to the more coarse forms of scaling that are often used in self–report measures. Reliability is improved when the measure requires less individual judgment. For example, multiple observers may agree more easily on how long an activity took than on whether the subject experienced difficulty. In addition, nonprofessional observers using a timed or counted measure may be more reliable than they would be using a measure that requires a trained eye for scoring.

Performance measures may be especially useful to detect preclinical changes at the highest level of function, thus expanding the range of assessment. There may be differences within a group of older adults that are best detected by very challenging tasks that are not spontaneously tested in everyday life. Thus, early aging effects may be revealed during a test of tandem walking. These subtle deficits may have no immediate clinical impact but may be important for detection and prevention of functional decline. Through increased precision and range, performance measures may be better than coarse measures at detecting the effects of treatment or following spontaneous change over time.

Performance measures also have disadvantages. There may be practical limitations resulting from limited time, space, equipment, or expertise. There may also be some inconvenience to subjects, including fatigue and possible injury. Another disadvantage is that performance measures do not reflect integrated function over time; they can reflect only actual function at the time of observation. For adults with fluctuating symptoms, like arthritis, performance today may not be indicative of performance yesterday or tomorrow.

The clinical meaning of performance measures can be lost if there is not a relationship between factors like difficulty and time. In some instance, the correlation may be well substantiated; for example, trouble with walking and walking speed seem to be strongly related. However, it is less clear whether there is a meaningful relationship between the relative difficulty of other tasks and the time required for their completion.

More investigation may be required into the factors that influence performance. Measures of balance, mobility, and gait may be influenced by attributes of the individual undergoing testing, the individual performing the testing, and the context of the testing. Subject characteristics that could affect performance include cognition, attention, cautiousness, prior experience, and motivation. The tester can influence subject performance through inconsistent verbal instructions or nonverbal cues; the interpersonal relationship between tester and subject can also produce variability. Finally, the context of the testing, which includes the physical surroundings, the timing, and the sequence of the testing, can affect the results. Definitive information is not available on the magnitude of these effects.

The idea that physical performance measures are better than self–reports has been challenged. In a recent study, Myers, Holliday, Harvey, and Hutchinson (1993) compared the scores of 14 performance tasks with the responses on a 50 item instrumental activities of daily living questionnaire. They did not demonstrate any advantage of performance–based assessment over self–report.

Even if physical performance measures are not proven superior to self–report, they may still be useful complements. Performance–based measures of balance, mobility, and gait are providing good ways to determine function and predict outcomes among the elderly. Clearly, we need to further develop and characterize these measures and to continue investigating the factors that influence test performance. If these issues are resolved, performance–based measures should have the potential for providing clinicians with increasingly useful information.

ACKNOWLEDGMENT

This work was Supported by the National Institute on Aging, Claude D. Pepper Older Americans Independence Center Grant #5 P60 AG 11268.

REFERENCES

Applegate, W. B., Blass, J. P., & Williams, T. F. (1990). Instruments for the functional assessment of older patients. *New England Journal of Medicine, 322,* 1207–1214.

Belenkii, Y. Y., Gurfinkel, V., and Paltsev, Y. (1967). Elements of control of voluntary movements. *Biofizika, 12,* 135–141.

Berg, K. (1992) Berg balance scale. Unpublished doctoral dissertation, McGill University, Montreal.

Berg, K., Maki, B., Williams, J. I., Holliday, P., & Wood-Dauphinee, S. L. (1992). Clinical and laboratory measures of postural balance in an elderly population. *Archives of Physical Medicine Rehabilitation, 73,* 1073–1080.

Berg, K., Wood-Dauphinee, S., Williams, J. I., & Gayton, D. (1989). Measuring balance in the elderly: Preliminary development of an instrument. *Physiotherapy Canada, 41,* 304–311.

Black, F. O., Wall, C., Rockette, H. E., & Kitch, R. (1982). Normal subjects postural sway during the Romberg test. *American Journal of Otolaryngology, 3,* 309–319.

Blanke, D., & Hatgeman, P. (1989) Comparison of gait of young and elderly men. *Physical Therapy, 69,* 144–148.

Bohannon, R. W., & Larkin, P. (1984). Decrease in timed balance test scores with aging. *Physical Therapy, 64,* 1067–1070.

Bouisset, S., & Zattara, M. (1986). Chronometric analysis of the posturo-kinetic programming of voluntary movement. *Journal of Motor Behavior, 18,* 215–223.

Bouisset, S., & Zattara, M. (1987). Biomechanical study of the programming of anticipatory postural adjustments associated with voluntary movement. *Journal of Biomechanics, 20,* 735–742.

Campbell, A. J., Borrie, M. J., & Spears, G.F. (1989). Risk factors for falls in a community based prospective study of people 70 years and older. *Journals of Gerontology: Medical Sciences, 44,* M112–M117.

Campbell, A. J., Reinken, J., Allen, B. C., & Martinez, G. S. (1981). Falls in old age: A study of frequent and related factors. *Age and Aging, 10,* 264–270.

Cerny, K. (1983). A clinical method of quantitative gait analysis. *Physical Therapy, 63,* 1125–1126.

Chandler, J., Duncan, P. W., & Studenski, S. (1990). Balance performance on the postural stress test: Comparison of young adults, healthy elderly, and fallers. *Physical Therapy, 70,* 410–415.

Duncan, P. W., Studenski, S., Chandler, J., & Prescott, B. (1992). Functional reach: Predictive validity in a sample of elderly male veterans. *Journals of Gerontology: Medical Sciences, 47,* M93–M98.

Duncan, P. W., Weiner, D. K., Chandler, J., & Studenski, S. (1990). Functional reach: A new clinical measure of balance. *Journals of Gerontology: Medical Sciences, 45,* M192–M197.

Feinstein, A.R. (1987). *Clinimetrics.* New Haven: Yale University Press.

Granger, C. (1990). *Guide for use of the uniform data set for medical rehabilitation version 3.0,* State University of New York at Buffalo, Research Foundation, State University of New York.

Gryfe, C. I., Amies, A., & Ashley, M. J. (1977). A longitudinal study of falls in the elderly population. I. Incidence and morbidity. *Age and Aging, 6,* 201–210.

Guralnik, J., Simonsick, E. M., Ferrucci, L., Glynn, R. J., Berkman, L. F., Blazer, D. G., Scherr, P. A., & Wallace, R. B. (in press). A short physical performance battery assessing lower extemity function: Association with self-reported disability and prediction of mortality and nursing home admission. *Journals of Gerontology: Medical Sciences.*

Guyatt, G.H., Sullivan, M. J., & Thompson, P. J. (1985). The 6-minute walk: A new measure of exercise capacity in patients with chronic heart failure. *Canadian Medical Association Journal, 132,* 919–923.

Guyatt, G., Walter, J., & Normal, G. (1987) Measuring change over time: Assessing the usefulness of evaluative instruments. *Journal of Chronic Diseases, 40,* 171–178.

Heitmann, D., Gossman, M. R., & Shaddeau, S. A. (1989). Balance performance and width in non–institutionalized elderly, female, fallers and nonfallers. *Physical Therapy, 69,* 923–931.

Hill, K., Vandervoort, A., & Kramer, J. (1990). Reproducibility of performance on a test of postural responses in healthy elderly females. *Physiotherapy Canada, 42,* 61–66.

Hogue, C. C., Studenski, S., Duncan, P. W. (1990). Assessing mobility: The first step in falls prevention. In S. G. Funk, E. M. Tornquist, M. P. Champagne, L. A. Copp, & R. A. Weise, (Eds). *Key aspects of recovery: Improving nutrition, rest, and mobility.* (pp. 275–280) New York: Springer.

Horak, F. B., Shupert, C. L., & Mirka, A. (1989). Components of postural dyscontrol in the elderly: A review. *Neurology of Aging, 10,* 727–738.

Kirshner, B. and Guyatt, G. H. (1985). A methodological framework for assessing health indices. *Journal of Chronic Disease, 38,* 27–36.

Lichenstein, M. J., Burger, C., Shields, S. L., & Shiavi, R.G. (1990). Comparison of biomechanics platform measures of balance and taped measures of gait with a clinical mobility scale in elderly women. *Journals of Gerontology: Medical Sciences, 45,* M49–M54.

Mathias, S., Mayak, U. S. L., & Isaacs, B. (1986). Balance in elderly patients: The Get Up and Go Test. *Archives of Physical Medicine and Rehabilitation, 67,* 387–389.

Myers, A., Holliday, P. J., Harvey, K. A., & Hutchinson, K. S. (1993). Functional performance measures: Are they superior to self–assessments? *Journals of Gerontology: Medical Sciences, 48,* M196–M206.

Nevitt, M. C., Cummings, S. R., Kidd, S., & Black, D. (1989). Risk factors for recurrent nonsyncopal falls. *Journal of the American Medical Association, 261,* 2663–2668.

Oberg, T., Karsznia, A., & Oberg, K. (1993). Basic gait parameters: Reference data for normal subjects, 10–79 years. *Journal of Rehabilitation Research and Development, 30,* 210–223.

Overstall, P. W., Smith, A. N., Imms, F. J., & Johnson, A. L. (1974). Falls in the elderly related to postural imbalance. *British Medical Journal, 1,* 261–264.

Podsiadlo, D. & Richardson, S. (1991). The timed "up and go," a test of basic mobility for frail elderly persons. *Journal of the American Geriatrics Society, 39,* 142–148.

Potvin, A. R., Syndulko, K., Tourtellotte, W. W., Lemmon, J. A., & Potvin, J. H. (1980). Human neurologic function and the aging process. *Journal of the American Geriatrics Society, 28,* 1–9.

Reuben, D. & Siu, A. (1990). An objective measure of physical function of elderly outpatients: The physical performance test. *Journal of the American Geriatrics Society, 38,* 1105–1112.

Robbins, A. S., Rubenstein, L. Z., Josephson, K. R., Schulman, B. L., Osterweil, D., & Fine G. (1989). Predictors of falls among elderly people: Results of two population–based studies. *Archives of Internal Medicine, 149,* 1628–1633.

Robinson, J. L. & Smidt G. L. (1981). Quantitative gait evaluation in the clinic. *Physical Therapy, 61,* 351–353.

Romberg, M. H. (1853). *Manual of nervous diseases of man.* London: Sudenham Society (pp. 395–401).

Stelmach, G. E. & Worringham, C. J. (1985). Sensorimotor deficits related to postural stability. *Clinics in Geriatric Medicine, 1,* 679–692.

Stewart, A. L., & Ware, J. E. (Eds.) (1992). Measuring functioning and well-being: The Medical Outcomes Study approach. Durham, NC: Duke University Press.

Studenski. S., Duncan, P. W., Chandler, J., Samsa, G., Prescott, B., Hogue, C., & Bearon, L. (in press). Predicting falls: The role of mobility and nonphysical factors. *Journal of the American Geriatrics Society.*

Tinetti, M. E. (1986). Performance oriented assessment of mobility problems in elderly patients. *Journal of the American Geriatrics Society, 34,* 119–126.

Tinetti, M. E. (1987). Factors associated with serious injury during falls by ambulatory nursing home residents. *Journal of the American Geriatrics Society, 35,* 644–648.

Tinetti, M. E., Richman, D., & Powell, L. (1990). Falls efficacy as a measure of fear of falling. *Journal of Gerontology: Psychological Sciences, 45,* P239–P243.

Tinetti, M. E., Speechley, M., & Ginter, S. F. (1988). Risk factors for falls among elderly persons living in the community. *New England Journal of Medicine, 319,* 1701–1707.

Tinetti, M. E., Williams, T. F., & Mayewski, R. (1986). Falls risk index for elderly patients based on number of chronic disabilities. *American Journal of Medicine, 80,* 428–434.

Weiner, D. K., Bongiorni, D. R., Studenski, S., Duncan, P. W., & Kochersberger, G. (1993). Does functional reach improve with rehabilitation? *Archives of Physical Medicine and Rehabilitation, 74,* 796–800.

Weiner, D. K., Duncan, P. W., Chandler, J., & Studenski, S. (1992). Functional reach: A marker of physical frailty. *Journal of the American Geriatrics Society, 40,* 203–207.

Weiner, W. J., Nora, L. M., & Glantz, R. H. (1984). Elderly inpatients' postural reflex impairment. *Neurology, 34,* 945–947.

Wild, D., Mayak, U. S. L., & Isaacs, B. (1981). Prognosis of falls in old people at home. *Journal of Epidemiology and Community Health, 35,* 200–204.

Winograd, C. H., Lemski, C. M., Nevitt, M. C., Nordstrom, T. M., Stewart, A. L., Miller, C. J., & Bloch, P. A. (1994). Development of a Physical Performance and Mobility Examination (PPME). Department of Medicine, Stanford University, and Department of Veterans Affairs Medical Center, Palo Alto, CA (Manuscript). Submitted for publication.

Winter, D. (1991). *The biomechanics and motor control of human gait: Normal, elderly and pathological.* (2nd ed.). Waterloo, Ontario: University of Waterloo Press.

Wolfson, L. I., Whipple, R., Amerman, P., & Kleinberg, A. (1986). Stressing the postural response: A quantitative method for testing balance. *Journal of the American Geriatrics Society, 34,* 845–850.

Wolfson, L. I., Whipple, R., Amerman, P., & Tobin, J. (1990). Gait assessment in the elderly: A gait abnormality rating scale and its relation to falls. *Journals of Gerontology: Medical Sciences, 45,* M12–M19.

Woollacott, M. H. (1990). Changes in posture and voluntary control in the elderly. Research findings and rehabilitation. *Topics in Geriatric Rehabilitation, 5,* 1–11.

CHAPTER 5

Brief Assessments of Cognitive Function in the Elderly

MARILYN S. ALBERT
DEPARTMENT OF PSYCHIATRY AND NEUROLOGY
MASSACHUSETTS GENERAL HOSPITAL, BOSTON

Cognitive impairment increases substantially as people age. Current estimates of the prevalence of cognitive impairment vary from 5% to 10% among those over the age of 65; among those over 85 estimates of cognitive impairment range from 25% to 48% (Evans et al., 1989; Molsa, Marttila, & Rinne, 1982). Despite the obvious differences in the prevalence rates produced by these studies, they concur in finding that the prevalence of cognitive impairment increases substantially with age and, at the very oldest age range is seen in at least 1 in 4 individuals. These findings suggest that the clinical evaluation of an older person should include an assessment of cognitive status.

In addition, elderly patients (or their family members) coming to a clinician for evaluation frequently complain about changes in cognition. A clinician who sees a patient regularly may also become concerned about changes in mental ability that are observed over time. It is neither cost effective nor optimal for the patient's well-being for a detailed assessment to be conducted every time such concerns arise. Therefore, the clinician must develop the means for determining the necessity for further evaluation.

The ideal way to accomplish this is for clinicians to incorporate brief cognitive testing into their regular clinical evaluations as an initial means of assessing mental abilities in their patient. If this is done prior to complaints of cognitive change, the baseline evaluation can serve as a standard against which all other testing can be compared. Nonstandard testing, developed by the clinician, can be used for this purpose. Many clinicians prefer to assess patients by conversing with them about the adequacy of their daily functioning. Alternatively, there are a variety of standardized, but brief, mental status tests available.

The most widely used standardized mental status tests are relatively brief tests, administered face-to-face to the subject whose mental abilities are being measured. This chapter will review the most widely used mental status screening tests, discuss their strengths and weaknesses, and their sensitivity and specificity in relation to a diagnosis of dementia. Additional methods of evaluating mental abilities have recently been developed, including a telephone mental status test and an interview regarding change in mental abilities that can be administered to an informant; these will also be reviewed. Methods for assigning ratings to differing degrees of cognitive ability will also be discussed.

MENTAL STATUS TESTS USING IN-PERSON ADMINISTRATION

Mini-Mental State Examination (MMSE)

The Mini-Mental State Exam (MMSE) (Folstein, Folstein & McHugh, 1975) is probably the most widely used brief mental status test. It was first developed to provide the clinician with a means of assessing mental abilities at the bedside. It is currently the most commonly used mental status test in clinical settings. An added benefit to its use among clinicians is that there is widespread familiarity with the scoring system, which facilitates communication among clinicians.

The MMSE takes approximately 10 minutes to administer and covers a broad range of cognitive abilities. This includes an assessment of memory (i.e., delayed recall of three items and response to questions related to temporal orientation), language (i.e., naming common objects, repeating a linguistically difficult phrase, following a three-step command, and writing a sentence), spatial ability (i.e., copying a two-dimensional figure), and set-shifting (i.e., performing serial sevens or spelling the word "world" backwards). Scores on the MMSE range from 0–30. Each correct response receives 1 point, thus a perfect performance yields a score of 30.

Although first designed for clinical settings, the MMSE has also been widely used in epidemiologic studies. Thus there is considerable information about cutoff scores that can facilitate the identification of patients with cognitive dysfunction. Scores above 26 are generally considered to be excellent and reflective of normal cognitive function. Mildly impaired patients typically obtain scores of 20–26. Moderate impairment is reflected by scores of 11–20 and severe impairment by 10 or below. A cutoff score of 23 is generally recommended as indicative of cognitive dysfunction; however, the application of this cutoff must be modified by knowledge of the educational level of the patient. For example, subjects with a substantial amount of education can experience a considerable amount of cognitive decline before a score of 23 is achieved. On the other hand, persons with little education may obtain a score of 23 at baseline. This is because some items on the MMSE (or comparable screening tests) require a minimal educational background. For example, the serial sevens task, which contributes heavily to the score on the MMSE, is difficult for most very elderly individuals with limited education. This may lower their total score sufficiently that, with a few other minor errors, they fall below the cut-off point on the test.

Recent studies offer some guidelines for adjusting MMSE cutoff scores for the premorbid level of the patient. Murden, McRae, Kaner, & Bucknam (1991) recently administered the MMSE to 148 black and 100 white nondemented individuals, aged 60–99. Persons with an eighth-grade education or less had significantly poorer scores than persons with more than 8 years of education. Of those with lower levels of education, 25% received scores of 18–23 on the MMSE, scores usually thought to suggest dementia. By examining an additional population of demented patients, the authors were able to identify cutoff scores that appeared more appropriate for persons with low educational achievement. They reported that a cutoff of 17 produced a sensitivity of 81% and a specificity of 100% for dementia in persons with <8 years of education. Among those with >8 years of education, the standard cutoff score of 23 yielded a sensitivity of 93% and a specificity of 100%. There were no consistently significant differences between blacks and whites of equal education, indicating that education, but not race, is the important factor that influences test performance.

Hereen, Lagaay, Beek, Rooymans, & Hijmans (1990) also examined the impact of education. They focused on the MMSE performance of very elderly persons. Their epidemiologic study, conducted in the Netherlands, examined 1,258 persons over 85 years of age. These individuals were screened for the presence of neurologic and psychiatric disease, including dementias such as Alzheimer's disease (AD). They report the MMSE scores of the 532 persons whose assessments showed no evidence of neurologic or psychiatric disorders and whose educational levels were 4 years or greater. (Within this group there were 37 persons with poor hearing or vision whose data were analyzed separately.) The median MMSE score for this very elderly cohort was 28; the cutoff score for the lowest quartile was 26, for the subjects in their eighties, and 25, for subjects in their nineties. These results are comparable to another study in which 80-to 89-year-old subjects were examined (Bleeker, Colla–Wilson, Kawas, & Agnew, 1988). The high median scores of the elderly subjects are striking. There appears, nevertheless, a statistically significant difference with age. There was no statistically significant difference between the scores of persons taking psychoactive medications and those who were not. Taken together, these results indicate that, for a person of average education, a cutoff score of 23 is likely to be appropriate. For a person with >8 years of education, it is better to use a cutoff score of 17. For persons of very high levels of education (i.e., >16 years of school) cutoff scores of 27 may be appropriate. Recently, population-based norms for the MMSE have been published for differing age and educational levels, providing additional guidelines (Crum, Anthony, Bassett, & Folstein, 1993).

The MMSE has also been used in numerous studies in other countries. For example, it has been employed in studies of the prevalence of Alzheimer's disease in Finland, China and Great Britain (Salmon et al.,1989; Roth et al.,1986).

Blessed Dementia Scale (BDS)

The Blessed Dementia Scale (BDS) (Blessed, Tomlinson, & Roth, 1968) is one of the oldest mental status tests in wide use today. It was first developed to demonstrate the relationship between severe mental decline in the elderly and the presence of neurofibrillary tangles and neuritic plaques in autopsy tissue. More recently, it has been used in numerous epidemiologic studies.

The original version of the BDS contained two parts. The first part contained an evaluation of activities of daily living (ADL) and changes in personality, interests and drives. This yielded a score 0–28, sometimes refered to as the dementia score. The second part contained an assessment of orientation, memory, and concentration. The scores on the second part ranged from 0–37. The scoring scheme counts errors rather than correct responses, thus the higher the score the poorer the performance. A person who performs perfectly on the section that assesses mental abilties receives a score of 0.

The original version of BDS contained a number of questions about historical and current events that were particularly focused on British history and politics (e.g., the name of the prime minister and the name of the monarch). Therefore, changes were made when it was used in other countries. The original version also contained questions related to personal history (e.g., place of birth, school attended, and name of employers), that had to be validated by a collateral source, making the BDS difficult to use in epidemiologic studies. Because of these conditions, several altered versions have developed over time, complicating comparisons across site (Fuld, 1978; Berg et al., 1984).

A reduced six-item version appears to be the most widely used in epidemiologic settings (Katzman et al., 1983). This version retained the questions related to orientation (i.e., the year, the month, and the time within one hour), memory (i.e., delayed recall of an address) and concentration (i.e., counting backwards from 20–1 and saying the months in reverse order). It is sometimes known as the Blessed Orientation-Memory-Concentration Test (BOMC) to differentiate it from the longer version, which is sometimes refered to as the Blessed Information-Memory-Concentration Test (BIMC) (Blessed et al., 1968). The six-item version correlates highly with the longer version ($r = 0.96$). It also correlates with counts of neuritic plaques ($r = 0.60$) and neurofibrillary tangles ($r = 0.54$).

Comparisons between the BOMC and the MMSE indicate that there is a high correlation ($r = -0.83$; $r = -0.81$) between the tests (Fillenbaum, Heyman, Wilkinson, & Haynes, 1987; and Thal, Grundman, & Golden, 1986, respectively). Both show high test–retest reliability (0.77 and 0.89, respectively). The two tests differ, however, in their factor structure. The MMSE is best represented by two factors, one related to Memory-Attention and the other related to Verbal Comprehension (Zilmer, Fowler, Gutnick, Becker, 1990). The most recent study of the factor structure of the BOMC indicates that it is unidimensional. As a result, some authors have argued that the MMSE is a better tool for assessing elderly impaired patients (Zilmer et al., 1990).

Short Portable Mental Status Questionnaire (SPMSQ)

The Short Portable Mental Status Questionnaire (SPMSQ) (Pfeiffer, 1975) is also a widely used mental status test. It has been primarily used in epidemiologic studies, thus, there is considerable information about the cutoff scores for moderate and severe cognitive impairment.

The SPMSQ is a 10-item test which primarily assesses orientation to time and place (i.e., date, day, place) and general and personal knowledge (i.e., president, mother's maiden name, telephone number). One question assesses concentration and set-shifting (i.e., counting backwards by 3s). Like the BOMC, the scoring scheme of the SPMSQ counts errors rather than correct responses.

Five of the 10 items in the SPMSQ are identical to those in the earlier Mental Status Questionnaire (MSQ) (Kahn, Goldfarb, Pollack, & Peck, 1960). The primary difference between the two tests, apart from the items that do not overlap, pertains to the standardization procedures. The SPMSQ emphasizes gender and education norms, whereas the MSQ does not.

The first study using the SPMSQ (Pfeiffer, 1975) proposed three or more errors as an indication of some level of cognitive impairment. Some subsequent studies (Smyer, Hofland, & Jonas, 1979; Wolber, Romaniuk, Eastman, & Robinson, 1984) have reported close agreement between SPMSQ score and diagnosis of dementia. However, others (Fillenbaum, 1980; Haglund & Schuckit, 1976; Dalton, Pederson, Blom, & Holmes, 1987) have confirmed that use of the SPMSQ yields a low likelihood of saying that someone is demented when they are not (i.e., false positive rate = 4%) but that false negatives are high (45%).

Performance on the SPMSQ varies with age and education. A recent study examined the sensitivity and the specificity of the SPMSQ in comparison to a clinical diagnosis of AD in a representative selection of 402 community-dwelling individuals (Albert et al., 1991). The specificity decreased slightly among individuals over age 75 in comparison to persons aged 65–74 (88.8% vs. 96.2%, respectively). The SPMSQ more sensitively identified AD in individuals aged 75 and older than in the 65- to 75-years-old group (33.0% vs. 16.4%, respectively). The SPMSQ was slightly more specific in identifying individuals with AD among persons with more than 8 years of education in comparison to persons with 8 or fewer years of education (97.0% vs. 90.8%, respectively); however, specificity decreased among persons with more than 8 years of education in comparison to those with fewer years of education (17.8% vs 34.0%, respectively).

Perhaps as a result of these findings, the SPMSQ has been less widely used in recent years as a method for detecting persons with dementia in the community. However, it continues to be used to document levels of impairment among older individuals, especially in inpatient settings (e.g., Tennstedt, Skinner, Sullivan, & McKinlay, 1992; Elam et al., 1991).

Cambridge Cognitive Examination (CAMCOG)

The Cambridge Cognitive Examination (CAMCOG) is the cognitive section of a structured interview designed to identify cognitive impairment in individuals living in the community (Blessed, Block, Butter, & Kay, 1991; Roth et al., 1986). It is a 57-item scale that takes approximately 20 minutes to administer. It assesses a wide range of mental abilities including memory, orientation, language, praxis, attention, abstract thinking, perception, and calculation. Of the 57 items on the CAMCOG, 14 overlap with the MMSE (5 of the MMSE items are not included in the CAMCOG). Scores on the CAMCOG range from 0–106. Each correct response receives 1 point, thus, a perfect performance yields a score of 106.

Correlation between the CAMCOG and the MMSE is high, both when all of the items, including those that are on the MMSE, are included ($r = .87$) and when the overlaping items are omitted ($r = 0.8$). A cutoff score of <70 yields a sensitivity of 97% and a specificity of 91% when compared with a computer-generated diagnosis of dementia based on the structured interview (without reference to the CAMCOG). This cut-off is equivalent to an MMSE cutoff of approximately <20. Thus, like the other mental status tests cited above, the CAMCOG is sensitive to moderate-to-severe levels of cognitive impairment.

Test for Severe Impairment (TSI) and Severe Impairment Battery (SIB)

The screening tests described above have, in general, been designed for the assessment of demented patients with mild-to-moderate cognitive impairments. The recent focus on Alzheimer's disease has created a greater interest in managing and following demented patients throughout the course of their illness. It has, therefore, increased the importance of objectively assessing patients with severe cognitive dysfunction.

The quantification of cognitive abilities in severely impaired patients can serve a variety of needs. It can provide an indication of spared abilities that health care professionals can use in the development of management strategies. It can establish a measure of current function that can be used in following patients throughout an intervention trial or some other specified period of time. It can also be used to examine the relationship between postmortem neurochemical and neuropathological findings and cognitive status shortly before death.

The Severe Impairment Battery (SIB) is a test designed specifically for severely impaired patients (Saxton, McGonigle-Gibson, Swihart, Miller, & Boller, 1990). It contains six subscales (Attention, Orientation, Language, Memory, Visuoperception, and Construction) and also briefly assesses social skills and praxis. Scores range from 0–152, and it takes approximately 20 minutes to administer. It is significantly correlated with the Mini-Mental State Exam (r = .74) and test-retest reliability for the scale as a whole is good (r = .85). Subscale test-retest reliabilities range from .22 to .79 (two subscales were not significantly correlated between Time 1 and Time 2).

The Test for Severe Impairment (TSI) was also developed for patients with severe cognitive impairments (Albert & Cohen, 1992). It includes subsections that assess language, memory, conceptualization and motor performance and takes approximately 10 minutes to administer. Scores range from 0–24. The TSI is significantly correlated with the Mini Mental State Exam (r = 0.83) and test-retest reliability is high (r = .96). The test-retest reliabilities of the subsections range from .74 to .97. The internal reliability of the test is also good ($\alpha = 0.90$). Preliminary results of a factor analysis suggest that factor scores can be derived that relate to Memory, Language Production, and Knowledge of Body Parts.

ALTERNATE APPROACHES TO EVALUATING MENTAL STATUS

Telephone Interview for Cognition (TICS)

The Telephone Interview for Cognition Scale (TICS) (Brandt, Spencer, & Folstein, 1988) is a screening test designed to be administered over the phone. It therefore should be applicable in a variety of research settings, such as acquiring cognitive information on participants in an epidemiologic study, or following the cognitive status over time of participants who had previously been examined in a laboratory setting. Although it was designed primarily with research goals in mind, as health care practice evolves it may someday be used in clinical settings.

The TICS is an 11-item scale that takes approximately 10 minutes to administer. It assesses orientation (i.e., date, place), memory (i.e., immediate recall of a 10 word list), language (i.e., naming, comprehension, repetition), concentration and set shifting (i.e., serial sevens), and concept formation (i.e., word opposites). Scores on the TICS range from 0–41. Each correct response receives 1 point; thus, a perfect performance yields a score of 41.

Scores on the TICS correlate highly with the MMSE (r = .94). Test-retest reliability was high (.97). When comparing clearcut cases of Alzheimer's disease (n = 121) and controls (n = 33), there was a sensitivity of 94% and a specificity of 100%, using a cutoff of <30. It is likely that a population with a more distributed level of ability, such as that seen in the community, would have sensitivity and specificity levels similar to the MMSE (Brandt et al., 1988).

Information Questionnaire of Cognitive Decline in the Elderly (IQCode)

The Information Questionnaire of Cognitive Decline in the Elderly, which is known as the IQCode, represents an alternative approach to quantifying cognitive status (Jorm & Jacomb, 1989). It is a questionnaire that quantifies the likelihood that an older individual has experienced significant cognitive decline. This approach differs from that of most scales which have been designed to quantify level of cognitive function, rather than decline. At the present time, standard rating scales can only establish decline by longitudinal evaluation. The IQCode evaluates the presence or absence of declines by asking questions regarding declines in performance over the last 10 years in a variety of functional domains, such as the capacity to follow a story on television or in a book or the ability to remember family addresses. Thus, it requires a cooperative informant who has known the subject for 10 years. It could be administered over the telephone, although the investigators do not report having done this, thereby greatly facilitating the screening of large numbers of persons, as well as permitting the screening of subjects who are geographically distant from one another. It should be noted, however, that it is unclear whether the 10-year frame of reference employed in the questionnaire will permit it to be used in a longitudinal fashion, for example, to screen for symptoms of incident disease in a person who was evaluated 1–2 years earlier.

The 26 items on the IQCODE can be broadly grouped into questions that deal with retrieval of previously learned information and questions that deal with acquisition of new information. For each area of inquiry, the informant is asked to state whether, "compared with 10 years ago," the subject is much better (1), a bit better (2), shows not much change (3), a bit worse (4), or much worse (5). The ratings are then summed for a maximum score of 130, with higher scores representing more decline. The internal consistency of the questionnaire is high (α = .95). Test-retest reliability over 1 year is adequate (.75). The correlation between the IQCODE and the MMSE is good ($r = -.74$). Correlation with education is poor, suggesting that the test results are not affected by differences in premorbid ability.

A recent study (Jorm, Scott, Cullen, & MacKinnon, 1991) compared IQCODE scores to clinical diagnosis. Using a cutoff of >3.60, the investigators report a sensitivity of 69% and a specificity of 82%, when compared to clinicians' DSM–III–R diagnoses. Using a cutoff of <23, the MMSE administered to the same individuals produced a sensitivity of 64% and a specificity of 75%. A comparison with the ICD–10 diagnoses (produced by a structured interview) yielded a sensitivity and specificity of 80% and 82% for the IQCODE and 76% and 73% for the MMSE, respectively. It should be noted that the patient sample in the study was a heterogeneous one, containing normals, patients with dementia of the Alzheimer type (AD), depression, etc. Thus, the IQCODE performed at least as well as the MMSE, and possibly better when compared with the ICD–10 diagnoses.

MENTAL STATUS RATING SCALES

Clinical Dementia Rating Scale (CDR)

The Clinical Dementia Rating Scale (CDR) (Hughes, Berg, Danziger, Coben, & Martin, 1982) provides a method for rating dementia. The original version rated cognitive function along a 5-point scale (0 = none, 0.5 = questionable, 1 = mild, 2 = moderate, 3 = severe). More recently (Heyman et al., 1987) two additional levels of severity were added to the scale (4 = profound and 5 = terminal). To obtain an overall rating of severity, each person first receives a rating in six areas of ability, based on information concerning how they function in daily life. These six areas include memory, orientation, judgment and problem solving, community affairs, home and hobbies, and personal care. An overall dementia rating is then generated, based on the ratings in each of the six areas. However, each of the six areas is not weighted equally; memory impairment carries more weight in determining the overall rating than the other areas. For example, an individual with 1.0 on memory and 0.5 on personal care will receive an overall CDR rating of 1.0, however a rating of 1.0 on personal care and 0.5 on memory will yield a CDR rating of 0.5.

The CDR rating system does not dictate the method by which the ratings are achieved. The investigators who designed the CDR generally utilize a structured interview to generate the ratings (Berg et al., 1984); however, any information-gathering scheme that addresses the six areas of interest in a meaningful manner can be employed.

The interrater reliability of the scale is .91 (Burke et al., 1988). The performance of persons rated as mildly, moderately or severely impaired can be differentiated psychometrically, thereby providing independent validation for the scale (Berg et al., 1984).

Global Deterioration Scale (GDS)

The Global Deterioration Scale (Reisberg, Ferris, de Leon, & Crook, 1982) rates cognitive impairment along a 7-point scale (1 = none, 2 = very mild, 3 = mild, 4 = moderate, 5 = moderate, 6 = severe, 7 = very severe). The individual receives an overall rating based on the general profile of an individual in the stage in question. For example, the description of Stage 3 outlines the individual's memory difficulty, word finding problems, psychiatric symptoms, and performance on psychometric tests, as well as the degree to which people in the environment are aware of the cognitive problems. The inclusion of psychometric test scores in the description suggests that these tests, or ones similar to them, should be used to assure adequate assignment of the ratings.

The GDS ratings are linked to, but not dependent upon, two other rating measures developed by Reisberg's team (Reisberg, Sclan, Franssen, Kluger, & Ferris, in press): The Brief Congnitive Rating Scale (BCRS) and the Functional Assessment Staging Technique (FAST). The BCRS has four axes: concentration, recent memory, remote memory and orientation. Each axis is rated on a 7-point continuum using semistructured clinical anchors. The FAST is also a 7-point scale of functional impairment. Its floor goes somewhat lower than the standard ADL scales. Together, the BCRS and the FAST provide more information on which to base GDS ratings, but the three-instrument set also requires more professional time in return for its possibly greater validity.

According to the authors of the GDS, the presence or absence of a specific symptom or score does not dictate the decision regarding the rating. Instead, the rater is asked to allow a general impression of the patient across all areas of function (cognitive, functional and behavioral) to guide the decision. In this sense, the GDS differs from the CDR, in that the CDR provides a series of rules regarding the relative weights that should be assigned to difficulties in each area of function.

Three different reliability studies have examined the interrater reliability of the GDS. One study examined ambulatory outpatients and found that the intraclass correlation between two raters was .82 (Gottlieb, Gur, & Gur, 1988). The two raters were within 1 point of each other for 41 of 43 cases, and there was complete concordance for 30 of the 43 cases (70%). A second study examined two sets of 20 patients each in a long-term care facility and found correlations of .97 and .92 (Foster, Sclan, Welkowitz, Boksay, & Seeland, 1988). A third study examined a group of subjects, approximately half of whom were cognitively normal (Reisberg et al., 1989). Test-retest reliability of the GDS at 7-day to 4-month intervals was .92.

The validation of the rating scheme is based on its correlation with neurophysiological measures in the subjects. There is a significant correlation between GDS level and ratings of degree of ventricular dilatation on computerized tomography scans ($r = 0.62$), and glucose utilization on positron emission tomography scans ($r = 0.69$).

CONCLUSION

Tests that briefly assess cognitive ability in the elderly are a considerable asset. They provide a means for quantifying cognitive performance in a standardized and reliable manner. The clinician can incorporate such tests into regular evaluations of patients and the epidemiologist can use them to identify individuals who are likely to be cognitively impaired and those who are not.

The most widely used brief test of cognitive function is the Mini-Mental State Exam. It has been very widely used in epidemiologic studies, and there is an increasing body of normative data providing guidelines for use (Crum et al., 1993). It is also used increasingly by clinicians. Widespread use of the MMSE provides a common means of communication among individuals who work with the elderly and, if for no other reason, suggests that the MMSE should be widely adopted.

However, the MMSE, as well as all other brief tests of cognitive function, has substantive limitations and it is important to keep them in mind. First, the accuracy with which the mental status screening tests identify persons with cognitive dysfunction is greatly altered by the age and educational level of the individuals being assessed. The racial background of the target population also alters the utility of the instrument being applied. Recent results suggest that the commonly used screening tests operate less efficiently for Hispanics and African Americans than for whites (Fillenbaum, Heyman, Prosnitz, & Burchett, 1990; Gurland, Wilder, Cross, Teresi, & Barrett, 1992). The discrepancy between test results and diagnosis by a clinician appears to be greatest for Hispanics (Gurland et al, 1992).

Among very elderly and impaired populations, such as those in chronic care facilities, there are additional considerations (Teresi, Lawton, Ory, & Holmes, in press). Many physically frail and/or vision-impaired individuals cannot complete some test items because of physical disability rather than cognitive dysfunction. In addition, individuals with focal cognitive deficits affecting language (e.g., aphasia) will score poorly on most standard screening tests because the tests are heavily language dependent.

Brief tests of cognitive ability must, therefore, be applied with these limitations in mind. Their results should not be confused with a diagnosis of disease which would preserve evaluations of the patient by skilled clinicians detailed.

None of the commonly used brief tests of mental ability require test-specific training. They do, however, require general skill and knowledge of test administration. As in any testing evaluation, the test environment should be quiet and well lit. With the elderly, perhaps more than any other group, it is important to establish a friendly and nonthreatening environment. As a group, the elderly are less educated than the young and are more intimidated by cognitive testing. It is also important to minimize failures, if they occur, so that embarrassment and exasperation do not cause the individual to give up. Naturally, one must be thoroughly familiar with the scoring rules of the test being administered.

Mental status rating scales, on the other hand, presume a detailed evaluation of the patient by a skilled clinician and primarily provide a broad means of classifying disability into stages. As their use expands, they may become useful for communicating degree of dysfunction among clinicians and caregivers.

REFERENCES

Albert, M., & Cohen, C. (1992). The test for severe impairment: An instrument for the assessment of patients with severe cognitive dysfunction. *Journal of the American Geriatrics Society, 40*, 449–453.

Albert, M., Smith, L., Scherr, P., Taylor, J., Funkenstein, H., & Evans, D. (1991). Use of brief cognitive tests to identify individuals in the community with clinically diagnosed Alzheimer's disease. *International Journal of the Neurosciences, 57*, 167–178.

Berg, L., Danziger, W., Storandt, M., Coben, L., Gado, M., Hughes, C., Knesevich, J., & Botwinick, J. (1984). Predictive features in mild senile dementia of the Alzheimer type. *Neurology, 34*, 563–569.

Bleeker, M.L., Colla–Wilson, K., Kawas, C., & Agnew, J. (1988). Age-specific norms for the Mini-Mental State Exam. *Neurology, 38*, 1565–1568.

Blessed, G., Tomlinson, B. E., & Roth, M. (1968). The association between quantitative measures of dementia and of senile changes in the cerebral gray matter of elderly subjects. *British Journal of Psychiatry, 114*, 797–811.

Blessed, G., Black. S., Butler, T., & Kay, D. (1991). The diagnosis of dementia in the elderly: A comparison of CAMCOG (the Cognitive Section of the CAMDEX), the AGECAT Program, DSM–III, the Mini-Mental State Examination and some short rating scales. *British Journal of Psychiatry, 159*, 193–198.

Brandt, J., Spencer, M., & Folstein M. (1988). The telephone interview for cognitive status. *Neuropsychiatry, Neuropsychology, and Behavioral Neurology, 1*, 111–117.

Burke, W., Miller, J., Rubin, E., Morris, J., Coben, L., Duchek, J., Wittels, G., & Berg, L. (1988). Reliability of the Washington University Clinical Dementia Rating. *Archives of Neurology, 45*, 31–32.

Crum, R., Anthony, J., Bassett, S., & Folstein, M. (1993). Population-based norms for the Mini-Mental State Examination by age and educational level. *Journal of the American Medical Association, 269*, 2386–2391.

Dalton, J., Pederson, S., Blom, B., & Holmes, N. (1987). Diagnostic errors using the Short Portable Mental Questionnaire with a mixed clinical population. *Journal of Gerontology, 42*, 512–514.

Elam, J., Graney, M., Beaver, T., El Derwi, D., Applegate, W.,& Miller, S. (1991). Comparison of subjective ratings of function with observed functional ability of frail older persons. *American Journal of Public Health, 81*, 1127–1130.

Evans, D., Funkenstein, H., Albert, M., Scherr, P., Cook, N., Chown, M., Hebert, L., Hennekens, C., & Taylor, J. (1989). Prevalence of Alzheimer's disease in a community population of older persons. *Journal of the American Medical Association, 262*, 2551–2556.

Fillenbaum, G. (1980). Comparison of two brief tests of organic brain impairment, the MSQ and the Short Portable MSQ. *Journal of the American Geriatrics Society, 28*, 381–384.

Fillenbaum, G., Heyman, A., Wilkinson, W., & Haynes, C. (1987). Comparison of two screening tests in Alzheimer's disease. *Archives of Neurology, 44*, 924–927.

Fillenbaum, G., Heyman, A., Prosnitz, B., & Burchett, B. (1990). Sensitivity and specificity of standardized screens of cognitive impairment and dementia among elderly black and white community residents. *Journal of Clinical Epidemiology, 43*, 651–660.

Folstein, M., Folstein, S., & McHugh, P. (1975). 'Mini-Mental State': A practical method for grading cognitive state of patients for the clinician. *Journal of Psychiatric Research, 12*, 189–198.

Foster, J., Sclan, S., Welkowitz, J., Boksay, I., & Seeland, I. (1988). Psychiatric assessment in medical long-term care facilities: Reliability of commonly used rating scales. *International Journal of Geriatric Psychiaty, 3,* 229–233.

Fuld, P. (1978). Psychological testing in the differential diagnosis of dementias. In R. Katzman, R. Terry, & K. Bick (Eds.), *Alzheimer's disease: Senile dementias and related disorders*. (pp. 185–193). New York: Raven Press.

Gottlieb, G., Gur, R., & Gur, R. (1988). Reliability of psychiatric scales in patients with dementia of the Alzheimer type. *American Journal of Psychiatry, 45*, 857–859.

Gurland, B., Wilder, D., Cross, P., Teresi, J., & Barrett, V. (1992). Screening scales for dementia: Toward reconciliation of conflicting cross-cultural findings. *International Journal of Geriatric Psychiatry, 7*, 105–113.

Haglund, R., & Schuckit, M. (1976). A clinical comparison of tests of organicity in elderly patients. *Journal of Gerontology, 31*, 654–659.

Heeren, T., Lagaay, A., Beek, W., Rooymans, H., & Hijmans, W. (1990). Reference values for the Mini-Mental State Examination (MMSE) in octo- and nonagenerians. *Journal of the American Geriatrics Society, 38*, 1093–1096.

Heyman, A., Wilkinson, W. E., Hurwitz, B. J., Helms, M. J., Haynes, C. S., Utley, C. M., & Gwyther, L. P. (1987). Early-onset Alzheimer disease: Clinical predictors of institutionalization and death. *Neurology, 37*, 980–984.

Hughes, C., Berg, L., Danziger, W., Coben, L., & Martin R. (1982). A new clinical scale for the staging of dementia. *British Journal of Psychiatry, 140*, 566–572.

Jorm, A., Scott, R., Cullen, J., & MacKinnon, A. (1991). Performance of the Informant Questionnaire on Cognitive Decline in the Elderly (IQCODE) as a screening test for dementia. *Psychological Medicine 21*, 785–790.

Jorm, A., & Jacomb, P. (1989). The Informant Questionnaire on Cognitive Decline in the Elderly (IQCODE): Sociodemographic correlates, reliability, validity and some norms. *Psychological Medicine, 19*, 1015–1022.

Kahn, R., Goldfarb, A., Pollack, M., & Peck, A. (1960). Brief objective measures for the determination of mental status in the aged. *American Journal of Psychiatry, 117*, 326–328.

Katzman, R., Brown, T., Fuld, P., Peck, A., Schecter, R., & Schimmel, H. (1983). Validation of a short orientation-memory-concentration test of cognitive impairment. *American Journal of Psychiatry, 140,* 734–739.

Molsa, P., Marttila, R., & Rinne, U. (1982). Epidemiology of dementia in a Finnish population. *Acta Neurologica Scandinavica, 65*, 541–552.

Murden, R., McRae, T., Kaner, S., & Bucknam, M. (1991). Mini-Mental State Exam scores vary with education in blacks and whites. *Journal of the American Geriatrics Society, 39*, 149–155.

Pfeiffer, E. (1975). SPMSQ: Short Portable Mental Status Questionnaire. *Journal of the American Geriatrics Society, 23,* 433–441.

Reisberg, B., Ferris, S., de Leon, M., & Crook, T. (1982). The Global Deterioration Scale for assessment of primary degenerative dementia. *American Journal of Psychiatry, 139*, 1136–1139.

Reisberg, B., Ferris, S., Steinberg, G., Shulman, E., de Leon, M., & Sinaiko, E. (1989). Longitudinal study of dementia patients and aged controls. In M. P., Lawton, & A. R., Herzog (Eds.), *Special research methods for gerontology* (pp. 195–231). Amityville, NY: Baywood.

Reisberg, B., Sclan, S. G., Franssen, E., Kluger, A., & Ferris, S. (in press). Dementia staging in chronic care populations. *Alzheimer's Disease and Associated Disorders.*

Roth, M., Tym, E., Mountjoy, C., Huppert, F., Hendrie, H., Verma, S., & Goddard, R. (1986). CAMDEX: A standardized instrument for the diagnosis of mental disorder in the elderly with special reference to the early detection of dementia. *British Journal of Psychiatry, 149*, 698–709.

Salmon, D., Riekkinen, P., Katzman, R., Zhang, M., Jin, H., & Yu, E. (1989). Cross-cultural studies of dementia. *Archives of Neurology, 146*, 769–772.

Saxton, J., McGonigle-Gibson, K., Swihart, A., Miller, V., & Boller, F. (1990). Assessment of the severely impaired patient: Description and validation of a new neuropsychological test battery. *Psychological Assessment, 12*, 298–303.

Smyer, M., Hofland, B., & Jonas, E. (1979). Validity study of the Short Portable Mental Status Questionnaire for the elderly. *Journal of the American Geriatrics Society, 27*, 263–269.

Tennstedt, S., Skinner, K., Sullivan, L., McKinlay, J. (1992). Response comparability of family and staff proxies for nursing home residents. *American Journal of Public Health, 82*, 747–749.

Teresi, J., Lawton, P., Ory, M., & Holmes, D. (in press) Measurement issues in chronic care populations: Dementia special care. *Alzheimer's Disease and Associated Disorders.*

Thal, L., Grundman, M., & Golden, R. (1986). Alzheimer's disease: a correlational analysis of the Blessed Information-Memory-Concentration Test and the Mini-Mental State Exam. *Neurology, 36*, 262–264.

Wolber, G., Romaniuk, M., Eastman, E., & Robinson, C. (1984). Validity of the Short Portable Mental Status Questionnare with elderly psychiatric patients. *Journal of Consulting and Clinical Psychology, 52*, 712–713.

Zilmer, E., Fowler, P., Gutnick, H., & Becker, E. (1990). Comparison of two cognitive bedside screening instruments in nursing home residents: A factor analytic study. *Journals of Gerontology: Psychological Science, 45*, P69–P74.

CHAPTER 6

Assessment of Behavioral Disturbance in Older Adults

LINDA TERI

AND

REBECCA G. LOGSDON
DEPARTMENT OF PSAYCHIATRY AND BEHAVIORAL SCIENCES
UNIVERSITY OF WASHINGTON MEDICAL CENTER, SEATTLE

Behavioral disturbance is a prevalent and pervasive aspect of many of the cognitive and emotional disorders afflicting older adults. For example, Alzheimer's disease (AD), one of the most common neurological diseases of aging, has been characterized as "a disease of cognition and behavior" (Teri, Rabins, et al., 1992). Numerous clinical and empirical writings have identified a plethora of behavioral problems characteristic of patients with AD (Swearer, Drachman, O'Donnell, & Mitchell, 1988; Teri, Borson, Kiyak, & Yamagishi, 1989; Teri, Larson, & Reifler, 1988; Zarit, Orr, & Zarit, 1985). Such problems include, depression, agitation, wandering, and aggression and are certainly not unique to any one diagnostic group. Individuals with severe and/or chronic mental disorders, such as schizophrenia and depression, also exhibit an array of behavior problems, commonly referred to as symptoms. These behavior problems can span a gamut of psychotic-like actions, including bizarre speech and hallucinations to disturbances of sleep, verbalizations of sadness, of guilt, and of worthlessness, and overt actions of violence toward oneself or others. For many patients, these problems occur on a daily basis with serious intra- and interpersonal consequences impeding effective care and quality of life (Deimling & Bass, 1986; Drinka, Smith & Drinka, 1987; Rabins, Mace, & Lucas, 1982; Reisberg, Franssen, Sclan, Kluger & Ferris, 1989, Roth, 1979; Teeter, Garetz, Miller, & Heiland, 1976; Rovner, Kafonek, Filipp, Lucas, & Folstein, 1986; Teri et al., 1988; Teri et al., 1989).

Because of this diversity of etiology and presentation, the term "behavioral disturbance" does not represent a unitary or uniform phenomenon. Rather, it represents a broad category, often multifactorial, multiform, and dynamic. Measures to assess behavioral disturbances, therefore, also vary. Some measures encompass a large range of problems; others focus on one or more specific areas. Some require little or no training to complete; others require trained clinicians. Some utilize paper and pencil informant report; others rely on structured interviews. Some employ direct observation. Whatever strategy is employed, the accurate assessment of behavioral disturbance has far-reaching implications for clinical research and care. Accurate assessment is often the precursor to effective intervention and is essential to clinical and research endeavors in both pharmacologic and nonpharmacologic spheres.

The purpose of this chapter is to provide readers with an overview of measures currently available for the assessment of behavioral disturbance in older adults. The breadth of the term "behavioral disturbance" is reflected in a recent computerized search of Medline Database from 1983–1993, and the PsychINFO database from 1967 to 1993 that revealed over 150 behavioral disturbance measurement citations. The number of available measures has more than doubled in the last 5 years.

To accommodate this array of information this chapter will focus on measures that meet three criteria:

1. The measure must be specifically designed for and used in the assessment of behavioral disturbance in older adults. The majority of these measures have also been designed for use with dementia patients and can be classified into three areas of measurement: (a) general behavioral problems, (b) agitation and aggression, and (c) depression.
2. The measure must be accessible and easily implemented. We specifically selected published instruments with clear, comprehensive instructions for administration, scoring, and interpretation. They can be completed by personnel with diverse backgrounds and training and are potentially useful in a variety of clinical and research endeavors with both institutionalized and community-dwelling adults. Measures requiring sophisticated diagnostic strategies or professional diagnosticians have been omitted.
3. The measure must have published or readily available psychometric data. Adequate reliability, validity, and standardized information on administration and scoring were all taken into account. We also selected measures that seem to be growing in popularity, so that more data will be available in the near future.

There are a number of measures available that do not meet these criteria but that the reader may find of interest. These, and the measures reviewed here, are listed in Table 6.1. In addition, the interested reader is referred to other recent reviews of this area (Kluger & Ferris, 1991; Niederehe, 1988; Overall & Rhoades, 1988; Teri et al., 1992).

TABLE 6.1 Measures Assessing Behavioral Disturbance in Older Adults[1]

Scale Name	*Primary References[1]*	*Rater Source*	*Sample*
1. Alzheimer's Disease Assessment Scale (ADAS)	Mohs et al., 1983; Rosen et al., 1984.	Clinician[(2)] (interview with patient)	Alzheimer's patients
2. Behavioral and Emotional Activities Manifested in Dementia (BEAM-D)	Sinha et al., 1992.	Psychiatrist/Psychologist (interview with patient and caregiver)	Alzheimer's patients
3. Behavioral Pathology in Alzheimer's Disease Rating Scale (BEHAVE-AD)	Reisberg et al., 1987.	Clinician (interview with patient and caregiver)	Alzheimer's patients
4. Brief Agitation Rating Scale (BARS)	Finkel et al., 1993.	Nursing staff	Nursing home residents
5. Brief Psychiatric Rating Scale (BPRS)	Overall & Gorham, 1962; Overall & Beller, 1984.	Caregiver (interview with patients	Dementia outpatients Geropsychiatric inpatients
6. Caregiver Obstreperous Behavior Rating Assessment Scale (COBRA)	Drachman et al., 1992.	Caregiver (questionnaire)	Dementia outpatients Nursing home residents
7. Consortium to Establish Registry in Alzheimer's Disease—Behavior Rating Scale for Dementia (BRSD)	Tariot et al., 1991.	Clinician (interview with caregiver)	Alzheimer's patients
8. Clinical Assessment of Psychopathology Among Elderly Residents (CAPER)	Reichenfeld et al., 1992.	Psychiatrist (interview with patient)	Nursing home residents
9. Cohen-Mansfield Agitation Inventory (CMAI)	Cohen-Mansfield et al., 1989.	Nursing staff	Nursing home patients

TABLE 6.1 (Continued)

	Scale Name	*Primary References*[1]	*Rater Source*	*Sample*
10.	Columbia University Scale for Psychopathology in Alzheimer's Disease (CUSPAD)	Devanand et al., 1992.	Clinician (interview with caregiver)	Alzheimer's patients
11.	Cornell Scale for Depression in Dementia (CSDD)	Alexopoulos et al., 1988.	Clinician (interview with patient and caregiver)	Alzheimer's patients
12.	Dementia Behavior Disturbance Scale (DBD)	Baumgarten et al., 1990.	Clinician (interview with caregiver) or caregiver questionnaire	Dementia outpatients
13.	Dementia Mood Assessment Scale (DMAS)	Sunderland et al., 1988.	Nursing staff	Alzheimer's patients
14.	Disruptive Behavior Rating Scales (DBRS)	Mungas et al., 1989.	Nursing staff	Nursing home residents
15.	Geriatric Evaluation by Relative's Rating Instrument (GERRI)	Schwartz 1983.	Caregiver/relative (questionnaire)	Alzheimer's patients
16.	Geriatric Mental State Schedule (GMS)	Copeland et al., 1976; Gurland et al., 1976.	Clinician (interview with patient)	Older adults
17.	Global Assessment of Psychiatric Symptoms (GAPS)	Raskin, 1985.	Mental health professional (patient interview)	Geriatric psychiatric patients
18.	Multidimensional Observation Scale for Elderly Subjects (MOSES)	Helmes et al., 1987.	Nursing staff	Nursing home residents

19.	Neurobehavioral Rating Scale	Levin et al., 1987; Seltzer et al., 1992.	Physician (interview with patient)	Brain injury patients Dementia outpatients
20.	Nurse-Oriented Scale for Inpatient Evaluation (NOSIE-30)	Ravensborg & Willenson, 1969.	Nursing staff	Psychiatric inpatients
21.	Nursing Home Behavior Problem Scale (NHBPS)	Ray et al., 1992.	Nursing Staff	Nursing home residents
22.	Pleasant Events Schedule – AD (PES-AD)	Teri & Logsdon, 1991.	Caregiver (questionnaire)	Alzheimer's outpatients
23.	Physical and Mental Impairment-of-Function Evaluation (PAMIE)	Gurel et al., 1972.	Nursing staff	Geriatric medical patients
24.	Relative's Assessment of Global Symptomatology (RAGS)	Raskin & Crook, 1988.	Caregiver (questionnaire)	Geropsychiatric patients
25.	Revised Memory and Behavior Problems Checklist (RMBPC)	Teri, Truax, et al., 1992.	Caregiver (questionnaire)	Dementia outpatients
26.	Ryden Aggression Scale (RAS)	Ryden, 1988.	Caregiver (questionnaire)	Alzheimer's outpatients
27.	Sandoz Clinical Assessment—Geriatric (SCAG)	Shader et al., 1974.	Clinician (interview with patient)	Geriatric patients
28.	Texas Research Institute Mental Studies-Behavioral Problem Checklist (TRIMS-BPC)	Niederehe, 1988.	Caregiver (questionnaire)	Dementia patients

[1]When psychometric data are presented in an article subsequent to the original citation, two references are given.
[2]The term clinician refers to a range of professionals, such as social workers, nurses, research staff, and others.

METHODOLOGICAL OVERVIEW

The assessment of behavioral disturbance in older adults has undergone a relatively rapid evolution. Early measures were often developed as part of a larger study and included items of interest to that particular study with no attempt to explain their selection, balance the array of items included, or focus item content in any systematic or theoretical way. These measures were idiosyncratic in nature, responding to an immediate need of a particular study, with published reports providing little or no psychometric or descriptive information. Although recent measures remain atheoretical and idiosyncratic in many ways, there is a clear movement toward more methodologically sound measurement development. Considerably more attention is being paid to describing the measure, its rational for item selection, its method of administration and scoring, and its psychometric characteristics. Currently, however, measures of behavioral disturbance vary considerably. Item content, method of assessment, and format are often dramatically different.

Item content across measures varies by how the behavior is defined. Some measures focus on the presence or absence of a given behavior; some examine the frequency of occurrence; some investigate severity; some do a composite of all three. The time referent for assessment varies as well, with some measures indicating an indefinite time period (for example, "Did this happen?"); others specify a period of time (for example, "In the last two weeks . . . "). Some focus on the problem alone; others include the problem and the reporters' reactions to the problem. Last but not least, the method of measurement also varies. Some measures use a yes/no format, whereas others use a Likert scale, and still others employ categorical scaling. Different measures tap different behaviors, and the degree of overlap, agreement, or disagreement among measures is largely unknown.

Informant report, structured interviews, and direct observation have all been used to assess behavioral disturbances in older adults. Informant report is a substitute for the traditional self-report format, since individuals with cognitive and behavioral problems are often unable to complete assessment forms themselves. The informant is, therefore, asked to report on behaviors of the patient. This circumstance make the assessment of behavioral disturbance unique. To the best of our knowledge, no true self-report form of behavioral disturbance exists. Indeed, if it did, its utility would be limited.

Some structured interviews require that time be spent with the patient as well as with the informant. The information gleaned from the patient, however, may be minimal, and the information from the informant heavily influences the final assessment. Thus, interviews often reflect the same biases as informant reports. Indeed, in two recent studies, interview data were highly correlated with direct informant report data (Teri & Wagner, 1992; Logsdon & Teri, 1993).

Direct observation offers the opportunity for the rater to observe the patient objectively, avoiding problems associated with informant reporting. Unfortunately, direct observational strategies are rarely employed. Often, measures that are labeled "observational" are not really observational measures. Rather, they ask informants to rate how often they think they have observed different behaviors over a specified time period. This is in contrast to true observational strategies that require the actual recording of behavior as it occurs. Needless to say, this method of ongoing direct observation is much more labor intensive and time consuming than either interview or informant report. Consequently, direct observations are usually scheduled to occur during a given time period using various time-sampling methods. Disturbances, however, are often episodic and unscheduled. They may not necessarily occur (and therefore will not be observed) during a designated assessment period. Further, the effect of an observer on the behavior disturbance is unknown. It is thus no surprise that direct observational strategies are rarely employed, and when they are, tend to occur in institutional settings.

Given this reliance on information provided by an informant to assess the behavior of a given patient, one would think that the instrument would specify who is appropriate to provide this information. Studies often do not detail how informants were selected, what degree of familiarity they have with the patient, or how much direct observation of the behavioral disturbance they have. Therefore, the informant may or may not be able to make an accurate assessment. The factors that influence informant report data, whether obtained by questionnaire or interview, are largely unknown.

Measures

General Behavioral Problems

Table 6.1 summarizes some of the large array of measures designed to evaluate behavior problems in older adults. We focus our discussion here on measures that meet the criteria identified earlier. In addition, the measures reviewed here were specifically designed to evaluate the spectrum of behavioral disturbances in demented older adults, and thus represent a solid assessment of general behavioral disturbance. They include measures developed for use with community-residing samples, institutionalized samples, inpatients, and outpatients.

The CERAD Behavior Rating Scale for Dementia (BRSD). The Consortium to Establish a Registry for Alzheimer's Disease (CERAD) scale (Tariot et al., under review) was designed to assess behavioral symptoms in patients with dementia and uses a number of items from the BEHAVE-AD (Reisberg et al., 1987), described in the next section. It is administrated in an interview with the patient's primary caregiver, and consists of 51 items rated according to frequency of occurrence on a scale of 1 (has not occurred) to 4 (occurred on 16 or more days in the past month). Items cover a wide range of behaviors, including anxiety and fearfulness, depressive behaviors, restlessness, memory-related problems, socially inappropriate behavior, hallucinations, and delusions.

Since it has been incorporated into the battery of clinical and neuropsychological instruments administered by CERAD, the BRSD is being used nationally. In a sample of 303 subjects from 16 sites, the BRSD has demonstrated good interrater reliability (kappas ranging from .77 to 1.00). It yields 8 factors: Depressive Features, Psychotic Features, Defective Self-Regulation, Irritability/Agitation, Vegetative Features, Aggressions, and Affective Lability (Tariot et al., under review). Additional investigations are currently under way to further refine the item content and wording. The BRSD requires about 45 minutes to administer, and provides a comprehensive evaluation of the frequency of a wide spectrum of behavior problems in AD patients. It is, however, limited in the range of frequency assessed. The frequency rating scale does not distinguish between behaviors that occur several times a day and those that occur once every one or two days. It also does not provide an assessment of severity. These properties may limit its usefulness in detecting subtle changes or treatment effects.

The Behavioral Pathology in Alzheimer's Disease (BEHAVE-AD). This 25-item scale (Reisberg et al., 1987) was originally designed to evaluate changes in behavior of patients with Alzheimer's disease as a result of pharmacological intervention. It rates severity of behavior problems on a scale of O (not present) to 3 (most severe). Subscales include Paranoid and Delusional Ideation, Hallucinations, Activity Disturbances, Aggressiveness, Diurnal Rhythm Disturbances, Affective Disturbance, Anxieties and Phobias, and a global rating of the impact of all behavior problems on the caregiver and patient. In one study of 34 AD patients, interrater reliability was found to be good, with kappas ranging from .62 to 1.00 (Patterson et al., 1990).

The BEHAVE-AD has been found useful with outpatients and nursing home residents, and appears particularly useful for identifying behavioral disturbance in patients who are moderately to severely demented (Reisberg et al., 1989). It also has been reported to be useful in longitudinal and cross-sectional descriptive studies of behavioral disturbance in AD patients (Reisberg et al., 1992). Research to clarify psychometric properties and level of training needed by the interviewer to accurately complete the measure is needed, as are investigations of its sensitivity to change in treatment outcomes studies.

The Columbia University Scale for Psychopathology in Alzheimer's Disease (CUSPAD). A semistructured interview assessment of behavior problems that occur during the progressive course of Alzheimer's disease, CUSPAD (Devanand et al., 1992) emphasizes delusions, misidentifications, and hallucinations, but also includes a brief assessment of other behavioral disturbances (e.g., agitation and depression). In an investigation of 91 AD outpatients, interrater reliability between a psychiatrist and trained lay interviewer was high (kappas ranging from .74 to 1.0) (Devanand et al., 1992).

The CUSPAD was designed as a screening instrument to be administrated by a trained lay interviewer. It appears to be particularly useful for assessing psychotic features in AD patients, and provides standard definitional criteria for the presence and nature of these symptoms. Because it does not provide a detailed assessment of agitation or depression, it may need to be administered in conjunction with other measures when these behaviors are of interest.

The Revised Memory and Behavior Problems Checklist (RMBPC). The RMBPC (Teri et al., 1992) is a 24-item informant report measure of observable behavior problems in dementia patients, based on an earlier checklist (Zarit, Reever, & Bach-Peterson, 1980). It is different from the preceding three measures in that it is not interviewer administered. Rather, it is a self-administered questionnaire, on which the informant rates (a) the frequency of each behavior problem during the past week (1=not in the past week to 4=daily or more often) and (b) his or her reaction to each behavior (i.e., how bothered or upset the caregiver feels when the behavior occurs with 0=not at all to 4=extremely). In a sample of 201 geriatric outpatients and their caregivers, the RMBPC was found to be internally consistent, with mean α coefficients of .75 for frequency ratings and .87 for reaction ratings. Factors analysis yielded three subscales: memory-related behavior problems, depressive behaviors, and disruptive behaviors. The subscales showed good construct validity when compared with measures assessing comparable problems, and caregiver reaction ratings were significantly correlated with both caregiver depression and burden.

The RMBPC provides a method of assessing overall level of behavior problems, as well as specific areas of problems (memory, depression, disruption), and caregiver reactivity associated with these behaviors. It is unique in providing this latter dimension. It is also easy to use and easy to score. Currently, it is being used in a series of longitudinal investigations and treatment outcome studies.

The Caregiver Obstreperous-Behavior Rating Assessment Scale (COBRA). Drachman, Swearer, O'Donnell, Mitchell, & Maloon's (1992) scale is also a caregiver self-report questionnaire. It consists of 30 items in which behaviors are classified into four categories: aggressive/assaultive, mechanical/motor, ideas/personality, and vegetative. The frequency of occurrence of each behavior is rated on a scale of 0 (has not occurred in the last 3 months) to 4 (occurred daily or more often), and the severity of each behavior is rated on a scale of 0 (no disruption) to 4 (significant danger). Summary scores for frequency and severity can be obtained for each category of behavior problems. In a subsample of 25 outpatients diagnosed with dementia, the COBRA was found to have variable test-retest reliability over a one-week period, with correlations of the 12 summary scores ranging from .44 to .95. Interrater reliability on seven nursing home residents rated by two raters (nurses' aides) was also variable, with correlations on summary scores ranging from .30 to .99.

The COBRA provides instructions and a videotape of the behaviors to be rated.

It provides an assessment of both frequency and severity of a broad range of dementia-related behavior problems. Although the sample size of the study cited above is small and additional psychometric data are needed, further research using the COBRA will help clarify its utility.

*The Nursing Home Behavior Problem Scale (NHBPS).*The NHBPS (Ray, Taylor, Lichtenstein, & Meador, 1992) assesses the frequency of serious behavior problems in nursing home patients. It was designed for use in investigations of the efficacy of nonpharmacologic behavior management strategies and antipsychotic drug use in decreasing these behavior problems. The NHBPS consists of 29 items that most often precipitated antipsychotic medication or physical restraint of nursing home residents. The scale is completed by nurses, nursing assistants, or other care providers who know the resident. The rater reports the frequency of each behavior in the past 3 days on a 5-point scale (0=never to 4=always). Interrater reliability correlations range from .75 to .83 in samples (total *N*=553) from six sites in two different states, although it was noted that there did appear to be systematic differences among some raters (Ray et al., 1992). Cluster analysis revealed six subscales: Uncooperative or Aggressive behavior, Irrational or Restless Behavior, Sleep Problems, Annoying Behavior, Inappropriate Behavior, and Dangerous Behavior. The NHBPS correlated highly with other scales measuring similar behaviors and with increased physical and chemical restraint use (Ray et al., 1992).

Additional research with the NHBPS is needed to clarify causes of differences among raters and to study its sensitivity to changes in behavioral disturbance. It is currently being investigated as an outcome measure to assess the effect of interventions designed to decrease the frequency of behavior problems (Ray, et al., 1992).

The Multidimensional Observation Scale for Elderly Subjects (MOSES). MOSES (Helmes, Csapo, & Short, 1987) is a 40-item scale that assesses five areas of functioning: self-care, disoriented behavior, depressed or anxious mood, irritable behavior, and withdrawn behavior. Items are rated on a 4- or 5-point scale, (1 = unimpaired to 4 or 5 = severely impaired). It was standardized on over 2,300 elderly residents of hospitals and residential settings in Canada. Ratings, based on observations during the preceding week, are completed by a member of the nursing staff who is familiar with the subject. Interrater reliabilities for subscales ranged from .58 for depression to .97 for self-care, averaging .77 for the instrument as a whole. Internal consistency was excellent, with an average coefficient α of .81. The MOSES was found to correlate significantly with other rating scales that measures similar constructs, not to correlate with scales that measures different constructs, and to discriminate among patients in different settings who require different levels of care. It has been shown to be sensitive to change over time (Dillene & Longley, 1982), and has been recommended for use in assessment, treatment, and program evaluation research in a range of settings including nursing homes, continuing care facilities, and psychiatric facilities. Given its relatively low interrater reliability for depression, the MOSES may be inadequate for assessing mood, but useful in other areas.

Agitation

Agitation is a general term that typically describes a group of behaviors that occur in connection with a cognitive or psychiatric disturbance. It has been perhaps most broadly and objectively defined as follows: "Agitation is . . . inappropriate verbal, vocal, or motor activity that is not explained by needs or confusion per se. It includes behaviors such as aimless wandering, pacing, cursing, screaming, biting, and fighting" (Cohen-Mansfield & Billig, 1986, p. 712). For this chapter, two measures of agitation will be described in detail—one that focuses on agitation in nursing home residents (a typically more severely impaired group), and one that is designed for outpatients. It should be noted that most of the measures described in the preceding section also include an item or group of items that assess agitation.

The Cohen-Mansfield Agitation Inventory. The CMAI (Cohen-Mansfield, Marx, & Rosenthal, 1989) was developed to measure agitation in nursing home residents. It consists of 29 observable agitated behaviors, rated by a nurse on a 7-point Likert-type scale according to frequency of occurrence during the prior 2 weeks (0 = never occurred to 7 = occurred several times an hour). Interrater agreement was high, with agreement among three sets of raters (nurses on different shifts rating the same resident) ranging from .88 to .92. Factor analysis of the CMAI administered to 308 nursing home residents yielded four factors: Aggressive Behavior, Physically Nonaggressive Behavior, Verbally Agitated Behavior, and Hiding and Hoarding. Specific examples of aggressive behavior include hitting, kicking, pushing, and cursing or verbal aggression. Examples of physically nonaggressive behavior include pacing, inappropriate robing or disrobing, repetitious questions or mannerisms, and general restlessness. Verbally agitated behaviors include complaining, inappropriate requests for attention, and screaming. The CMAI is a promising instrument for rating agitation in demented patients, especially in institutional settings, and a version of it is currently being piloted in an outpatient sample as part of the Alzheimer's Disease Cooperative Study (Thal et al., 1993).

The Ryden Aggression Scale (RAS)

Ryden (1988) designed the RAS to assess aggression in dementia patients who live in the community with family caregivers. It is a 25-item Likert-type scale that rates the frequency of occurrence of aggressive behaviors (0 = less than the once a year to 5 = one or more times daily). It is designed as a paper-and-pencil questionnaire to be completed by caregivers about their dementia patient and is based on behavior during the past year. It consists of three a priori derived subscales: Physically Aggressive Behavior (e.g., threatening gestures, pushing, and throwing an object), Verbal Aggression (accusatory language, cursing, verbal threats, and name calling), and Sexual Aggression (unwanted hugging, kissing, touching body parts, intercourse, and obscene gestures). In 183 community residing subjects, the RAS yielded α of .88 for the overall scale, and .90–.74 for the subscales. Test-retest reliability after an interval of 8–12 weeks was .86.

Although it has not been widely used, the RAS shows promise for evaluation of aggression in community-residing dementia patients. It may be particularly useful in individuals for whom inappropriate sexual behavior is a problem, as it includes a number of item that measure sexual aggression.

Depression Measures

Twenty to thirty percent of patients with dementia are also depressed (Teri & Wagner, 1992) and 20% of patients with depression exhibit cognitive impairment severe enough to be diagnosed demented (LaRue, D'Elia, Clark, Spar, & Jarvik, 1986). The accurate assessment of depression in patients with dementia poses some unique problems. Traditional assessment of depression in the nondemented elderly relies on the patients' reports of mood and current behavior. Since patients with dementia cannot be relied upon to provide such information, measures of depression in demented patients rely more heavily on an informant, much the same as measures of other behavioral disturbances. Although traditional measures of depression (such as the Hamilton Depression Rating Scale) have been used successfully in assessing depression in demented patients, we will focus here on measures specifically designed for dementia. (For a more detailed discussion of the assessment of depression and dementia, the reader is referred to Teri and Wagner, 1992. (Also see chapter 9 on affect by Schulz, O'Brien, and Tompkins and chapter 11 on depression by Pachana, Gallagher-Tompson, and Thompson.)

The Cornell Scale for Depression in Dementia. The Cornell Scale (Alexopoulos, Abrams, Young, & Shamoian, 1988) is a 19-item clinician-rated scale of depressive symptoms designed for assessing dementia patients. It uses information from separate interviews with both the demented patient and a family member or nursing staff member who cares for the patient. The interviews require a total of about 30 minutes, after which the clinician completes the rating. More items are rated based on their presence during the past week. Each item is rated according to a 3-point scale: absent, mild or intermittent, and severe.

In demented subjects from psychiatric hospitals and nursing homes, the Cornell Scales was found to have good interrater reliability (weighted $K = .67$) and internal consistency ($\alpha = 0.84$). It significantly differentiated subjects meeting research diagnostic criteria (RDC) for no depression, minor, probable major, and definite major depression; it correlated well with RDC depression subtype ($r = .80$–0.89); and it performed equally well in rating depressive symptoms in dementia patients regardless of level of severity of cognitive impairment (Alexopoulos, et al., 1988).

In an investigation of 76 community-dwelling depressed Alzheimer's disease patients with family caregivers, the Cornell Scale was found to be internally consistent ($\alpha = .68$) and to correlate well with the Hamilton Depression Rating Scale ($r = .62$) Logsdon & Teri, 1993).

The Cornell Scale may not, however, be appropriate for use with medically ill populations (Agrell & Dehlin, 1989). The instructions for the scale indicate that no score should be given if symptoms result from physical disability or illness; thus, it may be difficult to interpret the presence or absence of symptoms in patients with medical problems that overlap the depression symptoms.

The National Institute for Mental Health (NIMH) Dementia Mood Assessment Scale

DMAS (Sunderland, et al., 1988; Sunderland, Hill, Lawlor, & Molchan, 1988) was also designed for assessing depression in dementia patients. It is completed based on clinical observation of the patient's behavior over the past week and a semi-structured interview with the patient. The total scale consists of 24 items: The first 17 items assess depressive symptoms and the last 7 assess overall dementia severity. Most items are scaled from 0 (within normal limits) to 6 (severe). The Mood Assessment Scale score is the sum of the first 17 items. In an investigation of 21 AD patients, the 17-item depression assessment has been demonstrated to have good interrater reliability, with intraclass correlation coefficients among raters of .69 to .74 (Sunderland et al., 1988). Scores on the DMAS were significantly correlated with global ratings of depression ($r = .73$), sadness ($r = 0.65$), and the Hamilton Depression Rating Scale ($r = .47$) (Sunderland, et al., 1988). Factor analysis of the 17-item scale on the DMAS in a sample of 54 AD patients yielded 4 factors: Depression, Social Interaction, Anxiety, and Vegetative Symptoms (Sunderland, et al., 1988).

The DMAS has not been widely used, and reported sample sizes are small, but it is a promising instrument for measuring the severity of depressive symptoms in dementia patients. Investigations of its usefulness have been conducted with with hospitalized mildly to moderately demented research patients at NIMH; further investigations with dementia patients residing in nursing homes and with patients still living in the community are needed to confirm its usefulness in these groups.

The Pleasant Events Schedule-AD (PES-AD)

This scale (Teri & Logsdon, 1991) differs from the other measures presented in this chapter, in that it assesses positive events in the lives of patients with AD rather than rating behavior disturbance. It was developed as part of an ongoing depression treatment outcome study designed to identify activities that AD patients enjoy and in which they can participate. It is an easy-to-use, 54-item inventory of pleasant experiences that is completed by caregivers about their patient. Each item is rated 3 times: first, on its frequency during the last month; second, on its availability; and third, on its enjoyability. Caregivers are typically able to complete the inventory in less than 30 minutes, and it provides valuable information about potentially pleasant activities for use in treating depressed AD patients. In a recent investigation comparing depressed and nondepressed AD patients' scores, the measure was found to have good internal consistency (alphas of .88 for frequency, .90 for availability, and .94 for enjoyability) and to significantly differentiate depressed and nondepressed patients. As with the other caregiver report measures, the PES-AD requires an informant who is familiar with the patient and who has some knowledge of what the patient enjoys now and what activities the patient enjoyed in the past. Many caregivers report that simply completing the inventory gives them ideas for activities they had forgotten about or never tried.

DISCUSSION

There has been a great deal of interest and activity in the last 5 years regarding the assessment and treatment of behavioral disturbance in older adults, particularly in older adults with dementia. Many new instruments have been proposed, and a few older standard instruments are still used. Studies to establish the validity, reliability, factor structure, and clinical and empirical utility of these instruments are largely in their infancy. Many questions as to the most effective and efficient way of assessing the myriad behavior problems that occur in dementia patients remain to be answered. There is, however, no question that the assessment of behavior disturbance is important conceptually and pragmatically. Our understanding of the relationship between behavior, cognition, function, and affect cannot advance unless we have adequate methods of assessment. Our understanding and identification of patients and careproviders who need intervention relies on accurate assessments, as does the determination of treatment efficacy.

This chapter has provided an overview of measures of behavioral disturbance in older adults. Different measures have different strenghts and weaknesses, but they all share several common characteristics: relatively clear instructions for administration and scoring, the ability (or potential ability) to be administered or completed by nonprofessional research assistants or care providers, proven usefulness with the older adult population, and at least some psychometric data supporting their use. There are many more potentially excellent instruments available that were not included in our discussion because they require administration by a skilled clinician (e.g., the Neurobehavioral Rating Scale, Leving et al., 1987) or because they include a significant component of cognitive assessment as well as behavioral disturbance (e.g., the Alzeimer's Disease Assessment Scale, ADAS, Mohs, Rosen, & Davis, 1983). Clearly all are needed, and the determination as to which measure is the best depends on the needs of the individual considering its use. Our knowledge of behavioral disturbance in older adults can only be aided by the continued refinement of the measures discussed here as well as the development of new ones.

The clinician or researcher seeking an appropriate measure has a broad array to choose from, each measure offering different advantages and disadvantages. On the other hand, there is no one measure that will serve all needs. Rather, the decision to select a measure of behavioral disturbance in older adults (comparable to the decision to select other measures) must be tempered by the needs of the particular project, patient group, clinician, or researcher.

ACKNOWLEDGMENT

Preparation of this article was supported in part by National Institute of Aging Grants AG 10845 and AG05136.

We which to extend our appreciation to Lauren Maxim, who assisted with the literature search.

REFERENCES

Agrell, B., & Dehlin, O. (1989). Comparison of six depression rating scales in geriatric stroke patients. *Stroke, 20,* 1190–1194.

Alexopoulos, G. S., Abrams, R. C., Young, R. C., & Shamoian, C. A. (1988). Cornell scale for depression in dementia. *Biological Psychiatry, 23,* 271–284.

Baumgarten, M., Becker, R., & Gauthier, S. (1990). Validity and reliability of the Dementia Behavior Disturbance Scale. *Journal of the American Geriatrics Society, 38,* 221–226.

Cohen-Mansfield, J., & Billig, N. (1986). Agitated behavior in the elderly. 1. A conceptual review. *Journal of the American Geriatrics Society, 34,* 711–721.

Cohen-Mensfield, J., Marx, M. S., & Rosenthal, A. S. (1989). A description of agitation in a nursing home. *Journal of Gerontology, 44,* 77–84.

Copeland, JU, R., Kelleher, M. J., Kellett, J. M., Hourlay, A. J., Gurland, B. J., Fleiss, J. L., & Sharpe, L. (1976). A semi-structured clinical interview for the assessment of diagnosis and mental state in the elderly: The Geriatric Mental State Schedule: I. Development and reliability. *Psychological Medicine, 6,* 439–449.

Deimling, G. T., & Bass, D. M. (1986). Symptoms of mental impairment among elderly adults and their effects on family caregivers. *Journal of Gerontology, 41,* 778–784.

Dillane, W., & Longley, G. (1982). Use in a longitudinal study. In R. W. Hopkins (Ed.), *Proceedings of the Ninth Annual Meeting of the Ontario Psychogeriatric Association,* 279–285.

Devanand, D. P., Miller, L., Richards, M., Marder, K., Bell, K., Mayeux, R., & Stern, Y. (1992). The Columbia University Scale for Psychopathology in Alzheimer's Disease. *Archives of Neurology, 49,* 371–376.

Drachman, D. A., Swearer, J. M., O'Donnell, B. F., Mitchell, A. L., & Maloon, A. (1992). The Caretaker Obstreperous-Behavior Rating Assessment (COBRA) Scale. *Journal of the American Geriatrics Society, 40,* 463–480.

Drinka, J. K., Smith, J. C., & Drinka, P. J. (1987). Correlates of depression and burden for informal caregivers of patients in a geriatrics referral clinic. *Journal of the American Geriatrics Society, 35,* 522–525.

Finkel, S. I., Lyons, J. S., & Anderson, R. L. (1993). A brief agitation ration scale (BARS) for nursing home elderly. *Journal of the American Geriatrics Society, 41*, 50–52.

Gurel, L, L., Linn, M. W., & Linn, B. S. (1972). Physical and Mental Impairment-of-Function Evaluation in the aged: The PAMIE scale. *Journal of Gerontology, 27*, 83–90.

Gurland, B. J., Fleiss, J. L., Goldberg, K., Sharpe, L., Copeland, J. R., Kelleher, M. J., & Kellett, J. M. (1976). A semi-structured clinical interview for the assessment of diagnosis and mental state in the elderly: The Geriatric Mental State Schedule II. A factor analysis. *Psychological Medicine, 6*, 451–459.

Helmes, E., Csapo, K. G., & Short, J. A. (1987). Standardization and validation of the Multidimensional Observation Scale for Elderly Subjects (MOSES). *Journal of Gerontology, 42*, 395–405.

Kluger, A., & Ferris, S. H. (1991). Scales for the assessment of Alzheimer's disease. *Psychiatric Clinics of North America, 14*, 309–326.

LaRue, A., D'Elia, L. F., Clark, E. O., Spar, J. E., & Jarvik, L. F. (1986). Clinical tests of memory in dementia, depression and healthy aging.. *Psychology and Aging, 1*, 69–77.

Levin, H. S., High, W. M., Goethe, K. E., Sisson, R. A., Overall, J. E., Rhoades, H. M., Eisenberg, H. M., Kalisky, Z., & Gary, H. E. (1987). The Neurobehavioral Rating Scale: Assessment of the behavioral sequelae of head injury by the clinician. *Journal of Neurology, Neurosurgery, & Psychiatry, 50*, 183–193.

Logsdon, R. G., & Teri, L. (1993). Depression in Alzheimer's disease: A comparison of measures. *The Gerontologist, 33*, 312.

Mohs, R. C., Rosen, W. G., & Davis, K. L. (1983). The Alzheimer's Disease Assessment Scale: An instrument for assessment treatment efficacy. *Psychopharmacology Bulletin, 19*, 448–450.

Mungas, D., Weiler, P., Franzi, C., & Henry, R. (1989). Assessment of disruptive behavior associated with dementia: The Disruptive Behavior Rating Scales. *Journal of Geriatric Psychiatry and Neurology, 2*, 196–202.

Niederehe, G. (1988). TRIMS Behavioral Problem Checklist (BPC). *Psychopharmacology Bulletin, 24*, 771–773.

Overall, J. E., Beller, S. A. (1984). The Brief Psychiatric Rating Scale (BPRS) in geropsychiatric research: I. Factor structure on an inpatient unit. *Journal of Gerontology, 39*, 187–193.

Overall, J. E., & Gorham, D. R. (1962). The Brief Psychiatric Rating Scale. *Psychological Reports, 10*, 799–812.

Overall, J. E., & Rhoades, H. M. (1988). Clinician-rated scales for multidimensional assessment of psychopathology in the elderly. *Psychopharmacology Bulletin, 24*, 587–594.

Patterson, M. B., Schnell, A. H., Martin, R. J., Mendez, M. F., Smyth, K. A., & Whitehouse, P. J. (1990). Assessment of behavioral and affective symptoms in Alzheimer's disease. *Journal of Geriatric Psychiatry and Neurology, 3*, 21–30.

Rabins, P. V., Mace, N. L., & Lucas, M. J. (1982). The impact of dementia on the family. *Journal of the American Medical Association, 248*, 333–335.

Raskin, A. (1985). Validation of a battery of tests designed to assess psychopathology in the elderly. In G. D. Burrows, T. R. Norman, & L. Dennerstein (Eds.), *Clinical and pharmacological studies in psychiatric disorders* (pp. 337–343). London: John Libbey.

Raskin, A., & Crook, T. (1988). Relatives' assessment of global symptomatology (RAGS). *Psychopharmacology Bulletin, 24*, 759–763.

Ravensborg, M. R., Willenson, D. (1969). Use of the NOSIE-30 Behavioral rating scale in hospitals for the mentally ill and retarded. *Journal of Clinical Psychology, 25,* 453–454.

Ray, W. A., Taylor, J. A., Lichtenstein, M. J., & Meador, K. G. (1992). The Nursing Home Behavior Problem Scale. *Journals of Gerontology: Medical Sciences, 47,* M9-M16.

Reichenfeld, H. F., Bazile, E., Khan, B. B., & Raman, S. (1992). Clinical assessment of psychopathology among elderly residents (CAPER): Development and pilot testing of a screening instrument to detect the presence of psychiatric disorders among residents of long-term institutions. *International Journal of Geriatric Psychiatry, 7,* 399–406.

Reisberg, B., Borenstein, J., Salob, S. P., Ferris, S. H., Franssen, E., & Georgotas, A. (1987). Behavioral symptoms in Alzheimer's disease: Phenomenology and treatment. *Journal of Clinical Psychiatry, 48,*(Suppl.), 9–15.

Reisberg, B., Ferris, S. H., Torossian, C., Kluger, A., & Monteiro, I. (1992). Pharmacologic treatment of Alzheimer's disease: A methodologic critique based upon current knowledge of symptomatology and relevance for drug trials. *International Psychogeriatrics, 4*(Suppl.), 9–42.

Reisberg, B., Franssen, E. Sclan, S. G., Kluger, A. & Ferris, S. H. (1989). Stage specific incidence of potentially remediable behavioral symptoms in aging and Alzheimer's disease: A study of 120 patients using the BEHAVE-AD. *Bulletin of Clinical Neuroscience, 54,* 95–112.

Rosen, W. G., Mohs, R. C., Davis, K. L. (1984). A new rating scale for Alzheimier's disease. *American Journal of Psychiatry, 14,* 1356–1364.

Roth, M. (1979). The psychiatric disorders of later life. *Psychiatric Annals, 6,* 57–101.

Rovner, B. W., Kafonek, S., Filipp, L., Lucas, M. J., & Folstein, M. F. (1986). Prevalence of mental illness in a community nursing home. *American Journal of Psychiatry, 143,* 1446–1449.

Ryden, M. (1988). Aggressive behavior in persons with dementia who live in the community. *Alzheimier's Disease and Associated Disorders, 2,* 342–355.

Schwartz, G. E. (1983). Development and validation of the Geriatric Evaluation by Relative's Rating Instrument (GERRI). *Psychological Reports,* 479–488.

Seltzer, D. L., Levin, H. S., Mahler, M. E., High, W. M., Cummings, J. L. (1992). Assessment of cognitive, psychiatric, and behavioral disturbance in patients with dementia: The Neurobehavioral Rating Scale. *Journal of the American Geriatrics Society, 40,* 549–555.

Shader, R. I., Harmatz, J. S., & Salzman, C. (1974). A new scale for assessment in geriatric populations: Sandoz Clinical Assessment-Geriatric (SCAG). *Journal of the American Geriatrics Society, 22,* 107–113.

Sinha, D., Zemlan, F. P., Nelson, S., Bienenfeld, D., Thienhaus, O., Ramaswamy, G., & Hamilton, S. (1992). A new scale for assessing behavioral agitation in dementia. *Psychiatry Research, 41,* 73–88.

Sunderland, T., Alterman, I. S., Yount, D., Hill, J. L., Tariot, P. N., Newhouse, P. A., Mueller, E. A., Mellow, A. M., & Cohen, R. M. (1988). A new scale for the assessment of depressed mood in demented patients. *American Journal of Psychiatry, 145,* 955–959.

Sunderland, T., Hill, J. L., Lawlor, B. A., & Molchan, S. E. (1988). NIMH Dementia Mood Assessment Scale (DMAS). *Psychopharmacology Bulletin, 24,* 747–751.

Sunderland, T., & Silver, M. A. (1988). Neuroleptics in the treatment of dementia. *International Journal of Geriatric Psychiatry, 3,* 79–88.

Swearer, J. M., Drachman, D. A., O'Donnell, B. F., & Mitchell, A. L. (1988). Troublesome and disruptive behaviors in dementia: Relationships to diagnosis and disease severity. *Journal of the American Geriatrics Society, 36,* 784–790.

Tariot, P. Blazina, L., Mack, J., & Patterson, M. (1991). CERAD Behavior Rating Scale for Dementia administration manual. Unpublished manual available from the Consortium to Establish a Registry for Alaheimer's (CERAD), St. Louis, Mo. (716)274–7508.

Tariot, P., Mack, J., Patterson, M., Edland, S. D., Weiner, M. F., Fillenbaum, G., Blazina, L., Teri, L., Rubin, E., Mortimer, J. A., & Stern, Y. (under review). CERAD Behavior Rating Scale for Dementia (BRSD).

Teeter, R. B., Garetz, F. K., Miller, W. R., & Heiland, W. F. (1976). Psychiatric disturbances of aged patients in skilled nursing homes. *American Journal of Psychiatry, 133,* 1430–1434.

Teri, L., Borson, S., Kiyak, A., & Yamagishi, M. (1989). Behavioral disturbance, cognitive dysfunction, and functional skill. *Journal of the American Geriatrics Society, 37,* 109–116.

Teri, L., Larson, E., & Raifler, B. V. (1988). Behavioral disturbance in dementia of the Alzheimier's type. *Journal of the American Geriatrics Society, 36,* 1–6.

Teri, L., & Logsdon, R. G. (1991). Identifying pleasant activities for Alzheimer's disease patients: The Pleasant Events Schedule-AD. *The Gerontologist, 31,* 124–127.

Teri, L., Rabins, P., Whitehouse, P., Berg, L., Reisberg, B., Sunderland, T., Eichelmen, B., & Phelps, C. Management of behavior disturbance in Alzheimer's disease: Current knowledge and future directions. *Alzheimer's Disease and Associated Disorders, 6,* 77–88.

Teri, L., Truax, P., Logsdon, R., Uomoto, J., Zarit, S., & Vitaliano, P. P. (1992). Assessment of behavioral problems in dementia: The Revised Memory and Behavior Problems Checklist. *Psychology and Aging, 7,* 622–631.

Teri, L., & Wagner, A., (1992). Alzheimer's disease and depression. *Journal of Consulting and Clinical Psychology, 3,* 379–391.

Thal, L., Ferris, S. H., Schneider, L., Mohs, R., Whitehouse, P., Weiner, M. F., Galasko, D., Schmitt, F., & Sano, M. (1993). *Alzheimer's disease cooperative study, instrument protocol training manual.* Unpublished manuscript, University of California, San Diego.

Zarit, S. H., Orr, N. K., & Zarit, J. M. (1985). *The hidden victims of Alzheimer's disease: Families under stress.* New York: New York University Press.

Zarit, S. H., Reever, K. E., & Bach-Peterson, J. (1980). Relatives of the impaired elderly: Correlates of the feeling of burden. *The Gerontologist, 20,* 649–655.

CHAPTER 7

Leisure and Productive Activity

ROGER C. MANNELL
DEPARTMENT OF RECREATIONAL AND LEISURE STUDIES
UNIVERSITY OF WATERLOO, ONTARIO

AND

SHERRY L. DUPUIS
DEPARTMENT OF FAMILY STUDIES
UNIVERSITY OF GUELPH, ONTARIO

INTRODUCTION

In spite of substantial research support for the hypothesis that the more active older adults are in their leisure, the greater their subjective well-being, reviews of leisure research in aging have suggested that such research has developed slowly (Kelly & Ross, 1989; Lawton, 1985). Bull (1982) concluded that there were considerable descriptive data available about the leisure activities of older persons, but that much work was needed on the development of leisure constructs and their measurement. While some progress in the application of new methods, constructs, and measures has occurred since Bull's review, the leisure and aging research is still dominated by an activity-oriented or behavioral approach to conceptualizing and measuring leisure.

In contrast, with the dominance of the social psychological approach in the general field of leisure studies during the past decade (Mannell, 1984a; Iso-Ahola & Mannell, 1985; Iso-Ahola, 1991), a much more diverse set of leisure constructs, measures, and research methods have been developed and used by researchers. Consistent with the social psychological approach, the unit of analysis has been the individual and leisure has been viewed as an important aspect of individual behavior and experience. Researchers have taken the position that the role of leisure in people's lives can only be understood if the quality as well as the quantity of their leisure is examined. The social psychological approach has also been fostered by the belief that leisure is an individual problem. Many researchers studying leisure have had a strong applied focus with a commitment to providing knowledge to those who typically work with individuals who are unable to participate or find satisfaction in their leisure.

The social psychological framework that has guided a great deal of the leisure research is *interactionism.* While there are a number of versions of interactionism, generally, the individual's leisure behavior and experience are seen to be a function of the interplay between internal psychological dispositions (attitudes, needs, perceptions, and personality traits) and situational influences in the social and physical environment (Iso-Ahola & Mannell, 1985). Consequently, while researchers continue to use inventories and time-budget diaries to measure observable leisure behavior, measures of leisure experiences, satisfactions, attitudes, leisure-specific personality traits, and perceived constraints have been developed. However, these constructs have received only limited attention in both the gerontological and leisure research concerned with older adults.

In this chapter, we will provide a brief overview of the leisure constructs and measures that have been used to study leisure and aging issues, as well as those constructs found in the general leisure studies literature that could be usefully applied. For the sake of brevity, only the most recent and representative references to this literature will be cited.

LEISURE BEHAVIOR AND TIME

While specific leisure activities, such as the use of shopping centers by older adults for sociability reasons (Graham, Graham, & MacLean, 1991) and contract bridge (Scott & Godbey, 1992) have been examined, researchers have typically been interested in overall patterns of leisure activity engagement and time usage—what we might call *leisure lifestyle.* Operationalizing leisure as behavior and time has been characterized as the *objective* approach (Neulinger, 1974) and allows the assessment of what Lawton (1993) has called the *denotative meaning* of leisure. This approach involves measuring the specific or general types of activities in which individuals participate, the frequency of participation in these activities, and the amount of time involved.

Similar to studies of the general population, two data collection strategies predominate in the research on the leisure behavior of older adults. *Leisure behavior inventories,* the most frequently used approach, are lists of leisure activities in which respondents are asked to check whether or not they have participated during a specified time period, or to identify frequency of participation on Likert scales. Researchers typically custom design inventories to suit their research purposes. Consequently, no widely used, standardized scales for use with older adults have been developed thus far, making comparisons between studies difficult (Bull, 1982).

One of the most comprehensive leisure behavior inventories available is the Leisure Activities Blank (LAB; McKechnie, 1974, 1975) developed for use with the general population. The LAB includes 120 leisure activities; however, many of the activities are not applicable to older adults and the instrument can be difficult to administer and to tabulate. Thus, few researchers or practitioners use the scale with older adults today, and those who do use the scale tend to modify it for their own purposes (e.g., Lounsbury & Hoopes, 1988; Ragheb & Griffith, 1982).

Recently, Stones and Kozma (1986) have attempted to bring some standardization to inventory instrumentation for use with older adults with the development of the Memorial University of Newfoundland Activity Inventory. Utilizing interviews with older adults, Stones and Kozma (1986) created a composite index comprising five general activity dimensions: household independence, family involvement, solitary activity, community involvement, and homemaker activity. They also provided some evidence for the construct validity of the measure. With the purpose of developing an index that could be used with both younger and older adults, Arbuckle, Sissons, and Harsany (1986) generated an instrument consisting of three activity dimensions: intellectual activity, physical activity, and social activity. However, a review of the literature suggests that these scales are rarely used.

The *time-budget diary* is another method used to measure leisure behavior and lifestyle; however, it is not widely used with older- adult samples. This approach allows the researcher to estimate the amount of time spent in various daily activities by having respondents carry a diary in which they record their activities and time of participation (Zuzanek & Box, 1988). Other researchers (e.g., Moss & Lawton, 1982) have collected data resembling the time-budget diary by asking respondents to recount each sequential activity in which they were engaged during the previous day.

The measures obtained with both inventories and diaries have been described as crude indicators of leisure behavior and lifestyle for a variety of reasons. There is no standard list of activities that researchers agree constitutes leisure, and inventories differ substantially on the specificity of the activities they include. Some researchers use a large number of very specific activities (e.g., Ouellette, 1986), whereas in other studies of older adults, researchers have used only very broad activity categories such as social activities (Heinemann, Colorez, Frank, & Taylor, 1988). Also, when analyzing data gathered with leisure behavior inventories and time-budget diaries, it is standard practice to group specific leisure activities into a smaller, more manageable number of broad activity classifications. There has been a lack of consistency, however, in how researchers have done this grouping. With respect to time-budget data, Zuzanek (1991) points out that the major rationale for classification has been tradition and convenience. As well as tradition and convenience, Lawton (1993) found that factor analysis of participation data collected with inventories was the most common strategy. He concluded that there was "little empirical evidence for a common set of activity categories" (p. 27).

Researchers have also tended to ignore the subjective meanings that older adults associate with the activities in which they engage, and have generally assumed that specific activities have a common meaning for all older adults. However, the sets of activities that constitute leisure for various groups of people are likely to show cultural and subcultural differences, and perhaps age differences. For some individuals, the same activity has been found to be leisure when asked at one occurrence, and something else at a second occurrence, depending on the context and underlying meaning of the activity (Shaw, 1984).

In spite of the problems identified, carefully designed inventories and time-budget methods continue to be useful research strategies and provide a quantified picture of how older adults structure their lives with activity. Time-budget diaries are less susceptible to the recall inaccuracies that can accompany inventories (Chase & Godbey, 1983). In fact, there is evidence to suggest that this reduced demand on memory recall may be particularly important for collecting accurate data when studying older adult populations (Romsa & Blenman, 1989). However, researchers investigating the comparability of data gathered with the time-budget diary relative to the behavioral inventory suggest that infrequent activities may be more accurately measured by survey methods than by time-budget diary approaches (Cosper & Shaw, 1985). When measuring daily or frequently occurring activities and socially desirable activities (e.g., exercising), the time-budget diary appears to be the superior approach (Zuzanek, 1991).

LEISURE STATES AND EXPERIENCE

In response to the limitations of treating leisure only as behavior, researchers have focused on measuring leisure from the subjective perspective of the participant (Mannell & Iso-Ahola, 1987). This perspective has led to the use of a variety of new methods and measurement instruments. Most leisure for most people is sandwiched between the many and varied obligatory activities of daily life, and, in fact, leisure may be experienced a great deal of the time in nonrecreational activities and settings. Consequently, researchers have been attempting to identify the criteria that people use in deciding if they are experiencing leisure rather than imposing academic definitions.

Iso-Ahola (1980) had his university student respondents imagine themselves in situations he presented to them that were varied according to factors predicted to influence the likelihood of an engagement being defined as leisure by the participant. He then had them judge whether the situation would be leisure for them. Gunter (1979) asked various groups of university students to describe in writing their most memorable and enjoyable leisure experiences. He then analyzed these stories to discover if the leisure experiences that stood out in their minds shared similar characteristics. Henderson and Rannells (1988), through extensive interviews with middle-aged to older adult farm women, examined what was leisure for them and the role it played in their lives. Similarly, Allen and Chin-Sang (1990) employed in-depth qualitative interviews to examine the context and meanings of leisure for older adult African American women.

Researchers have also used methods that involve monitoring people's daily behavior. Shaw (1984) used a modified time-budget diary approach to examine the factors that determine whether individuals define a given situation or activity as leisure or nonleisure during the course of their daily lives. After the completion of the time-budget diaries, during a follow-up interview, her research participants were asked to classify all the activities they had listed in their diaries as "work," "leisure", "a mixture of work and leisure," or "neither work nor leisure". Shaw found that some activities, such as cooking, home chores, and child care were more frequently defined as leisure by males than by females.

Knowing how the people being studied personally define leisure, rather than relying on researcher imposed judgments, provides a more sensitive approach to measuring the quantity and quality of leisure experienced and may better allow researchers to establish the relationship between leisure and other aspects of life, such as mental health, the quality of life, work, successful retirement, and so on. Shaw (1985) found significant differences in the amount of leisure reported by her respondents when their psychological definitions of leisure were used compared to an objective activity definition.

Researchers have also gone to the recreation setting itself to study the quality, duration, intensity, and memorability of leisure experiences (Mannell, 1980). Following extensive interviews with people in a variety of leisure pursuits, Csikszentmihalyi (1975) developed his flow model, which has provided insight into how the activities of everyday life come to be invested with meaning and experienced as optimal. He identified the characteristics of those experiences which his working-aged, adult subjects reported to be leisure at its best. Episodes that provided intensely absorbing experiences, challenges that matched participants' skills, and in which the participants lost track of the time and their awareness of themselves, were best remembered and most rewarding.

Out of this research Larson and Csikszentmihalyi (1983) have developed the *experiential sampling method* (ESM). Typically, respondents carry electronic pagers with them and are randomly signalled throughout the day for a period of one week. Each time the pager emits a signal (an audible beep), the respondents take out a booklet of brief questionnaires, called experiential sampling forms (ESF), and complete a series of open- and closed-ended items indicating their current activity, the social and physical context of their activity, and psychological state.

While the ESF has been varied slightly across studies, the types of variables and scales included have been fairly standard. The ESF includes items that require respondents to write in the time of the pager signal and the time that they actually filled out the ESF (usually the questionnaire data are dropped if too much time elapses between signal and response); record what they were thinking about at the time of the signal; record the main thing/activity they were doing; check on a list who they were with; rate on Likert scales several items that measure the level of psychological involvement in the activity (e.g., level of concentration, personal skills and challenge, perception of the passage of time); rate mood states on semantic differential scales assessing affect and arousal; and check reasons or motivations for participation. Some researchers have included additional scales or items on the ESF, for example, self-esteem (Wells, 1988), leisureliness (Samdahl, 1988), and willingness to engage in alternative activities (Mannell & Zuzanek, 1991). The reliability of the multiple-item mood scales have been shown to be consistently high in most studies reported. In analyses of the psychometric properties of the ESF measures over a week of repeated use, the subjects' responses have been shown to change only slightly from the first to the second half of the study week. Differences between individuals were also found to be stable (Csikszentmihalyi & Larson, 1984; Wells, 1988).

The ESM has been used to address a number of leisure-related research questions (see Mannell & Zuzanek, 1991). However, only a few studies have examined the leisure experience of older adults. Studies using older-adult samples have examined the experience of loneliness among older adults (Larson, Zuzanek, & Mannell, 1985), leisure as a context for social relationships (Larson, Mannell, & Zuzanek, 1986), and the influence of freedom of choice and commitment on optimal experiences during leisure (Mannell, Zuzanek, & Larson, 1988). The frequency of optimal leisure experiences as measured with the ESM has been found to be positively related to life satisfaction (Mannell, 1992). Researchers have also used ESM in long term care facilities and the findings from these studies suggest that, with some modification, the method can be implemented to assess the daily experiences of older adults living in these settings (Voelkl & Birkel, 1988; Voelkl & Brown, 1989; Voelkl, 1990; Voelkl & Nicholson, 1992). The ESM appears to be a reliable and valid method of obtaining information from a variety of groups, including older adults (Hnatiuk, 1991). Samdahl and Jekubovich (1993), in a study of adults between the ages of 30 and 65, have recently suggested that using qualitative interviews to complement the ESM data collection strategy can elicit a deeper and more comprehensive understanding of the leisure experience.

LEISURE SATISFACTION

The construct of leisure satisfaction has been popular in leisure research and various terms—motivations, preferences, psychological outcomes, experience expectations, and benefits—have been used. Leisure satisfaction has been studied to provide explanations for why people engage in leisure activities and lead the leisure life styles they do. Leisure satisfaction has also been used as a summary measure of the quality of leisure life styles and as an alternative measure to frequency of leisure participation in research attempts to identify the relationships among leisure, work, family, and general quality of life. Service providers have been interested in the satisfactions people seek in their leisure so that they can provide the same activities and opportunities. Measures of leisure satisfaction vary substantially in terms of (a) the extent to which they are conceptualized as being based on acquired expectations or an explicit theory of human needs, (b) the level of specificity of the domain of leisure behavior with which they are associated, and (c) the use of single-item or standardized multi-item scales (see Mannell, 1989).

The expectancy approach to conceptualizing and measuring satisfaction has emerged from the extensive research that has been done over the past several decades on the subjective well-being of working-aged and older adults. From this perspective, satisfaction "implies an act of judgment, a comparison of what people have to what they think they deserve, expect, or may reasonably aspire to" (Campbell, 1980, p. 22). With respect to leisure, researchers have been concerned with satisfaction with the whole leisure domain. Single-item measures are frequently used and the domain of behavior has been identified in different ways. Subjects have been asked to rate satisfaction with their "present level of leisure participation" (Guin, 1980, p. 200), "amount of spare time" (Lounsbury, Gordon, Bergermaier, & Francesco,1982, p. 290), and "leisure in general" (Iso-Ahola & Weissinger, 1987, p. 360). Total leisure satisfaction has also been assessed by having subjects appraise various facets of their leisure and summing across these ratings. For example, Francken and van Raaij (1981) had older adult respondents rate their satisfaction with major categories of leisure activities and summed these. Backman and Mannell (1986) had the older adults in their study recall the leisure activities engaged in during the preceding week and rate their satisfaction with each recalled activity. Some researchers have been interested in measuring leisure satisfaction with only specific activities or subdomains of leisure behavior, such as a fishing trip (Graefe & Fedler, 1986).

The needs-based approach to leisure satisfaction has led to the development of several standardized multi-item scales. Researchers have identified differences in the need-satisfying characteristics or satisfactions that different recreational activities or settings provide to participants. The best known and tested instruments developed for this purpose are the Recreation Experience Preference scales (REP) developed by Driver, Brown, Stonkeg, and Gregoire (1987) and the Paragraphs About Leisure (PAL) developed by Tinsley, Colbs, Teaff, and Kaufmann (1987) and Tinsley and Tinsley (1988). A review of these two instruments has recently been provided by Driver, Tinsley and Manfredo (1991).

The REP scales were developed primarily to aid managers of parks and other natural resources in identifying the kinds of satisfactions people visiting outdoor recreation sites were seeking. The current instrument uses 43 scales to measure the extent to which specific satisfactions are desired and expected from leisure activities. These 43 scales reflect 19 general recreational experience preference domains (e.g., enjoyment of nature, tension reduction, sharing of similar values, independence, creativity, nostalgia, and achievement).

Although the PAL has not been widely used by other researchers, the reliability of the scale is quite respectable (Tinsley & Tinsley, 1988). Each scale of the PAL consists of a single paragraph which describes the gratification of a particular psychological need. Respondents are instructed to indicate the extent to which each paragraph is an accurate statement about the leisure activity they are describing. The PAL thus quantifies the perceived degree to which a designated leisure activity provides opportunities to obtain certain satisfactions. Forty-four psychological needs that may be satisfied by participation in leisure activities have been identified, comprising eight general types of leisure satisfactions (i.e., self-expression, companionship, power, compensation, security, service, intellectual aestheticism, solitude). The PAL has also been modified (Paragraphs About Leisure: Form E) and tested for use with older adults (see Tinsley, Colbs, Teaff, & Kaufman, 1987).

The only other standardized multi-item instrument reported in the literature that has received some use is the Leisure Satisfaction Scale developed by Beard and Ragheb (1980). This instrument was designed to assess satisfaction with the whole of the individual's leisure activities. This satisfaction scale has 51 statements divided into six subdomains or types of leisure satisfactions (psychological, educational, social, relaxation, physiological and aesthetic). The authors also report a 24-item version. Reliability has been shown to be quite high (e.g., Russell, 1987). Riddick (1986) found no age differences in leisure satisfaction as measured by the scale among 18 to 65 year olds. Several researchers have utilized the Beard and Ragheb scale to measure the leisure satisfaction of community-based older adults (e.g., Ragheb & Griffith, 1982; Sneegas, 1986) and of older adults living in institutionalized settings (e.g., Savell, 1991). Brown, Frankel, and Fennell (1991) used the Leisure Satisfaction Scale to develop a new shortened and simplified leisure satisfaction scale for their study involving adults 18 years of age and older. Respondents were asked to indicate on a 5-point Likert scale how satisfied they were with each of the 12 items (e.g., the challenge provided by your activities, the relaxations provided by your activities, the opportunity to be creative). The α reliability coefficient of this new scale was completely satisfactory.

Finally, a last scale to be mentioned is the Leisure Meaning Scale (Kelly, Steinkamp & Kelly, 1986). While it has not been used by other researchers and has undergone little psychometric testing, the scale was developed for use with adults 40 years of age and older. In relation to their two most important activities, respondents are asked to indicate on a scale of 1 to 5 the extent to which they agree that these activities are participated in for each of 21 reasons provided. These 21 items reflect seven types of leisure motivations (i.e., companionship in the activity, strengthening primary relationships, competence and skill-development, health and exercise, expression and personal development, meeting role expectations, and enjoyment).

LEISURE ATTITUDES

What people think of leisure in general can be regarded as a belief system or as a set of attitudes. Attitudes have been typically seen as having affective, cognitive, and behavioral components. When attitudes are studied, affect is typically measured. In applying Fishbein and Ajzen's (1975) conceptualization of attitude, Iso-Ahola (1980) has defined a leisure attitude "as the expressed amount of affect toward a given leisure-related object" (p. 251). A leisure attitude can be both general or specific depending on its object. The object of a leisure attitude can be the idea of leisure, everything done in free time, a specific recreational activity or program, or a place where leisure participation takes place.

Leisure attitude research has moved away from measuring general leisure attitudes or orientations. Given the weak relationships generally found between all types of attitudes and behavior, researchers have focused on developing models that predict much more specific types of behavior. Set in attitude change and persuasive communication frameworks, theories like the "theory of reasoned action" have been applied to understanding how to influence and manage people's behavior in a variety of recreational settings (see Manfredo, 1992). However, researchers still use measures of general leisure attitudes to assess people's orientation to leisure. For example, Iso-Ahola and Buttimer (1981) were interested in the effects of socialization on leisure and measured changes in the leisure attitudes of people ranging in age from adolescence to adulthood. With respect to older adults, Backman and Mannell (1986) measured changes in leisure attitudes due to a leisure counselling program.

Little recent research has been directed toward developing multi-item, standardized leisure attitudes scales and none have been specifically designed for older adults. While scales developed by Neulinger (1974) and Ragheb and Beard (1982) have not been used frequently, a scale created by Crandall and Slivken (1980) has been used most frequently when researchers want to assess people's overall attitudes toward leisure in general. For example, Iso-Ahola and Weissinger (1987) found that in a sample of working, unemployed, and retired people the more negative their leisure attitudes the more boredom they experienced in their free time. Weissinger, Caldwell, and Bandalos (1992) found leisure attitudes to be unrelated to overall leisure activity levels among a group of university students, while in a study of older adults, Searle and Iso-Ahola (1988) found that more positive leisure attitudes were associated with greater leisure participation. Riddick (1986), in a study of ten different age groups, found that leisure attitudes were "the second most influential determinant of leisure satisfaction" (p.263).

The Ragheb and Beard (1982) scale consists of 36 statements about leisure activities and free time divided into Cognitive, Affective, and Behavioral subscales. Crandall and Slivken's (1980) Leisure Ethic Scale is comprised of 10 statements that assess the importance of leisure, desire for leisure time, and enjoyment of leisure. Both scales have acceptable levels of reliability.

LEISURE-SPECIFIC PERSONALITY ORIENTATIONS

Following the social psychological tradition, researchers have explored the relationship between leisure and individual differences. Until the mid-1980s, individual differences, that is, the impact of personality on leisure behavior and experience, was all but ignored (Kleiber & Dirkin, 1985; Mannell, 1984b). Where personality research on leisure had been reported, it was highly simplistic, using an outmoded trait approach; only weak associations between personality traits and leisure behaviors were found (Iso-Ahola, 1976, 1980). However, in more recent research personality variables have been chosen because of their theoretical relevance to leisure behavior and they are being studied from the perspective of interactionism. For example, in an experiment, Mannell and Bradley (1986) found that under certain conditions their university student subjects' locus of control (Rotter, 1966) affected the amount of freedom of choice they perceived and consequently their psychological involvement and satisfaction in a leisure activity. Other theoretically relevant personality factors that have been investigated include extraversion, Type A-B personality, and shyness (see Iso-Ahola, 1991).

While general personality constructs may be used to aid in explaining leisure behavior, it has been argued that leisure researchers could profit from conceptualizing leisure-specific personality dimensions that are more germane to the use of free time and leisure (Mannell, 1984b). Leisure-specific personality scales that have been developed include a self-as-entertainment scale (Mannell, 1984b), an intrinsic leisure motivation scale (Weissinger & Iso-Ahola, 1984) and a leisure boredom measure (Iso-Ahola & Weissinger, 1987). Also a number of the subscales on the Leisure Diagnostic Battery (Ellis & Witt, 1986), which was designed to assess the leisure functioning of children and adults with disabilities, provide measures of individual differences.

These leisure-specific personality measures have been developed to help explain why and predict how people use and experience their free time and leisure differently even when their opportunities may be quite similar. Iso-Ahola and Weissinger's (1987, 1990) leisure boredom scale is a good example. The 16-item scale measures individual differences in perceptions of boredom in leisure and has been shown to have good reliability across several studies. In a study by Iso-Ahola and Crowley (1991), adolescents who experienced their leisure as boredom were more likely to be recreational drug users. The leisure-specific personality orientations of older adults have not been assessed and used in the study of leisure and aging issues.

BARRIERS AND CONSTRAINTS TO LEISURE

Research on barriers and constraints grew out of the assumption that leisure participation was good or better than nonparticipation and that more participation was better than less (Goodale & Witt, 1989). Thus, leisure researchers believed that if barriers or constraints to participation could be identified, they could be eliminated or, at least, minimized. Barriers have been defined as "any impediment to an individual's participation in an activity or use of a facility; the impediment may affect frequency, duration, or quality of participation or usage" (Smith, 1990, p. 39). However, most researchers have focused just on participation and have treated a constraint as "any factor which intervenes between the preference for an activity and participation in it" (Crawford & Godbey, 1987, p. 120).

Constraints, like leisure behavior, are typically measured by having respondents check off or rate a list of constraints presented to them on a questionnaire. These constraints are typically classified into different types. Several different classification systems of constraints have been proposed (see Jackson, 1988; Smith, 1990). Jackson, Crawford and Godbey (1992) have identified and suggested that intrapersonal, interpersonal, and structural constraints form a hierarchy of importance. Constraints at each level must be overcome before a person encounters the next level of constraint. In these models personality, attitudes, and interests can be constraints.

The idea of constraints negotiation has also been suggested. People are seen to actively negotiate barriers to participation and maintain some level of leisure involvement in spite of being constrained. Researchers are just beginning to examine this process and develop typologies of negotiation strategies (see Jackson & Rucks, 1993). As yet, no standardized scale for measuring constraints or negotiation strategies has been developed.

The research on the leisure constraints experienced by older adults has been primarily descriptive and atheoretical. Researchers have examined the constraints to participation experienced by older adults from several different perspectives. The most widely used approach has been to examine the constraints or barriers to leisure participation in general (e.g., DeGroot, 1976; McAvoy, 1976; McGuire, 1979, 1984; Scott & Zoernick, 1977). Another approach has addressed the constraints or barriers which have impeded participation in a specific activity or activity type such as physically active leisure or outdoor recreation (e.g., Buchanan & Allen, 1985; Mannell & Zuzanek, 1991; Strain & Chappell, 1982). Other researchers have employed a life span perspective to identify changes in perceived constraints at different life cycle stages (e.g., Buchanan & Allen, 1985; McGuire, Dottavio & O'Leary, 1986).

McGuire (1984) has developed the only constraints measure for older adults. This instrument includes a list of 30 different constraints identified in the literature and through interviews conducted prior to the study. Using factor analysis, McGuire identified five different categories of leisure constraints (External Resources, Time, Lack of Approval, Lack of Abilities and Health-Related). A review of the literature suggests that this scale has seldom been used in constraints research. Blazey (1987) adapted McGuire's scale to examine the constraints to travel for older adults.

Survey methods continue to be almost the only approach used in studies concerned with leisure constraints. They are subject to the same limitations discussed earlier for measures of leisure behavior. Mannell and Zuzanek (1991) have examined older adults' leisure constraints using the experiential sampling method in an attempt to overcome some of these difficulties.

CONCLUSIONS

Instruments specifically designed for measuring leisure-related phenomena with respect to older adults are in short supply. Our review also suggests that some of the measures of leisure behavior, experience, psychological outcomes, functioning, and individual differences being developed by leisure researchers may be usefully applied to aging and leisure issues. There is tremendous variation, however in the extent to which these measures operationalize well-understood phenomena, reflect standardization, report psychometric assessment for reliability and validity, and appear in aging and leisure applications.

Improved and standardized leisure behavior inventories are still needed, not only for the study of aging and leisure issues, but, also for the study of leisure generally. Advances have been made in efforts to assess subjective leisure with the development of modified time-budget and experiential sampling method approaches. These strategies allow the measurement of respondents' own definitions of leisure, and of the experience and meaning of leisure in daily life. Some research has already been stimulated and these approaches hold a great deal of promise for the study of aging and leisure.

Leisure satisfaction and attitude measurements could be used in aging and leisure research more than they have been to allow researchers to go beyond operationalizing leisure as only what older adults do in their free time. How older adults value leisure and the psychological outcomes they derive from it are also important indicators of leisure life style. Individual differences in how older adults relate to leisure have not been examined. An examination of the general and leisure-specific personality differences that are currently being explored in the leisure studies field may prove useful in understanding the diverse ways in which older adults respond to changes in their abilities, resources, and leisure opportunities.

REFERENCES

Allen, K. R., & Chin-Sang, V. (1990). A lifetime of work: The context and meanings of leisure for aging black women. *The Gerontologist*, *30*, 734–740.

Arbuckle, T. Y., Sissons, M. E., & Harsany, M. (1986). Development of a measure of intellectual, social, and physical activity for use with young and older adults. *Research Bulletins of the Centre for Research in Human Development, Concordia University*, *5*, 4.

Backman, S. J., & Mannell, R. C. (1986). Removing attitudinal barriers to leisure behavior and satisfaction: A field experiment among the institutionalized elderly. *Therapeutic Recreation Journal*, *20*, 46–53.

Beard, J. G., & Ragheb, M. G. (1980). Measuring leisure satisfaction. *Journal of Leisure Research, 12*, 20–33.

Blazey, M.A. (1987). The differences between participants and non-participants in a senior travel program. *Journal of Travel Research, 26*, 7–12.

Brown, B. A., Frankel, G. G., & Fennell, M. (1991). Happiness through leisure: The impact of type of leisure activity, age, gender and leisure satisfaction on psychological well-being. *Journal of Applied Recreation Research, 16*, 367–391.

Buchanan, T., & Allen, L. R. (1985). Barriers to recreation participation in later life cycle stages. *Therapeutic Recreation Journal, 19*, 39–50.

Bull, C. N. (1982). Leisure activities. In D. J. Mangen & W. A. Peterson (Eds.), *Research instruments in social gerontology: Vol. 2 Social roles and social participation.* Minneapolis: University of Minnesota Press.

Campbell, A. P. (1980). *The sense of well-being in America.* New York: McGraw-Hill.

Chase, D. R., & Godbey, G. (1983). The accuracy of self-reported participation rates: A research note. *Leisure Studies, 2*, 231–235.

Cosper, R. L., & Shaw, S. M. (1985). The validity of time-budget studies: A comparison of frequency and diary data in Halifax, Canada. *Leisure Sciences, 7*, 205–225.

Crandall, R., & Slivken, K. (1980). Leisure attitudes and their measurement. In S. E. Iso-Ahola (Ed.), *Social psychological perspectives on leisure and recreation* (pp. 261–284). Springfield, IL: Thomas.

Crawford, D. W., & Godbey, G. C. (1987). Reconceptualizing barriers to family leisure. *Leisure Sciences, 9*, 119–127.

Csikszentmihalyi, M. (1975). *Beyond boredom and anxiety: The experience of play in work and games.* San Francisco: Jossey–Bass.

Csikszentmihalyi, M. & Larson, R. (1984). *Being adolescent: Conflict and growth in the teenage years.* New York: Basic Books.

DeGroot, W. L. (1976). Analysis of leisure time profiles of selected adult males. Unpublished doctoral dissertation, Arizona State University. *Disertation Abstracts International, 37*(3), 140A. DDJ76–19817.

Driver, B. L., Brown, P. J., Stankey, G. H., & Gregoire, T. G. (1987). The ROS planning system: evolution, basic concepts, and research needed. *Leisure Sciences, 9*, 201–212.

Driver, B. L., Tinsley, H. E. A., & Manfredo, M. J. (1991). The Paragraphs About Leisure and Recreation Experience Preference Scales: Results from two inventories designed to assess the breadth of the perceived psychological benefits of leisure. In B. L. Driver, P. J. Brown, & G. L. Peterson (Eds.), *Benefits of leisure* (pp. 263–286). State College, PA: Venture.

Ellis, G. D., & Witt, P. A. (1986). The Leisure Diagnostic Battery: Past, present, and future. *Therapeutic Recreation Journal, 20*, 31–47.

Fishbein, M., & Ajzen, I. (1975). *Belief, attitude, intention, and behavior: An introduction to theory and research.* Reading, MA: Addison-Wesley.

Francken, D. A., & van Raaij, W. F. (1981). Satisfaction with leisure time activities. *Journal of Leisure Research, 13*, 337–352.

Goodale, T. L., & Witt, P. A. (1989). Recreation non-participation and barriers to leisure. In E. L. Jackson, & T. L. Burton (Eds.), *Understanding leisure and recreation: Mapping the past, charting the future* (pp. 421–449). State College, PA: Venture Publishing, Inc.

Graefe, A. R., & Fedler, A. J. (1986). Situational and subjective determinants of satisfaction in marine recreational fishing. *Leisure Sciences, 8*, 275–295.

Graham, D. F., Graham, I., and MacLean, M. J. (1991). Going to the mall: A leisure activity of urban elderly people. *Canadian Journal on Aging, 10*, 345–358.

Guin, R. (1980). Early recreational vehicle tourists: Life satisfaction correlates of leisure satisfaction. *Journal of Leisure Research, 12*, 198–204.

Gunter, B. G. (1979). Properties of the leisure experience. In H. Ibrahim & R. Crandall (Eds.), *Leisure: A psychological approach* (pp. 63–91). Los Alamitos, CA: Hwong.

Heinemann, A. W., Colorez, A., Frank, S., & Taylor, D. (1988). Leisure activity participation of elderly individuals with low vision. *The Gerontologist, 28*, 181–184.

Henderson, K. A., & Rannells, J. S. (1988). Farm women and the meaning of work and leisure: An oral history perspective. *Leisure Sciences, 10*, 41–50.

Hnatiuk, S. H. (1991). Experience sampling with elderly persons: An exploration of the method. *International Journal of Aging and Human Development, 33*, 45–64.

Iso-Ahola, S. E. (1976). On the theoretical link between personality and leisure. *Psychological Reports, 39*, 3–10.

Iso-Ahola, S. E. (1980). *The social psychology of leisure and recreation*. Dubuque, Iowa: Brown.

Iso-Ahola, S. E. (1991). The social psychology of leisure. In L. A. Barnett (Ed.), *Research about leisure: Past, present, and future* (pp. 75–93). Champaign, IL: Sagamore.

Iso-Ahola, S. E., & Buttimer, K. J. (1981). The emergence of work and leisure ethic from early adolescence to early adulthood. *Journal of Leisure Research, 13*, 282–288.

Iso-Ahola, S. E., & Crowley, E. D. (1991). Adolescent substance abuse and leisure boredom. *Journal of Leisure Research, 23*, 260–271.

Iso-Ahola, S. E., & Mannell, R. C. (1985). Social and psychological constraints on leisure. In M. G. Wade (Ed.), *Constraints on leisure* (pp. 111–151). Springfield, IL: Thomas.

Iso-Ahola, S. E., & Weissinger, E. (1987). Leisure and boredom. *Journal of Social and Clinical Psychology, 5*, 356–364.

Iso-Ahola, S. E., & Weissinger, E. (1990). Perceptions of boredom in leisure: Conceptualization, reliability and validity of the Leisure Boredom Scale. *Journal of Leisure Research, 22*, 1–17.

Jackson, E. L. (1988). Leisure constraints: A survey of past research. *Leisure Sciences, 10*, 203–215.

Jackson, E. L., Crawford, D. W., & Godbey, G. (1992). Negotiation of leisure constraints. *Leisure Sciences, 15*, 1–12.

Jackson, E. L., & Rucks, V. C. (1993). Reasons for ceasing participation and barriers to participation: Further examination of constrained leisure as an internally homogeneous concept. *Leisure Sciences, 15*, 217–230.

Kelly, J. R., & Ross, J. (1989). Later-life leisure: Beginning a new agenda. *Leisure Sciences, 11*, 47–59.

Kelly, J. R., Steinkamp, M. W., & Kelly, J. R. (1987). Later-life satisfaction: Does leisure contribute? *Leisure Sciences, 9*, 189–200.

Kleiber, D. A., & Dirkin, G. R. (1985). Intrapersonal constraints to leisure. In M. G. Wade (Ed), *Constraints on leisure* (pp. 17–42). Springfield, IL: Thomas.

Larson, R. W., & Csikszentmihalyi, M. (1983). The experience sampling method. In H. T. Reis (Ed.), *Naturalistic approaches to studying social interaction* (pp. 41–56). San Fransisco: Jossey-Bass.

Larson, R. W., Mannell, R. C., & Zuzanek, J. (1986). Daily well-being of older adults with friends and family. *Psychology and Aging, 1*, 117–126.

Larson, R. W., Zuzanek, J., & Mannell, R. C. (1985). Being alone versus being with people: Disengagement in the daily experience of older adults. *Journal of Gerontology, 40*, 375–381.

Lawton, P. (1985). Activities and leisure. In C. Eisdorfer (Ed.), *Annual review of gerontology and geriatrics* (Vol. 5) (pp. 127–164). New York: Springer .

Lawton, M. P. (1993). The meaning of leisure. In J. Kelly (Ed.), *Activity and aging*. Newbury Park, CA: Sage.

Lounsbury, J. W., & Hoopes, L. L. (1988). Five-year stability of leisure activity and motivation factors. *Journal of Leisure Research, 20*, 118–134.

Lounsbury, J. W., Gordon, S. R., Bergermaier, R. L., & Francesco, A. M. (1982). Work and nonwork sources of satisfaction in relation to employee intention to turnover. *Journal of Leisure Research, 14*, 285–294.

Mannell, R. C. (1980). Social psychological techniques and strategies for studying leisure experiences. In S. E. Iso-Ahola (Ed.), *Social psychological perspectives on leisure and recreation* (pp. 62–88). Springfield, IL: C. Thomas.

Mannell, R. C. (1984a). A psychology of leisure research. *Society and Leisure, 7*, 13–21.

Mannell, R. C. (1984b). Personality in leisure theory: The self-as-entertainment construct. *Society and Leisure, 7*, 229–242.

Mannell, R. C. (1989). Leisure satisfaction. In E. L. Jackson, & T. L. Burton (Eds.), *Understanding leisure and recreation: Mapping the past, charting the future* (pp. 281–301). State College, PA: Venture.

Mannell, R. C. (1992). High-investment activity and life satisfaction among older adults: Committed, serious leisure, and flow activities. In J. R. Kelly (Ed.), *Activity and aging: Staying involved in later life*. Newbury Park, CA: Sage.

Mannell, R. C., & Bradley, W. (1986). Does greater freedom always lead to greater leisure? Testing a person X environment model of freedom and leisure. *Journal of Leisure Research, 18*, 215–230.

Mannell, R. C., & Iso-Ahola, S. E. (1987). Psychological nature of leisure and tourism experience. *Annals of Tourism Research, 14*, 314–331.

Mannell, R. C., & Zuzanek, J. (1991). The nature and variability of leisure constraints in daily life: The case of the physically active leisure of older adults. *Leisure Sciences, 13*, 337–351.

Mannell, R. C., Zuzanek, J., & Larson, R. W. (1988). Leisure states and "flow" experiences: Testing perceived freedom and intrinsic motivation hypotheses. *Journal of Leisure Research, 20*, 289–304.

Manfredo, M. J. (Ed.). (1992). *Influencing human behavior: Theory and applications in recreation, tourism, and natural resources management*. Champaign, IL: Sagamore.

McAvoy, L. H. (1976). Recreation preferences of the elderly in Minnesota. Unpublished doctoral dissertation, University of Minnesota. *Dissertation Abstracts International, 37(6)*, 38 98A.

McGuire, F. A. (1979). An exploratory study of leisure constraints advanced adulthood. Unpublished doctoral dissertation, University of Illinois. *Dissertation Abstracts International, 40(10)*, 55 88.

McGuire, F. A. (1984). A factor analytic study of leisure constraints in advanced adulthood. *Leisure Sciences, 6*, 313–326.

McGuire, F. A., Dottavio, D., & O'Leary, J. T. (1986). Constraints to participation in outdoor recreation across the life span. *The Gerontologist, 26*, 538–544.

McKechnie, G. E. (1974). The psychological structure of leisure: Past behavior. *Journal of Leisure Research, 6*, 27–45.

McKechnie, G. E. (1975). *Manual for the leisure activities blank*. Palo Alto, CA: Consulting Psychologists Press.

Moss, M. S. & Lawton, M. P. (1982). Time budgets of older people: A window on four lifestyles. *Journal of Gerontology, 37*, 115–123.

Neulinger, J. (1974). *The psychology of leisure*. Springfield, IL: Thomas.

Ouellette, P. (1986). The leisure participation and enjoyment patterns of French and English-speaking members of senior citizens' clubs in New Brunswick, Canada. *Canadian Journal on Aging, 5*, 257–268.

Ragheb, M. G., & Beard, J. G. (1982). Measuring leisure attitude. *Journal of Leisure Research, 14*, 155–167.

Ragheb, M. G., & Griffith, C. A. (1982). The contribution of leisure participation and leisure satisfaction to life satisfaction of older adults. *Journal of Leisure Research, 14*, 295–305.

Riddick, C. C. (1986). Leisure satisfaction precursors. *Journal of Leisure Research, 18*, 259–265.

Romsa, G. H. & Blenman, M. (1989). Recording activity patterns: Some comments from a southwestern Ontario study of retirees. *Journal of Applied Recreation Research, 8*, 393–401.

Rotter, J. B. (1966). Generalized expectancies for internal versus external control of reinforcement. *Psychological Monographs: General and Applied, 80*, 1–28.

Russell, R. V. (1987). The importance of recreation satisfaction and activity participation to the life satisfaction of age–segregated retirees. *Journal of Leisure Research, 19*, 273–283.

Samdahl, D. M. (1988). A symbolic interactionist model of leisure: Theory and empirical support. *Leisure Sciences, 10*, 27–39.

Samdahl, D. M., & Jekubovich, N. J. (1993). Patterns and characteristics of adult daily leisure. *Society and Leisure, 16*, 129–149.

Savell, K. S. (1991) Leisure, perceptions, perceptions of control and well-being: Implications for the institutionalized elderly. *Therapeutic Recreation Journal, 25*, 44–59.

Scott, D., & Godbey, G. C. (1992). An analysis of adult play groups: Social versus serious participation in contract bridge. *Leisure Sciences, 14*), 29–46.

Scott, E.O., & Zoernick, D.A. (1977). Exploring leisure needs of the aged. *Leisurability, 4*, 25–31.

Searle, M. S., & Iso-Ahola, S. E. (1988). Determinants of leisure behavior among retired adults. *Therapeutic Recreation Journal, 22*, 38–46.

Shaw, S. M. (1984). The measurement of leisure: A quality of life issue. *Society and Leisure, 7*, 91–107.

Shaw, S. M. (1985). The meaning of leisure in everyday life. *Leisure Sciences, 7*, 1–24.

Smith, S. L. J. (1990). *Dictionary of concepts in recreation and leisure studies*. New York: Greenwood Press.

Sneegas, J. J. (1986). Components of life satisfaction in middle and later life adults: Perceived social competence, leisure participation, and leisure satisfaction. *Journal of Leisure Research, 18*, 248–258.

Stones, M. J., & Kozma, A. (1986). Happiness and activities as propensities. *Journal of Gerontology, 41*, 85–90.

Strain, L. A., & Chappell, N. L. (1982). Outdoor recreation and the rural elderly: Participation, problems and needs. *Therapeutic Recreation Journal, 16*, 42–48.

Tinsley, H. E. A., Colbs, S. L., Teaff, J. D., & Kaufman, N. (1987). The relationship of age, gender, health and economic status to the psychological benefits older persons report from participation in leisure activities. *Leisure Sciences, 9*, 53–65.

Tinsley, H. E. A., & Tinsley, D. J. (1988). An expanded context for the study of career decisionmaking, development and maturity. In W.B. Walsh, & S.H. Osipow (Eds.), *Career decisionmaking* (pp. 213–264). Hillsdale, NJ: Erlbaum.

Voelkl, J. E. (1990). The challenge skill ratio of daily experiences among older adults residing in nursing homes. *Therapeutic Recreation Journal, 24*, 7–17.

Voelkl, J. E., & Birkel, R. C. (1988). Application of the experience sampling method to assess clients' daily experiences. *Therapeutic Recreation Journal, 22*, 23–33.

Voelkl, J. E., & Brown, B. B. (1989). Experience sampling method in therapeutic recreation research. *Therapeutic Recreation Journal, 23*, 35–46.

.Voelkl, J. E., & Nicholson, L. A. (1992). Perceptions of daily life among residents of a long term care facility. *Activities, Adaptation and Aging, 16*, 99–114.

Weissinger, E., & Iso-Ahola, S. E. (1984). Intrinsic leisure motivation, personality and physical health. *Society and Leisure, 7*, 217–228.

Weissinger, E., Caldwell, L. L., & Bandalos, D. L. (1992). Relation between intrinsic motivation and boredom in leisure time. *Leisure Sciences, 14*, 317–325.

Wells, A. J. (1988). Self-esteem and optimal experience. In M. Csikszentmihalyi & I. Csikszentmihalyi (Eds.), *Optimal experience: Psychological studies of flow in consciousness (pp. 327–341)*. Cambridge: Cambridge University Press.

Zuzanek, J. (1991). Time-budget research: Methodological problems and perspectives. In E. J. McCullough, & R. L. Calder (Eds.), *Time as a human resource* (pp. 243–250). Calgary, Alberta: the University of Calgary Press.

Zuzanek, J., & Box, S. J. (1988). Life course and the daily lives of older adults in Canada. In K. Altergott (Ed.), *Daily life in later life* (pp. 147–185). London: Sage.

CHAPTER 8

Assessing the Health-Related Dimensions of Older Adults' Social Relationships

KAREN S. ROOK
SCHOOL OF SOCIAL ECOLOGY
UNIVERSITY OF CALIFORNIA, IRVINE

Persuasive evidence indicates that informal social relationships significantly influence human health and well-being (see reviews by Burman & Margolin, 1992; Cohen, 1988; House, Umberson, & Landis, 1988). This work suggests that social bonds are no less important in late life than in other life stages, although the specific interpersonal factors that influence health may differ. For example, mortality and morbidity have been found to be less strongly linked to marital status (Sugisawa, Liang, & Liu, 1994; Rushing, Ritter, & Burton, 1992) and more strongly linked to peer ties among older adults than among younger age groups (Seeman, Kaplan, Knudsen, Cohen, & Guralnik, 1987). More generally, aspects of older adults' social involvement have been found to predict mortality, morbidity, health behaviors, treatment compliance and rehabilitation outcomes, psychological health, perceived quality of life, risk of institutionalization, and adaptation to a variety of serious life stresses (see reviews by Antonucci, 1985, 1990; Oxman & Berkman, 1990; Schulz & Rau, 1985; Wan, 1982). The strength of these associations is impressive, as evidenced by the fact that interpersonal variables predict mortality and morbidity nearly as well as do more conventional risk factors, such as smoking (House et al., 1988). In addition, neither social selection nor reverse causation appear to account fully for these effects (e.g., Gove, Hughes, & Style, 1983; Johnson, 1991; Krause, Liang, & Yatomi, 1989).

Although a considerable consensus exists regarding the importance of social ties for health, less consensus exists regarding the best way to measure or assess these ties. This is not surprising, given that the question of how social bonds influence emotional and physical health is exceedingly complex and subsumes a host of narrower, interrelated questions, each of which may require researchers to employ somewhat different measurement strategies and research designs. Thus, it seems unlikely that a single measure will be found the best for studying the health effects of informal social ties in late life. The goal of this chapter, therefore, is not to advocate the superiority of a particular measure but, rather, to discuss the conceptual underpinnings of current measurement approaches and to describe the characteristics of measures that have been used with elderly populations (see also Heitzmann & Kaplan, 1988; House & Kahn, 1985; Krause, 1989; O'Reilly, 1988; Orth-Gomer & Unden, 1987; Oxman & Berkman, 1990; Sarason, Sarason, & Pierce, 1990; Vaux, 1992, for discussions of measurement issues and evaluations of specific measures). Comprehensive conceptual models presented elsewhere can help link measurement to theory (e.g., Burman & Margolin, 1992; Cohen, 1988; Schwarzer & Leppin, 1991) and to statistical analysis (e.g., Barrera, 1986; Lin, 1986; Wheaton, 1985); this chapter focuses more narrowly on the rationale for and methods of assessing several health-related dimensions of older adults' social relationships.

Existing measurement approaches generally vary in their emphasis on one or more of three conceptually distinct aspects of older adults' social relationships (cf. Dunkel-Schetter & Bennett, 1990; Oxman & Berkman, 1990; Schwarzer & Leppin, 1991): (a) *social integration*, or the extent of older adults' social network ties and the structural properties of these ties, (b) *relational content*, or the substantive (functional) content of older adults' positive and negative transactions with members of their social networks, (c) *network evaluations*, or older adults' evaluations of quantitative and qualitative aspects of their transactions with social network members (see Figure 8.1). The chapter discusses the conceptual rationale for and means of operationalizing these different emphases. Wherever possible, the chapter attempts to illustrate the kinds of research problems for which different measurement approaches may have particular relevance.

The chapter emphasizes older adults' informal ties to members of their social networks, even though religious and organizational affiliations (e.g., Bryant & Rakowski, 1992; Maton, 1989) and formal support systems (Litwak & Messeri, 1989) clearly may help to sustain older adults' well-being. In addition, although the literature on caregiving has spawned a great deal of research on the psychosocial resources, including social support, that help to reduce caregiving burdens, a review of approaches to conceptualizing and assessing support in the specific context of caregiving is beyond the scope of the chapter (see DeLongis & O'Brien, 1990; Stephens, 1990). Assessment strategies in which older adults are viewed as the recipients, or targets, of social network members' actions are emphasized, even though older adults often function as the initiators or providers of various forms of social contact and support (Antonucci, 1985, 1990; Spitze & Logan, 1992). This focus on the recipient role dovetails with the predominant theoretical orientation of the literature; it is not intended to imply that older adults rarely provide support and companionship to others or that such activities are inconsequential for their health and well-being. Finally, in view of the fact that older adults' social relationships have been linked to a wide variety of health-related outcomes, the term *health* is used broadly in this chapter to subsume emotional health and physical health. Taking such a broad view does not belie the importance of differentiating

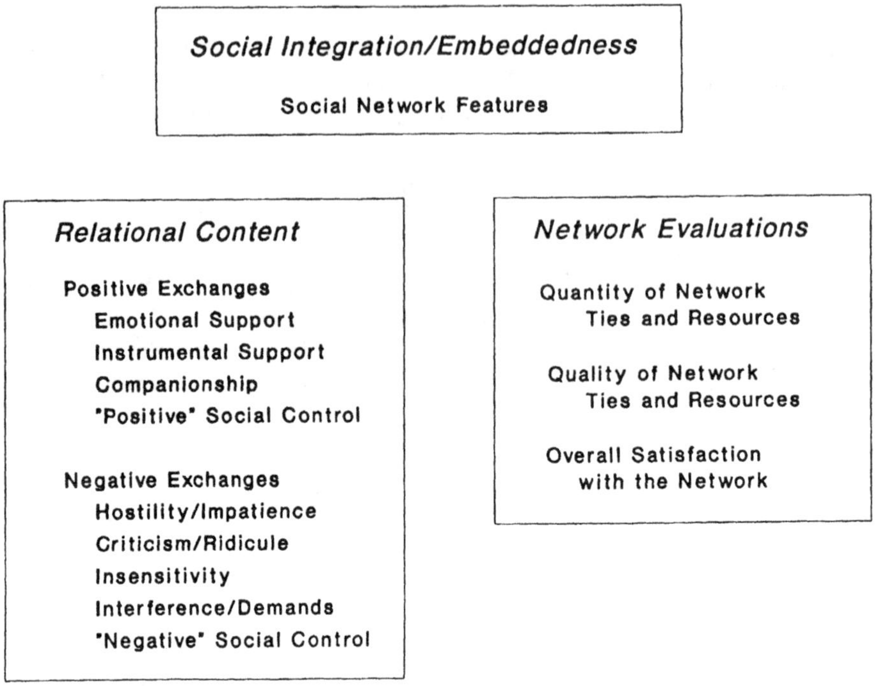

FIGURE 8.1 Three Aspects of scoial relationships.

among health problems and stages of illness or recovery (e.g., Cohen, 1988; Litwak & Messeri, 1989; Monroe & Johnson, 1992).

SOCIAL INTEGRATION/EMBEDDEDNESS

Social integration, or social embeddedness, is commonly regarded as the extent to which individuals belong to a network of informal social ties (House et al., 1988). Theorists view social embeddedness as protecting health by reducing feelings of isolation and alienation and by restraining deviant or self-injurious behavior (e.g., Durkheim, 1897/1951; Gove, 1973; Hughes & Gove, 1981). Measures of social integration typically assess relatively concrete or objective aspects of a person's informal social involvement, such as marital status, the number of ties to kin and nonkin, the frequency of contact with kin and nonkin, and the presence or absence of a confidant in the social network (Oxman & Berkman, 1990). Brief measures such as these have been criticized by some as too limited or uninformative, yet it is important to bear in mind that such measures have demonstrated impressive associations with significant health outcomes in well-controlled prospective studies (House et al., 1988). Thus, these simple measures may be adequate for researchers who wish to predict which older adults are at increased risk for adverse health outcomes. Use of these abbreviated measures may have more limited value, in contrast, for researchers who seek to explain why interpersonal factors influence risk status. In addition, emerging evidence suggests that simple measures of embeddedness more successfully predict outcomes for men than for women, whereas measures that capture the quality of social network involvement (discussed later) more successfully predict outcomes for women (e.g., Johnson, 1991).

Analysis of the characteristics of social networks, including characteristics of specific dyadic relationships and of the network as a whole, represents an extension of the social integration approach. Social network properties presumably influence the flow of supportive resources through a network, thus providing an indication of the potential responsiveness of a network in times of need (e.g., Hall & Wellman, 1985; Granovetter, 1973; Wellman & Wortley, 1990). Network properties frequently cited in connection to health and well-being are described below, and arguments bearing on the utility of network assessment are addressed.

Social Network Properties

Properties of specific dyadic relationships (between a focal person and his or her network members) that have been emphasized by network theorists include the nature of the role relationship (e.g., spouse, adult child, friend), geographic proximity, frequency of contact, duration of the relationship, degree of reciprocity, multiplexity (the number of different resources provided by a particular network member), and strength (e.g., importance, closeness). Properties of social networks as a whole that have been emphasized include size, homogeneity (the extent to which members of a network share similar attributes), density (the extent to which members of a network know each other), and composition (e.g., the proportion of kin versus friends) (see Hall & Wellman, 1985, for an overview). Additional network measures, can be derived as well by aggregating dyadic measures across the multiple dyads that comprise the network. This procedure yields composite measures, such as the average frequency of contact with network members, average duration of network relationships, and average proximity to network members. The implications of alternative methods of aggregation have yet to be fully explored, but Milardo (1988) argues that investigator-based aggregation usually produces more accurate data than respondent-based aggregation (in which interviewees estimate their average frequency of contact with others).

Social network properties, such as size and multiplexity, have been linked empirically to well-being in some studies of older adults (e.g., Felton & Berry, 1992; Schoenbach, Kaplan, Fredman, & Kleinbaum, 1986; Wan, 1982) but not in others (e.g., Auslander & Litwin, 1991; Shahtamasebi, Davis, & Wegner, 1992). A similar pattern of mixed findings in studies of other age groups has led some researchers to question whether the overall yield of such work has been sufficient to justify the effort needed to assess network properties (e.g., Sarason et al., 1990; Turner, 1992). Assessment of network characteristics can be fairly labor intensive, but conclusions about the utility of this approach may be premature, because the empirical work conducted to date has not always specified network analysts' predictions correctly. Network analysts typically emphasize the role of network characteristics in influencing the exchange of support and other resources within a network. They less often hypothesize direct links between network properties and health outcomes, yet failure to find such direct links in previous work has been construed as evidence of the limited yield of the network approach.

Some studies have demonstrated that network properties do predict access to support resources (e.g., Haines & Hurlbert, 1992; Wellman & Wortley, 1990), although strong and consistent patterns have been difficult to discern. For example, recent analyses of a large, representative sample of adults revealed that only some network characteristics predicted subjects' perceived access to social support, and the associations varied considerably for different kinds of support and for men versus women (Haines & Hurlbert, 1992). Mixed results similarly have emerged in studies of caregivers (e.g., Suitor & Pillemer, 1993) and urban older adults (e.g., Felton & Berry, 1992).

A recent elaboration of the network perspective proposes that social network properties influence exposure to stress as well as access to social support. For example, Haines and Hurlbert (1992) found that greater network size was associated with greater stress among women, a finding that converges with emerging ideas about the psychological costs of social network involvement for women (e.g., Riley & Eckenrode, 1986; Kessler, McLeod, & Wethington, 1985). Similarly, in a study of female caregivers, variables such as proximity, similarity, and the nature of the role relationship (e.g., sibling versus friend) predicted the degree of strain in caregivers' relationships with individual network members (Suitor & Pillemer; 1993). Thus, a better understanding of the role of network variables in influencing health and well-being may emerge as researchers examine indirect as well as direct links with these outcomes.

Assessment of Social Networks: Existing Approaches. Two primary methods have been developed for formally defining older adults' social networks and assessing their characteristics, as summarized in Table 8.1. One approach (Antonucci & Akiyama, 1987)involves first defining network membership on the basis of sentiments (e.g., identifying the people "who are so close that its hard to imagine life without them"), and then determining who among these individuals provide various types of social support. The second approach (Fischer, 1982a; McCallister & Fischer, 1978) first determines who provides various types of support (e.g., "Is there anyone to whom you could turn to for help if you became ill and needed assistance with meal preparation or house care?"), and then uses the pooled set of names to define network membership. The number of questions used to elicit network membership with this latter approach varies across studies, as does the number of names coded

TABLE 8.1 Measures of Social Network Size and Characteristics used with Older Adults

Measure	*Illustrative Studies Using this Measure*[a]	*Description*	*Reliability and Validity*[b]	*Comments*
Social Networks in Adult Life Survey (Kahn & Antonucci, 1980)[c]	Antonucci & Akiyama, 1987; Antonucci & Israel, 1986; Depner & Ingersoll-Dayton, 1988; Levitt et al., 1993	Respondents identify persons who are "close and important" to them at each of three levels depicted by concentric circles; additional questions for a subset of 10 network members determine who provides support (affect, aid, affirmation) and assess properties of the relationships with these individuals; interview format	Measures correlate in expected direction with psychological health; Reasonable degree of convergence between respondents' and significant others' reports of support (Antonucci & Israel, 1986)	Social network membership is defined on the basis of sentiment (closeness, importance)
Social Network Interview (Fischer, 1982a; McCallister & Fischer, 1978)[c]	Used in adapted form by Finch & Zautra, 1992; Finch et al., 1989; Rook, 1984; Stephens et al., 1987; Suitor & Pillemer, 1993	12 questions identify persons (up to a maximum of six per question) who could provide emotional and instrumental aid and companionship; additional questions assess properties of the relationships with and sentiments (e.g., closeness) felt toward the network members; interview format	Measures correlate in expected direction with sociodemographic factors and psychological health; pilot research suggests good test-retest reliability; reliability is greatest for "core" network members	Social network membership is defined on the basis of participation in social exchanges

(continued)

TABLE 8.1 Continued

Measure	*Illustrative Studies Using this Measure*[a]	*Description*	*Reliability and Validity*[b]	*Comments*
Social Network Questionnaire (Seeman & Berkman, 1988; adapted from Berkman & Syme, 1979)[c]	Seeman & Berkman, 1988 Weinberger et al., 1987	Questions assess number of ties with children, other relatives, friends; number of monthly in-person and indirect (phone calls, letters) contacts; whether or not network can be counted on to provide emotional support or instrumental support when needed; interview format	Measure predicts 9-year mortality (Berkman & Syme, 1979)	Network membership size determined primarily on the basis of role relations (e.g., kin, friend status)
Network Analysis Profile (Cohen et al., 1985)	Cohen et al., 1985; Cohen et al., 1988a; Cohen et al., 1988b	Items assess material and emotional support exchanged with others, network size, frequency of contact, features of the network and of the relationships with network members; designed to yield separate measures of interactional and structural aspects of network involvement reflecting; interview format	Interrater reliability for subsections of the profile = .83–.92; factor analyses demonstrate independence of many structural measures; some measures health outcomes among inner-city older adults	Semistructured interview suitable for use with vulnerable populations; likely to require highly skilled interviewers

[a]Gerontological studies
[b]Based on original validation research
[c]Also yields assessment of perceived support

in response to each question. As a check on the adequacy of the set of name-eliciting questions, respondents are sometimes asked to review a list of the names compiled and to indicate whether anyone important to them is missing from the list (e.g., Fischer, 1982a; Rook, 1984). To the extent that few additional names are offered, the set of name-eliciting questions can be considered to provide a good estimate of the respondent's (exchange-based) social network.

With both approaches, additional questions assess the features of the relationship with each network member (e.g., role relation, duration, frequency of contact, etc.). From this information, the size and characteristics of the overall network can be determined, as can the size and characteristics of "subnetworks" of potential interest to researchers, such as the kin network or the friend network. Although the latter of the two approaches described above defines network membership on the basis of participation in concrete behavioral exchanges, sentiments felt toward network members nonetheless can be assessed by asking respondents who, if anyone, from the list of compiled names they feel especially close to, especially fond of, etc. (e.g., Fischer, 1982a). This provides an efficient way to obtain information about respondents' views of their network members, although the typically dichotomous scoring of responses (e.g., 0=*not close*; 1=*close*) limits the kinds of data analyses that can be undertaken. (Requiring respondents to discriminate among multiple levels of closeness or importance for each network member can rapidly lead to fatigue, which is why simple dichotomous distinctions are often preferred.)

The two methods of network assessment yield analogous information, but they use different criteria to define network membership. Fischer and his colleagues (Fischer, 1982a; McCallister & Fischer, 1978; see also Milardo, 1988) believe that the exchange-based approach offers several advantages over the sentiment-based approach, although comparative studies with older adults have not been undertaken to evaluate their claims. They suggest that the use of exchange-based questions avoids the subjectivity and ambiguity inherent in the use of terms such as close or important, reduces recall problems by presenting concrete referents to trigger respondents' thoughts about network members, and provides a more comprehensive assessment of the active network by including a broad sample of the important social transactions in which people engage in the course of their daily lives.

Network data obtained through either of the two primary approaches allow the researcher to construct measures suitable for analysis at any of several levels: behavioral level (emphasizing the types of functions performed by network members, irrespective of the number of individuals who perform these functions, cf. House & Kahn, 1985), dyadic level (emphasizing the functions performed by particular network members and the characteristics of particular dyadic relationships), and network level (emphasizing the functions performed by the network as a whole and the characteristics of the overall network). Which level of analysis is most appropriate will be determined largely by the requirements of specific research projects (Marsden, 1990).

Both approaches to network assessment have been used successfully with older adults, and the exchange-based method of assessment has been extended in some studies to identify network members with whom respondents experience conflict or other difficulties as well as those with whom they find support and companionship (e.g., Finch, Okun, Barrera, Zautra, & Reich, 1989; Rook, 1984; Stephens, Kinney, Norris, & Ritchie, 1987). Both approaches offer advantages over assessments that simply ask people to estimate how many friends they have or how many relatives they can turn to for support, because the kind of mental calculus that underlies such estimates remains poorly understood (Milardo, 1988). Moreover, both approaches can be adapted to accommodate the goals of particular studies by modifying the set of questions asked. For example, researchers interested in caregiving could add questions that assess the provision by network members of support that is relevant to particular caregiving demands and burdens (cf. Suitor & Pillemer, 1993). It is important to recognize, however, that formal methods of assessing social networks, such as those described here, can consume considerable time, typically require the use of interviews, and may generate more detailed information about network membership and composition than is needed for a particular study.

Summary of Social Integration Measurement

This brief review suggests that simple measures of social embeddedness (e.g., marital status, number of friends, presence or absence of a confidant) have value in predicting which older adults (particularly which men) may be at increased risk for physical or emotional disorders. Such measures will be less useful, however, in helping to illuminate the underlying processes that account for any associations observed. More formal, social network measures may be helpful in predicting older adults' access to support and other social resources in times of need and, for women, may be helpful in predicting exposure to stress. The usefulness of network measures in predicting health outcomes directly remains uncertain. Of the numerous network measures available to researchers, those that have shown greatest promise thus far in studies of older adults include total network size (e.g., Schoenbach et al., 1986; Wan, 1982), network composition (Dean, Kolody, & Wood, 1990; Felton & Berry, 1992; Heller & Mansbach, 1984), proximity (Suitor & Pillemer, 1993), and frequency of contact (Oxman & Berkman, 1990).

Measures of social embeddedness and/or social network characteristics can, of course, be combined with measures of other interpersonal factors to yield richer information about the critical health-related dimensions of older adults' social ties (House & Kahn, 1985; Vaux, 1992). Such a strategy has proven valuable, for example, in clarifying the association between older adults' martial status and health. Specifically, assessing both marital status and the availability of a confidant has revealed that married individuals whose spouses do not function as confidants report more depression than do unmarried individuals (e.g., Dean et al., 1990). Measurement approaches that could supplement network assessment are discussed in the following sections.

CONTENT OF SOCIAL RELATIONSHIPS

Some approaches to social relationship emphasize the content of older adults' transactions with others, seeking to categorize and contrast the different social *functions* (see Lawton & Moss, 1987, for a discussion of this term) or *social provisions* (Weiss, 1974) that influence well-being. This work is generally guided by the view that universal (Weiss, 1974) or situation-specific (Cohen & Wills, 1985) needs exist for various social provisions and that deficits of key provisions create distinctive kinds of distress. Some theorists argue, further, that particular kinds of network members (e.g., family members vs. friends) are best-suited to offer particular resources (Litwak, 1985; Weiss, 1974). This position requires attention both to the sources of the provisions and the range of resources available from a social network.

Most research has investigated the positive functions of social ties, such as the support and companionship available from a person's social network. Other work has examined social networks as a source of conflict and stress, demonstrating that such negative transactions, although infrequent, can detract substantially from older adults' health and well-being (see review by Rook, 1990a). This section reviews researchers' efforts to conceptualize and assess older adults' positive and negative exchanges with network members.

Social Support

Many investigations of the health effects of positive social exchanges have been motivated by an interest in understanding how social support helps to protect, or buffer, people from the adverse effects of life stress (Cohen & Wills, 1985). Stress researchers have proposed numerous taxonomies of social support (see reviews by House, 1981; Wills, 1985), and, although variations exist, most taxonomies have included emotional support (empathy, reassurance, liking, respect), appraisal support (feedback relevant to self-evaluation), informational support (problem-solving advice and information), and instrumental support (services and other forms of tangible aid). The helpfulness of each type of support is believed to vary across stressors (Cohen & McKay, 1984; Cutrona & Russell, 1987; Wills, 1985) and across phases of the stress-adaptation process (Jacobson, 1986). Researchers, accordingly, have operationalized these conceptual distinctions in the form of measures containing subscales that tap the availability or receipt of different kinds of social support (e.g., see reviews by Heitzmann & Kaplan, 1988; Orth-Gomer & Unden, 1987; Sarason et al., 1990; Vaux, 1992).

Other researchers believe that emotional support (especially when construed in terms of intimacy and affirmation) is singularly important to well-being (Antonucci, 1985; House, 1981; Sarason et al., 1990), both because a wide variety of stressors arouse needs for reassurance of self-worth (Wills, 1985) and because intimacy represents an existential human need (House, 1981). From this perspective, assessment of emotional support has greater value than assessment of other types of support. Resolution of this debate will rest, in part, on evidence of the empirical distinctiveness of social support constructs.

Efforts to differentiate empirically among conceptually distinct forms of social support have met with some difficulties, most notably the problem of high intercorrelations among different support subscales (House & Kahn, 1985; Sarason, Shearin, Pierce, & Sarason, 1987; Sarason et al., 1990). Factor analyses of items believed to represent five or six conceptually distinct forms of support have often yielded evidence of fewer factors (e.g., Levitt, Weber, & Guacci, 1993; Sherbourne & Hays, 1990; though see Mancini & Blieszner, 1992). The factors that emerge most consistently from studies of older adults (e.g., Anderson & McCulloch, 1993) and other age groups reflect three types of social support: Emotional, Instrumental, and, to a lesser extent, Informational (see reviews by Krause, 1989; Orth-Gomer & Unden, 1987; Oxman & Berkman, 1990). Moreover, emotional support and instrumental support have been found to exhibit differing associations with health-related outcomes in studies of older adults (e.g., Russell & Cutrona, 1991; Ensel, 1991).

Thus, it has been difficult to substantiate theoretical distinctions among more closely related constructs, such as esteem support and appraisal support, but some distinctions do appear to be reliable and valid. Greater use of structural equation methods that permit examination of a higher order, global support factor as well as specific, intercorrelated support factors may yet yield evidence of the unique effects of additional support constructs that have been proposed (Newcomb, 1990; Russell & Cutrona, 1991). In the interim, distinguishing among emotional support, instrumental support, and (possibly) informational support appears to be warranted (cf. Ensel, 1991; Krause, 1986; Russell & Cutrona, 1991).

Assessment of Social Support: Existing Approaches. Dozens of formal and ad hoc measures of social support can be identified in the available literature, but only a subset of these have been developed or adapted for use with elderly populations. These measurement approaches vary in the extent to which they distinguish different types of support, differentiate among sources of support, emphasize support perceived to be available if needed (potential support) versus support actually received (enacted support), and assess general (everyday, or routine) support versus situation-specific (e.g., crisis- or treatment-specific) support (O'Reilly, 1988). Of these various points of differentiation among measures, the one that has sparked the greatest controversy among researchers concerns the merits of assessing perceived versus received support.

Many researchers favor efforts to document and evaluate the effects of support actually provided by network members, but others believe that perceptions of support available from their network members are more consequential for health (e.g., Sarason et al., 1987, 1990; Turner, 1992). Proponents of the latter view argue that assessing people's perceptions of the support available to them has greater value than assessing the support derived from actual transactions. Turner (1992) argued, for example, that "perceived support is . . . what matters for health and well-being and the central tool for identifying the most promising targets toward which . . . intervention efforts might be aimed" (p. 219). The phenomenological perspective was expressed succinctly by House (1981), who maintained that "social support is likely to be effective only to the extent perceived" (p. 27).

These researchers base their argument about the critical importance of perceived social support on several kinds of empirical evidence. First, perceptions of available social support have been found to relate only weakly to the amount of support received in a particular period (see review by Dunkel-Schetter & Bennett, 1990). Second, in studies that have examined both subjective and objective indicators of social support in relation to health outcomes, the subjective indicators often have exhibited stronger associations (e.g., Antonucci & Akiyama, 1987; Ward, Sherman, & La Gory, 1984). Research suggests, for example, that perceived social support more reliably buffers the adverse effects of life stress on psychological health than does received support (see reviews by Cohen & Wills, 1985; Kessler, 1992). Similarly, in a study that did not examine stress-buffering per se, Blazer (1982) found that perceived support was more strongly related to 30-month mortality in an elderly sample than were the frequency of interaction with friends and family or the existence of social ties (e.g., spouse, number of living children and siblings). Third, measures of perceived social support show impressive stability over time (Costa, Zonderman, & McCrae, 1985; Field & Minkler, 1988; Sarason et al., 1987), which should not be the case if such perceptions derive from dynamic, changing transactions with social network members (Vaux, 1992). Hence, perceptions of social support exhibit traitlike stability, leading some to propose that social support (particularly perceptions of being accepted and cared for by others) more closely resembles an enduring personality trait than a mirror of transactions occurring in the social environment (Sarason et al., 1990).

Considerable debate exists regarding the best interpretation of these empirical findings, and some researchers reject the inference that measures of received or enacted social support have limited utility (e.g., Vaux, 1992; Dunkel-Schetter & Bennett, 1990). Many of the studies that have found measures of perceived and received support to correlate weakly failed to determine the extent to which stress or other factors created needs for support (Dunkel-Schetter & Bennett, 1990; Ensel, 1991). It is doubtful that people attempt to access the full range of support perceived to be available through their social networks in the absence of a compelling reason to do so(e.g., the need to cope with a disruptive life event). Moreover, even in the context of a stressful situation, people may not seek to mobilize an entire network to assist with their coping efforts; rather, they may seek help selectively from a subset of their network ties, broadening their help-seeking efforts over time only as needed. Evidence for just such a hierarchical model of support seeking has emerged in studies of older adults (Cantor, 1979). From this perspective, measures of perceived support and received support would be expected to correlate weakly in many life contexts.

Additional research challenges the view that measures of received support rarely buffer people from the adverse effects of life stress. Studies in which large samples have been disaggregated to identify subsamples experiencing relatively homogeneous stressors have demonstrated that received support does buffer certain categories of stressors (e.g., Krause, 1986). Clear evidence of a buffering effect of received support emerged in a recent study of a representative sample of older adults that distinguished health-related from non-health-related stressors and that further distinguished support needed from support received (Ensel, 1991); received support alone did not predict well-being, but received support did predict well-being when considered in conjunction with the degree of need reported. In addition, stress-buffering studies that contrast baseline levels of perceived support and received support as predictors of subsequent adjustment to a stressor may not provide a fair test of the relative importance of the two types of support because baseline measures of received support fail to capture the support that may be mobilized once a stressor occurs (Alloway & Bebbington, 1987). Thus, some of the evidence that has been mustered to buttress the claim that measures of perceived support are superior to measures of received support may not bear up under close scrutiny.

The best interim resolution of this debate, given the available evidence, may be to conclude that perceived support and received support represent complementary, rather than competing, constructs that describe different facets of a genuinely complex problem (Schwarzer & Leppin, 1991; Vaux, 1992). Several psychometrically sound measures of both constructs have been used successfully with older adults.

Table 8.2 summarizes information about several different measures of perceived support that have been used with older adults. These measures assess respondents' views of the support resources available to them, as distinct from their evaluations of the adequacy of these resources (see preceding section on network evaluations). Some measures yield support subscales as well as an overall measure of support, but they vary in the particular kinds of support emphasized. Some measures emphasize respondents' perceptions of the number of people available to provide support, whereas others emphasize perceptions of the overall amount of support that can be expected from the network or the extent to which specific network members can be counted on to provide support when needed. The measures in Table 8.2 vary as well in length, suitability for questionnaire versus interview administration, and the extent to which they assess constructs other than support (e.g., network size and structure). The implications of these variations have not been fully explored in gerontological studies, although studies of young adults suggest that the measures correlate strongly despite variations in measure content and format (e.g., Sarason et al., 1987).

It should be noted that the methods of assessing social networks, described earlier, can also yield measures of the support perceived to be available from the network as a whole or from theoretically relevant subnetworks (e.g., the friend network vs. kin network). The set of name-eliciting questions used to define network membership can be structured so as to probe about specific types of support of interest to the researcher (e.g., emotional vs. instrumental support). Thus, although they are less often recognized as measures of perceived support, the methods of network assessment discussed previously should not be overlooked for their potential usefulness in assessing perceived support as well as network size and characteristics.

Measures of received support that have been used with older adults are summarized in Table 8.3. Like measures of perceived support, these measures vary in the extent to which they emphasize one or more distinct types of support, in their focus on the number of network members who provided support versus the frequency with which network members provided support, in their length, and in their suitability for questionnaire versus interview administration. In addition, measures of received support vary in the time frame specified for reporting occurrences of support (e.g., the past month or past 6 weeks). Ideally, the time frame specified should fit the problem under investigation (Cohen, 1988; Jacobsen, 1986). For example, researchers studying adaptation to stressful events occurring in the past month should probably assess support received during the same period (Krause, 1989). More generally, the time frame chosen should be neither so narrow as to exclude important instances of received support that may have occurred early in the course of adapting to a stressor nor so broad as to strain the limits of accurate recall.

Alpha coefficients are sometimes lower for measures of received support than for corresponding measures of perceived support (e.g., Rivera, Rose, Futterman, Lovett, & Gallagher-Thompson, 1991). Items assessing received support presumably tap the selective utilization of available support resources during a particular period of need and, as such, should not be expected to intercorrelate as highly as items assessing perceived (potential) support. Thus, indicators of reliability other than the conventional α coefficient become important in evaluating measures of received support.

Finally, in addition to deciding whether to assess perceived or received support and whether to differentiate among sources and types of support, researchers sometimes need to consider whether to assess general or stressor-specific support (i.e., support that has special relevance to particular tasks, transitions, or crises, O'Reilly, 1988). A measure of support that is specific to the respondent's life situation may be more useful than a general measure of support in some contexts. For example, Lopata (1979) studied the specific kinds of support needed by women who were coping with bereavement. Similarly, researchers studying compliance with diabetic treatment regimens among older adults have found it useful to assess both general and diabetes-specific support (e.g., Connell, Fisher, & Houston; 1992).

Companionship

A potentially important positive function of older adults' social ties that has received less attention than social support is companionship, or opportunities for pleasurable interaction and shared leisure. Stress researchers understandably have paid less attention to companionship than to problem-focused support, given their interest in social resources that aid adaptation to life stress. Yet people seek social

TABLE 8.2 Measures of Perceived Social Support Used with Older Adults

Measure	*Illustrative Studies Using this Measure*[a]	*Description*	*Reliability and Validity*[b]	*Comments*
Arizona Social Support Inventory Schedule (Barrera, 1981)[c,d,e,f]	Rivera et al., 1991; Thompson et al., 1993	For each of six types of support (material aid, physical assistance, intimate interaction, guidance, feedback, social participation), four questions identify who typically provides support, who provided support in the past month, how adequate the amount of support was, and how much support was needed; yields overall measure as well as subscales; interview or questionnaire format	Alphas = .33 for satisfaction and .52 for need; test-retest (2 days) $r = .88$ for network size; 74% overlap in supporters identified in retest; overall measure correlates in expected direction with psychological health	
Louisville Social Support Scale (Norris & Murrell, 1987)[c]	Kaniasty & Norris, 1993; Norris & Murrell, 1990	13 items assess the amount of contact with network members, feelings of closeness, and the amount of help expected to be available in an emergency from friends, family, and the community; interview format	Alpha = .82; test-retest (6 months) $r = .71$; measure correlates in expected direction with psychological health, self-esteem, and socioeconomic factors	Factor analyses have identified two subscales: social embeddedness, and support expectations
Norbeck Social Support Questionnaire (Norbeck et al., 1981)[c,d]	Auslander & Litwin, 1991	Respondent identifies up to 20 important social network members; 9 items assess which members could provide each of three types of support (affect, affirmation, aid); questionnaire format	Alphas = .69–.98; test-retest r's = .85–.92; measures correlate with other support measures; not confounded with social desirability	

Social Provisions Scale (Cutrona & Russell, 1987)	Cutrona et al., 1986; Connell et al., 1992; Felton & Berry, 1992; Holahan & Holahan, 1987; Mancini & Blieszner, 1992; Russell & Cutrona, 1991	24 items assess perceived access to each of six social provisions identified by Weiss (1974); designed to yield an overall measure of support as well as six subscales; interview format	Alpha for overall scale = .92; alphas for subscales = .64–.76; measures correlate with other support measures and with health outcomes; not confounded with social desirability	Subscale structure varies across studies; subscales intercorrelate highly; emotional and instrumental support subscales relate most strongly to health
Social Resources items in the Older Americans Resources and Services Instrument (Blazer, 1982)	Arling, 1987; Blazer, 1982; Roberts et al., 1994	11 items assess social roles and attachments, perceived social support, frequency of interaction with others; interview format	Predicts psychological distress (Arling, 1987; Roberts et al, 1994) and 30-month mortality (Blazer, 1982)	Part of a larger battery that assess older adults' functioning
Interview Schedule for Social Interaction (Henderson et al., 1980)[e]	Bergeman et al., 1990	52 items assess perceived availability and adequacy of attachment and social integration; interview format	Alpha = .67–.81; test-retest (18 days) $r = .75–.79$; measure exhibits predicted relation to psychological health; 9-item short form exhibits good psychometric properties (Bergeman et al., 1990)	
Social Networks in Adult Life Survey (see Table 8.1)[c]	see Table 8.1	6 items assess which network members could provide social support; interview format	see Table 8.1	
Social Network Inventory (see Table 8.1)[c]	see Table 8.1	12 items assess the number (and identities) of network members who could provide support and companionship; interview format		

[a]Gerontological studies
[b]Based on original validation research
[c]Also yields assessment of social network characteristics
[d]Also yields assessment of received support
[e]Also yields assessment of perceived adequacy of support
[f]Also yields assessment of conflict with network members

TABLE 8.3 Measures of Received Social Support Used with Older Adults

Measure	*Illustrative Studies Using this Measure*[a]	*Description*	*Reliability and Validity*[b]	*Comments*
Arizona Social Support Inventory Schedule (see Table 8.2)[c,d,e,f]	see Table 8.2	Questions identify people who provided six types of support in the past month; questionnaire format	see Table 8.2	Analyzed in terms of the number of people who provided support in a specified time period
Instrumental-Expressive Support Scale (Ensel & Woelfel, 1986)	Dean et al., 1989; Dean et al., 1990; Dean et al., 1992; Matt & Dean, 1993	26 items assess instrumental and expressive support received in past 6 months; yields overall measure as well as support subscales; sources of support are also distinguished (e.g., spouses, adult children, friends); interview format	Alphas = .89–.93; measures correlate in expected direction with psychological health	Analyzed in terms of frequency of receiving support within a specified time period
Inventory of Socially Supportive Behaviors (Barrera, 1981; Barrera et al., 1981)	Krause, 1986, 1987a, 1987b	40 items assess the frequency of receiving 4 types of support in the past month (emotional, informational, instrumental, socializing); interview format	Alpha = .93; test-retest (2 days) $r = .88$; correlates with other support measures and with emotional health	Subscale structure varies across studies; Krause (1986) adapted scale for use with older adults by extending the recall period, deleting items, and adding items that assess the provision of support to others
Norbeck Social Support Questionnaire (see Table 8.2)[ac,d]	see Table 8.2	Questions assess degree to which important social network members provided three types of support; questionnaire format	see Table 8.2	

[a]Gerontological studies
[b]Based on original validation research
[c]Also yields assessment of social network characteristics
[d]Also yields assessment of perceived support
[e]Also yields assessment of perceived adequacy of support
[f]Also yields assessment of conflict with network members

bonds not only for the aid and security they provide (Bowlby, 1977), but also for the intrinsic satisfactions they afford, such as shared recreation, humor, and fun (Gordon & Gaitz, 1976; Simmel, 1949, Weiss, 1974). The cultivation of the social environment to regulate affect, presumably including the production of positive affect, represents a central motive for social interaction, one that may become particularly important in late life (Carstensen, 1991).

Relatively few studies have explicitly differentiated companionship from support, and even fewer have done so with elderly samples. Nevertheless, the available evidence suggests that the two constructs can be meaningfully distinguished. Measures of social support and companionship (termed *belonging support*, *social participation*, or *social integration* in some studies) have been found to correlate only moderately (e.g., Rook, 1987), and items assessing these two constructs have formed separate factors in factor analyses of data from older adults (e.g., Mancini & Blieszner, 1992; Cutrona & Russell, 1987; Revicki & Mitchell, 1986) and younger age groups (e.g., Buunk, 1990; Wellman & Wortley, 1990).

Additional evidence suggests that companionship and social support make distinctive contributions to emotional health (Bolger & Eckenrode, 1991; Buunk, 1990; Haines & Hurlbert, 1992; Rook, 1987, 1990b) and friendship satisfaction (Fischer, 1982b; Hays, 1985). For example, companionship figured prominently as a source of relief from the burdens of caregiving in a recent study (Thompson, Futterman, Gallagher-Thompson, Rose, & Lovett, 1993). Comparisons of companionship and five types of social support revealed that companionship was most consistently related to the adaptational outcomes studied. Indeed, the five types of support studied were largely ineffectual in providing relief from caregiving burdens, leading the researchers to conclude that opportunities to socialize and engage in recreation with others more readily relieve emotional distress under conditions of chronic stress than do opportunities to obtain support. In a nationally representative sample of older adults, Steinbach (1992) found that a dichotomous measure of social activities (whether or not the participants had engaged in any of several social activities, such as visiting with friends or relatives, or going to a social event) predicted both the risk of institutionalization and mortality over a 2-year period, controlling for age, self-perceived health status, and other factors (cf. Berkman & Syme, 1979; Sugisawa et al., 1994). Similarly, social support and companionship exhibited differential associations with affect and life events (in this case, desirable events) in another longitudinal study of older adults (Murrell, Norris, & Chipley, 1992).

Further clues about the potential usefulness of assessing opportunities for companionship come from studies comparing the effects on older adults' morale of contact with friends versus family members. A surprising but robust finding from this research suggests that contact with family members contributes modestly or negligibly to older adults' morale, whereas contact with friends contributes significantly to morale (see review by Lee & Ishii-Kuntz, 1987). This difference has been attributed to the fact that family members routinely serve as support providers for older adults but less often serve as companions for leisure activities. Friends, in contrast, less often provide support to older adults but do function regularly as companions for leisure activities (e.g., Stoller & Earl, 1983). Larson, Mannell, and Zuzanek (1986) argued in this regard, "It is kin whom you confide in and count on; it is friends whom you enjoy" (p. 122). Consistent with this, research that has differentiated positive and negative affect suggests that older adults' contact with kin helps to relieve negative affect but does not foster positive affect, whereas contact with friends helps to foster positive but does little to alleviate negative affect (Lawton, 1983).

Thus, research provides evidence, albeit indirect, that companionship and social support may have different consequences for older adults' health and well-being (see also Connell et al., 1992; Kaniasty & Norris, 1993; Rook, 1990b). In addition, it suggests that some degree of relationship specialization tends to occur in older adults' social networks (cf. Felton & Berry, 1992; Litwak, 1985).

Assessment of Companionship: Existing Approaches. In contrast to the wide array of measures that have been developed to assess social support, far fewer measures have been developed to assess companionship. Some ad hoc measures have been developed (e.g., Buunk, 1990; Rook, 1987), which typically consist of items that assess the frequency with which respondents visit or are visited by others, chat by telephone, and take part in shared outings or activities. Companionship also appears as a subscale in some of the multidimensional measures of social support that have been used with older adults, as shown in Table 8.4.

As was true for measures of social support, measures of companionship can be worded to assess either companionship perceived to be available to the respondent or actually received (enacted) during a specified period of time. Similarly, some of the methodological complexities that arise in assessing enacted support arise in assessing enacted companionship. Alpha coefficients for measures of enacted companionship may be lower than corresponding coefficients for perceived companionship because the specific social activities undertaken to meet companionship needs within a particular time period (e.g, telephone calls, in-person visits, shared hobbies, joint outings) are apt to be less strongly intercorrelated than the set of social activities perceived to be potentially available though one's set network ties. In addition, the time frame specified by the measure requires consideration in the context of the goals of the study.

Social Control

Regulation by social network members, or social control, represents another little studied but potentially important health-related function of social ties (House et al., 1988, Rook, Thuras, & Lewis, 1990; Umberson, 1987). Social control exercised by social network members has the potential to protect health by dissuading target persons from engaging in health-damaging behaviors (e.g., smoking, excessive drinking, dangerous driving) and/or by encouraging target persons to engage in health-enhancing behaviors (e.g., exercise, sound dietary practices, compliance with prescribed medical regimens). Social control operates through network mem-

TABLE 8.4 Measures of Companionship Used with Older Adults

Measure	*Illustrative Studies Using this Measure*[a]	*Description*	*Reliability and Validity*[b]	*Comments*
Social Participation subscale of Arizona Social Support Inventory (see Table 8.2)[c]	see Table 8.2	Four questions about social participation (e.g., getting together to have fun or relax) assess who usually does this with the respondent, who did this in the past month, how adequate the amount of companionship was, how much companionship the respondent needed; questionnaire format	Subscale exhibits distinctive relation to emotional health outcomes (e.g., Thompson et al., 1993)	Can assess both companionship perceived to be available and companionship experienced in a specified time period
Social Integration subscale of the Social Provisions Scale (see Table 8.2)	see Table 8.2	Four items assess social integration (e.g., belonging to a group with similar interests, concerns, and recreational activities); interview format	Subscale alpha = .67; subscale exhibits distinctive relation to emotional health outcomes	Scale emphasizes companionship perceived to be available
Social Integration subscale of Expressive Support Scale (see Table 8.3)	Dean et al., 1989	Three items measure frequency of socializing, receiving visits, sharing meals with others in the past 6 months; sources of companionship are also distinguished (e.g., spouses, adult children, friends); interview format	Subscale alpha = .87; factor analyses support distinctiveness of this subscale from other support subscales	

[a]Gerontological studies
[b]Based on original validation research
[c]Also yields assessment of social network characteristics

bers' efforts to monitor, persuade, and reward or punish a focal person as well as through a focal person's self-restraint of risky behavior. Such self-restraint can be viewed as socially motivated to the extent that it arises from having important role obligations to others, obligations that would be compromised by engaging in unstable or self-destructive behavior (Umberson, 1987). For example, the parent of a young child may be motivated to refrain from substance abuse, at least in part, by the need to fulfill parental role responsibilities.

Interestingly, social control theorists postulate that social control has dual effects, deterring risky health practices while simultaneously provoking irritation or distress. "Constraint may be the source of considerable frustration; at the same time it tends to reduce the probability of problematic or maladaptive behaviors" (Hughes & Gove, 1981, p. 71). Attention to the hypothesized dual effects of social control may be of special interest to gerontologists because challenges to autonomy have been implicated as a source of tension in some studies of older adults' social relationships (e.g., Cicirelli, 1983; 1992).

Findings consistent with the social control perspective have appeared in studies that have contrasted people with different living arrangements (Hughes & Gove, 1981), marital statuses (Umberson, 1987, 1992), and parental statuses (Umberson, 1987). For example, married individuals have been found to engage in fewer health-compromising behaviors than unmarried individuals (e.g., Umberson, 1987), presumably because spouses can readily monitor and seek to influence the behavior of their partners.

Few studies, however, have attempted to examine social control processes directly. A preliminary effort to investigate social network-based social control in a small sample of community-residing older adults revealed that most participants could easily identify family members and friends who sought to influence or control their behavior, but the measures of social control exhibited few of the hypothesized associations with health risk taking and psychological distress (Rook, Thuras, & Lewis, 1990). In another sample, social role obligations predicted self-care behaviors among elderly diabetic women and metabolic control among elderly diabetic men (Connell et al., 1992).

Thus, empirical work on social control exercised by informal social networks, particularly in late life, is limited and not entirely consistent. Control and support, nevertheless, represent basic elements of many close relationships (Hogan, 1982; McAdams, 1988. Some research has linked social control to health behaviors and, in turn, health status. Thus, efforts to analyze the occurrence and conseqeunces of social control in older adults' lives appear warranted.

Assessment of Social Control: Existing Approaches. Approaches to measuring network-based social control that do not rely on comparisons of groups with different marital and/or parental statuses are sparse, as indicated by the limited number of entries in Table 8.5. Rook et al. (1990) embedded several questions about social control in a larger interview focused on older adults' social relationships. The

TABLE 8.5 Measures of Social Network-Based Control Used with Older Adults

Measure	*Illustrative Studies Using this Measure*[a]	*Description*	*Reliability and Validity*[b]	*Comments*
Social Control (Rook et al., 1990; approach adapted from Fischer, 1982a; see Table 8.1)[c]	Rook et al., 1990	Three questions identify persons who deter the respondent from unsound health practices and risky behaviors, prompt the respondent to engage in sound health practices, depend on the respondent on a regular basis for assistance or contact; no time frame specified; interview format	Individual items were weakly intercorrelated; items exhibited some expected associations with health behaviors and with marital status	Analyzed in terms of number of social control functions reported as well as number of persons involved in these control functions
Social Control (Umberson, 1992)	Umberson, 1992[d]	One item assesses how often people remind or tell the respondent to do something to protect his or her health; interview format	Measure exhibits some expected associations with health behaviors, gender, and marital status	Analyzed in terms frequency of exposure to social control attempts by others
Social Control (Lewis, 1992)	Lewis, 1992[d]	13 items assess how often network members seek to influence the respondent's health behaviors; subscales distinguish control attempts directed toward health-compromising versus health sources of control (e.g.,, spouse, family members, friends) are distinguished; questionnaire format	Alpha (overall scale) = .80; alpha for subscale focused on health-compromising behaviors = .65; alpha for subscale focused on health-enhancing behaviors = .75; exhibit some predicted associations with health behaviors and psychological distress	Analyzed in terms of average frequency of exposure to social control attempts by others

[a]Gerontological studies
[b]Based on original validation research
[c]Also yields assessment of social network characteristics
[d]Nongerontological study (included given scarcity of gerontological work)

brevity of this social control measure, however, undermines its psychometric properties and limits its usefulness in future research. In a recent study of a nationally representative sample of adults, Umberson (1992) assessed exposure to social control with a single question that asked how often others told or reminded the respondent to protect his/her health. Responses to this item covaried in the hypothesized direction with gender, marital status, and some health behaviors, but the potential unreliability of the single-item measure limits its potential usefulness. Lewis (1992) sought to improve upon these measurement approaches (albeit not with an elderly sample) by greatly expanding the number of items used to assess social control, by assessing social control in relation to a diverse set of health behaviors, and by distinguishing between social control aimed at the discontinuation of existing, health-compromising practices versus the initiation of new, health-enhancing practices. Her multi-item measures exhibited good psychometric properties and represent a distinct improvement over more abbreviated approaches, although their relevance to elderly samples remains to be determined. Moreover, neither Umberson (1992) nor Lewis (1992) attempted to assess the role obligations component of social control.

Social role obligations, particularly to vulnerable or dependent others (Umberson, 1987), presumably motivate adequate self-care and discourage risk taking so as not to jeopardize role performance. The association between social roles and health typically has been studied in early or middle adulthood, but evidence suggests that social roles continue to be consequential for health into late adulthood (e.g., Rushing et al., 1992; Antonucci, Akiyama, & Adelmann, 1990). Among older adults, however, some role obligations, such as those associated with caring for a disabled family member, entail so many burdens that self-care deteriorates rather than improves. Assessment of role obligations as a component of social control in late life, therefore, requires some special considerations. Both the number of roles that involve meaningful, ongoing obligations to others and the balance of rewards to burdens that such roles entail need to be evaluated. In addition, gerontologists should be alert to the possibility that social role obligations exhibit a curvilinear relationship to self-care, with both too few and too many obligations associated with deficient self-care.

More generally, the assessment of social network-based social control represents an area that is ripe for further development. There is a need for reliable and valid multi-item measures, suitable for use with older adults, that assess each of the theoretical components of the social control construct (deterrence of health-damaging behavior, promotion of health-enhancing behavior, role-motivated self-regulation of risk taking and self-care). Of particular importance are efforts to demonstrate that social control can be distinguished empirically from social support (an issue that has received little attention in existing studies) and efforts to assess exposure to social network-based social control through methods that do not rely solely on self-report. Self-reports of others' social control attempts are informative but may underestimate exposure to the extent that others employ subtle or artful influence strategies. Such control attempts may be effective but may go largely unnoticed by the target person, a phenomenon that been demonstrated in recent research on social support (Kessler, 1992). Moreover, informants' concerns about issues of control may lead to distorted reports of others' social control attempts. Measurement approaches that compare the perspectives of a focal person and one or more significant others would contribute greatly to our ability to assess and analyze social control processes in late life (cf. Antonucci & Israel, 1986).

Interpersonal Conflict and Stress

Social networks represent a source not only of support, companionship, and health-promoting social influence but also of conflict, disappointment, and, sometimes, health-damaging influence. Interest has grown in recent years in examining social ties as a source of distress, and much of this work has been conducted with older adults (see review by Rook, 1990a).

Measures of positive and negative interactions with social network members have been found to correlate only weakly or negligibly in many studies (see reviews by Barrera, Chassin, & Rogosch, 1993; Rook, 1990a), leading researchers to conclude that these represent relatively independent domains of social experience. Moderate inverse correlations have been reported in some studies that have assessed positive and negative exchanges within a particular dyadic relationship, such as a close network member (e.g., Abbey, Abramis, & Kaplan, 1985) or a family member (e.g., Barrera et al., 1993), but negligible correlations typically emerge when exchanges are aggregated across a set of relationships. Thus, knowledge of the extent to which an older person's social network provides social support and companionship tells us little about the extent to which the network may also generate tension and distress. This can be ascertained only by directly assessing the older person's negative as well as positive social network transactions.

Evidence suggests that negative exchanges detract significantly from older adults' well-being and, indeed, may be more consequential for well-being than positive exchanges. The results of studies that have assessed both negative and positive social exchanges have found negative exchanges to be related significantly to worse emotional health but have found positive exchanges to be related weakly or not significantly to emotional health (Rook, 1990a). Evidence of similar asymmetries has emerged in studies assessing dimensions of physical health, such as cardiovascular reactivity (e.g., Ewart, Taylor, Kraemer, & Agras, 1991) and immune function (Kiecolt-Glaser, Glaser, Gottman, Chee, & Malarkoy, 1992). The strong adverse effects of negative interaction reported in these studies do not appear to reflect a mere artifact of the participants' mental health or personality characteristics. Pagel, Erdly, and Becker (1987) demonstrated in a short-term longitudinal study of caregivers that negative social interactions predicted caregivers' depression at a 10-month follow-up. The study controlled for their initial depression levels as well as health and demographic factors (cf. Finch & Zautra,

1992). Moreover, baseline depression did not predict participants' subsequent reports of upsetting interactions. Effects of negative interactions have survived controls in other studies for neuroticism, extraversion, social desirability, physical health, and a variety of demographic characteristics (Finch & Zautra, 1992; Rook, 1992). Even if further research challenges the view that the detrimental effects of negative social interaction outweigh the beneficial effects of positive social interaction (Rook, 1992), a comprehensive understanding of the contributions to older adults' health of their social network involvement requires attention to the negative as well as the positive aspects of such involvement.

Assessment of Interpersonal Conflict and Stress: Existing Approaches. Approaches to measuring interpersonal conflict and stress that have been used with older adults are summarized in Table 8.6. As the entries in Table 8.6 indicate, the conceptualization of interpersonal conflict varies considerably across researchers, in part because efforts to develop theoretically meaningful taxonomies of negative social exchanges have lagged behind comparable efforts to develop taxonomies of supportive exchanges (Rook & Pietromonaco, 1987). Some have focused specifically on supportive transactions that go awry (e.g., Fiore, Becker, & Coppel, 1983), such as well-intentioned efforts to convey sympathy that aggravate rather than alleviate the recipient's distress (Wortman & Lehman, 1985). Other researchers have focused on diverse negative interactions (not limited to those arising from efforts to provide social support), such as criticism, exploitation, demands, betrayals, and invasion of privacy (e.g., Finch et al., 1989; Hansson, 1990; Krause & Jay, 1991; Rook, 1984). Research also implicates being let down by others in times of need (i.e., others' failure to provide expected support) as a factor that contributes to depression among older adults experiencing life stress (e.g., Dean et al., 1990). Such disappointments regarding expected support may have special relevance to older adults, given that many of the stressors with which older adults must contend are chronic in nature (Stephens, 1990) and that social support often erodes over time in the face of chronic stressors (e.g., Kaniasty & Norris, 1993).

In one of the first attempts to develop an empirically based taxonomy of negative social exchanges, Ruehlman and Karoly (1991) asked young adults to rate how often they had experienced each of 45 negative social exchanges on a list designed to reflect a broad range of negative experiences. Factor analyses of these ratings yielded four distinct and psychometrically sound factors: Hostility/Impatience, Insensitivity, Interference, and Criticism/Ridicule.

These factors dovetail fairly well with the categories of negative exchanges assessed in studies of older adults (see Table 8.6), although some researchers have also urged attention to negative social control, or social pressures and inducements by network members to engage in unhealthy rather than healthy behaviors (e.g., Antonucci, 1985; Rook & Pietromonaco, 1987). For example, whether intentionally or unintentionally, some older adults' family members and friends undoubtedly encourage excessive alcohol consumption or noncompliance with treatment regimens. Similarly, overly solicitous family members may interfere with older adults' efforts to recover from strokes or other disabling conditions by reinforcing complaints and dependent behavior (Kaplan & Toshima, 1990). Additionally, although social control theorists have tended to view social role obligations as promoting stable functioning and self-care, some role obligations in late life clearly have the potential to compromise health and self-care, as suggested by the substantial literature on caregiving strain (e.g., Cantor, 1983).

Comprehensive and psychometrically sound scales for use with older adults are only beginning to emerge, but the work just discussed suggests the following categories of negative exchanges that might usefully be assessed: support failures (e.g., clumsy gestures of support, failure to provide expected support), hostility/impatience, insensitivity and violations of trust, interference (e.g., intrusion into personal plans, invasion of privacy), criticism/ridicule, demands, and negative social control. Moreover, as has been true in studying social support (Felton & Berry, 1992; Dean et al., 1990), it may be useful to differentiate among spouses, adult children, other kin, and friends as sources of negative exchanges (Kaniasty & Norris, 1993; Krause & Jay, 1991).

Summary of Relational Content Measurement

As this brief review indicates, researchers who wish to assess the content and context of social network transactions that influence older adults' health and well-being face a number of difficult decisions for which the existing literature cannot as yet offer unambiguous guidance. Nonetheless, the research reviewed in these sections provides a basis for offering several tentative recommendations. First, it seems reasonable to propose that studies aimed at a general evaluation of the health-related effects of older adults' social ties should investigate positive as well as negative exchanges that older adults experience with others. Within the broad category of positive exchanges, attention to emotional support and instrumental support seems warranted, as does attention to companionship. Assessment of social control may be appropriate in studies that have a special focus on health behaviors (including preventive behaviors, high-risk behaviors, routine self-care, and compliance with treatment regimens). Within the broad category of negative exchanges, more theoretical and empirical work is needed to identify the kinds of exchanges that warrant assessment, but the work described above suggests that attention should be directed to support failures, hostility, insensitivity, interference, demands, criticism, and negative social control.

Finally, researchers who wish to analyze specific sources of support and conflict should heed House and Kahn's (1985) advice to use a measurement strategy that avoids confounding the number of positive and negative functions performed by the network and the number of people performing the functions. Researchers can then disentangle, for example, the effects of the number of conflictual exchanges

TABLE 8.6 Measures of Interpersonal Conflict and Stress Used with Older Adults

Measure	*Illustrative Using Studies this Measure*[a]	*Description*	*Reliability and Validity*[b]	*Comments*
Negative Social Ties (Finch et al., 1989; approach adapted from Fischer, 1982a, see Table 8.1)[d]	Finch et al., 1989; Finch & Zautra, 1992	Four questions identify number of people who were sources of negative experiences for the respondent in the past 6 months (criticize, break promises, take advantage of respondent, consistently provoke feelings of anger); interview format	Alpha = .79; test-retest (6 months), $r = .77$; factorial independence of measures of conflict and support well established; measure is not confounded with emotionality; measure correlates in expected direction with emotional health	Analyzed in terms of number of people who were a source of problems in a defined period of time
Problematic Social Ties and Exchanges (Rook, 1984; approach adapted from Fischer, 1982a, see Table 8.1)[c,d]	Rook, 1984	Five questions identify persons who are sources of negative experiences for the respondent (criticize, break promises, take advantage of respondent, invade privacy, provoke feelings of anger); no time frame specified; interview format	Measure correlates in expected direction with emotional health	Analyzed in terms of number of interpersonal problems, number of problematic network members, and frequency of contact with these network members; distinguishes network members who are a source of problems only from those who are a source of support and problems
Social Network Upset (Fiore et al., 1983; adapted from Hirsch, 1980)[c,d]	Fiore et al., 1983 Kiecolt-Glaser et al., 1988 Pagel et al., 1987	Respondents rate how upsetting (and how helpful) network members were with respect to five categories of social support (emotional support, tangible aid, cognitive guidance, self-disclosure, socializing); interview format	Measure is not confounded with social desirability; measure correlates in expected direction with depression	Analyzed in terms of average upsettingness of network interactions

Negative Interaction (approach adapted from Fischer, 1982a, see Table 8.1; Stephens et al., 1987)[c,d]	Norris et al., 1990; Stephens et al., 1987	10 questions identify persons who are sources of unhelpful and unwanted interactions in the past 2 months (e.g., unwanted advice or assistance) also assesses frequency of occurrence; interview format	Alpha = .67; test-retest (1 week) $r = .77$; measure correlates with morale and psychiatric symptoms	Analyzed in terms of average frequency of occurrence or number of social problems reported
Social Undermining (Vinokur & van Ryan, 1992; approach adapted from Abbey et al., 1985)[d]	Vinokur & Vinokur-Kaplan 1990	Six items assess how often the spouse (significant other) acts angry or unpleasant, makes life difficult, shows (s)he dislikes the respondent, makes the respondent feel unwanted, gets on the respondent's nerves, criticizes the respondent; six parallel items ask how often the respondent exhibits these negative behaviors toward the spouse (significant other); interview format	Alphas = .84–.86; measure predicts depression; husbands' and wives' reports of undermining by the spouse show moderate convergence (r's = .36–.58)	Emphasizes interactions that undermine sense of self-worth; typically assessed within marital relationships (or relationships involving significant others)
Negative Social Ties (Okun et al., 1990)[d]	Okun et al., 1990	One question asks respondents to identify people who make them feel very bad, unhappy, upset, or angry in the past 6 months; respondents also rate the quality of the interaction (from "terrific" to "terrible") for each person identified; interview format	Measure exhibits expected relationship to emotional health	Analyzed in terms of proportion of network members who were sources of negative interactions
Interpersonal Stress (Suitor & Pillemer, 1993; approach adapted from Fischer, see Table 8.1)[c,d]	Suitor & Pillemer, 1993	Five questions identify persons who created stress for caregivers by criticizing them, making care giving harder, failing to provide support, neglecting them, complaining about insufficient contact; sources of interpersonal stress are distinguished; interview format		Emphasizes interpersonal problems experienced by caregivers (cf. Poulshock & Deimling, 1984)

[a]Gerontological studies
[b]Based on original validation research
[c]Additional items yield assessment of social network characteristics
[d]Additional items yield assessment of perceived or received support

an older person experiences from the effects of the number of people with whom the older person engages in such exchanges.

NETWORK EVALUATIONS

Assessing older adults' evaluations of their social network ties and interactions represents another vantage point from which to investigate the health-related effects of social relationships in late life. Objective aspects of social network involvement typically exhibit only modest associations with subjective appraisals of such involvement (Dunkel-Schetter & Bennett, 1990); This curious finding motivates inquiry into each of the two domains separately and in relation to each other. Moreover, evaluations of the adequacy of existing support resources have been found to predict mortality in an elderly sample, independent of the number of social ties and frequency of social interaction (Blazer, 1982). For some researchers, such evidence makes the assessment and analysis of network evaluations of paramount importance.

Assessment of Network Evaluations: Existing Approaches. Approaches to assessing network evaluations generally reflect one of three emphases (Vaux, 1992): evaluations of the quantity of support and companionship available, evaluations of the quality of support and companionship available, and ratings of the overall satisfaction with the existing network ties or contacts. In addition, measures of loneliness represent another, closely related, form of global network evaluation, one that captures explicit feelings of disappointment with the existing network and a yearning for more contact. These emphases appear in several measurement approaches that have been used with older adults (see Table 8.7).

As indicated in Table 8.7, some measures direct respondents to evaluate the adequacy of their social network resources, ties, or contacts within a specified time period (e.g., Krause, 1989), whereas other measures call for more open-ended evaluations (e.g., Procidano & Heller, 1983). Some measures ask respondents to make their evaluations with reference to specific categories of network members (e.g., Procidano & Heller, 1983), whereas others essentially ask respondents to evaluate the network at large. Moreover, although the measures shown in Table 8.7 do not solicit evaluations of the quantity or quality of specific kinds of social provisions, such as emotional support or instrumental support, some measures used with younger age groups incorporate such differentiated evaluations (see review by Vaux, 1992). Measures of network evaluations used with elderly populations could be similarly adapted if such differentiation represented an important research goal.

CONCLUSION

This chapter has taken a deliberately broad view of the health-related aspects of older adults' informal social relationships, one that recognizes social relationships as a

Measure	*Illustrative Studies Using this Measure*[a]	*Description*	*Reliability and Validity*[b]	*Comments*
Satisfaction with Social Support (Krause et al., 1989)	Krause et al., 1989	Items assess whether or not respondent was satisfied with amount of support received in past month for each of three types of support (emotional, informational, tangible); interview format	Measure of satisfaction with support received predicts depression longitudinally	Measure emphasizes evaluation of quantity of support received
Perceived Social Support, Friend and Family Scales (Procidano & Heller, 1983)	Heller et al., 1991 Heller & Mansbach, 1984	20 items assess perceived supportiveness of friends; 20 items assess perceived supportiveness of family members; designed to yield two scales; questionnaire format	Alphas = .88–.90; test-retest (1 month) $r = .83$; factor analyses indicate unidimensional structure of each scale; scales correlate in expected direction with emotional health and with verbal behaviors (e.g., disclosure) assessed in the laboratory	Measure emphasizes evaluation of quality (helpfulness) of support resources; dichotomous scoring makes measure more sensitive to low-to-moderate range of support
Social Network Satisfaction (Pagel et al., 1987; approach adapted from Hirsch, 1980)[c]	Pagel et al., 1987	Items ask respondents to rate their overall satisfaction with the network as a whole on five dimensions (emotional support, tangible aid, cognitive guidance, self-disclosure, socializing)	Factor analysis suggests unidimensional structure; measure exhibits expected association with emotional health	Measure emphasizes overall satisfaction with the network
UCLA Loneliness Scale (Russell et al., 1980)	Cutrona et al., 1986; Hansson et al., 1986–87; Mullins et al., 1987; Rook, 1984	20 items assess how often the respondent feels isolated and misunderstood, how often (s)he wishes (s)he knew more people, etc.; interview or questionnaire format	Alpha = .90 or better for various populations; measure correlates in expected direction with number of social contacts and emotional health; discriminates from unrelated constructs (e.g., anxiety, embarrassment); 4-item short form of the scale also exhibits good psychometric properties	Measure emphasizes dissatisfaction with the current network and a yearning for more social contact

[a]Gerontological studies [b]Based on original validation research [c]Additional items yield assessment of network support and problems

source of support and companionship (positive) as well as of conflict and control (negative). This broad view has included, as well, attention both to objective dimensions of older adults' social network involvement (e.g., number and structure of network ties, frequency of contact, range of network resources available) and subjective dimensions (perceived adequacy/helpfulness of network ties, contacts, and resources). Such breadth seems essential in order to reflect the myriad streams of research that converge, often from very different theoretical perspectives, in suggesting that informal social ties influence older adults' health and well-being.

Taking such a broad view, however, necessarily defies simple or straightforward recommendations about optimal assessment strategies. Moreover, gerontologists have not yet amassed the kind of comparative data base that would substantiate strong claims about the relative merits of alternative measurement approaches. This chapter has tried to identify some of the key dimensions that researchers might wish to assess in studying the health implications of older adults' social relationships and has illustrated current strategies for assessing these dimensions. Future studies, particularly those that take on the arduous but critically important task of comparing the strengths and weaknesses of current measurement approaches, will provide researchers with a firmer empirical foundation upon which to base their assessment decisions. Ultimately, the choice of a measurement strategy must be guided by the specific objectives of a given research project. Such choices are apt to be less bewildering and more successful to the extent that they are linked to a clear conceptual model of the direct and indirect pathways by which interpersonal processes influence older adults' health and well-being. Fortunately, the emerging literature on social network involvement and health offers a rich array of conceptual models (e.g., Barrera, 1986; Burman & Margolin, 1992; Cohen, 1988; House et al., 1988; Lin, 1986; Schwarzer & Leppin, 1991; Wheaton, 1985). These models should help to guide our research questions and, consequently, our assessment efforts for many years to come.

REFERENCES

Abbey, A., Abramis, D. J., & Caplan, R. D. (1985). Effects of different sources of social support and social conflict on emotional well-being. *Basic and Applied Social Psychology, 6*, 111–129.

Alloway, R., & Bebbington, P. (1987). The buffer theory of social support: A review of the literature. *Psychological Medicine, 17*, 91–108.

Anderson, T. B., & McCulloch, B. J. (1993). Conjugal support: Factor structure for husbands and wives. *Journal of Gerontology: Social Sciences, 48*, S133–S142.

Antonucci, T.C. (1985). Personal characteristics, social support, and social behavior. In R. H. Binstock & E. Shanas (Eds.), *Handbook of aging and the social sciences* (2nd ed.) (pp. 94–128). New York: Van Nostrand-Reinhold.

Antonucci, T. C. (1990). Social supports and social relationships. In R. H. Binstock & L. K.

George (Eds.), *Handbook of aging and the social sciences* (pp. 205–226). San Diego: Academic Press.

Antonucci, T. C., & Akiyama, H. (1987). Social networks in adult life and a preliminary examination of the convoy model. *Journal of Gerontology, 42*, 519–527.

Antonucci, T. C., Akiyama, H., & Adelmann, P. (1990). Health behaviors and social roles among mature men and women. *Journal of Aging and Health, 2*, 3–14.

Antonucci, T. C., & Israel, B. A. (1986). Veridicality of social support: A comparison of principal and network members' responses. *Journal of Consulting and Clinical Psychology, 54*, 432–437.

Arling, G. (1987). Strain, social support, and distress in old age. *Journal of Gerontology, 42*, 107–113.

Auslander, G. K., & Litwin, H. (1991). Social networks, social support, and self-ratings of health among the elderly. *Journal of Aging and Health, 3*, 493–510.

Barrera, M., Jr. (1981). Social support in the adjustment of pregnant adolescents: Assessment issues. In B. H. Gottlieb (Ed.), *Social networks and social support* (pp. 69–96). Beverly Hills, CA: Sage.

Barrera, M., Jr. (1986). Distinctions between social support concepts, measures, and models. *American Journal of Community Psychology, 14*, 413–446.

Barrera, M., Jr., Chassin, L., & Rogosch, F. (1993). Effects of social support and conflict on adolescent children of alcoholic and nonalcoholic fathers. *Journal of Personality and Social Psychology, 64*, 602–612.

Barrera, M. Jr., Sandler, I. N., & Ramsay, T. B. (1981). Preliminary development of a scale of social support: Studies on college students. *American Journal of Community Psychology, 9*, 435–443.

Bergeman, C. S., Plomin, R., Pedersen, N. L., McClearn, G. E., & Nesselroade, J. R. (1990). Genetic and environmental influences on social support: The Swedish adoption/twin study of aging. *Journal of Gerontology: Psychological Sciences, 45*, P101–P106.

Berkman, L. F., & Syme, L. S. (1979). Social networks, host resistance, and mortality: A nine-year follow-up study of Alameda County residents. *American Journal of Epidemiology, 109*, 186–204.

Blazer, D. G. (1982). Social support and mortality in an elderly community population. *American Journal of Epidemiology, 115*, 684–694.

Bolger, N., & Eckenrode, J. (1991). Social relationships, personality, and anxiety during a major stressful event. *Journal of Personality and Social Psychology, 61*, 440–449.

Bowlby, J. (1977). The making and breaking of affectional bonds. I. Aetiology and psychopathology in the light of attachment theory. *British Journal of Psychiatry, 130*, 201–210.

Bryant, S., & Rakowski, W. (1992). Predictions of mortality among elderly African-Americans. *Research on Aging, 14*, 50–67.

Burman, B., & Margolin, G. (1992). Analysis of the association between marital relationships and health problems: An interactional perspective. *Psychological Bulletin, 112*, 39–63.

Buunk, B. (1990). Affiliation and helping interactions within organizations: A critical analysis of the role of social support with regard to occupational stress. In W. Stroebe & M. Hewstone (Eds.), *European review of social psychology* (Vol. 1, pp. 293–322). Chichester, England: Wiley.

Cantor, M. H. (1979). Neighbors and friends: An overlooked resource in the informal support system. *Research on Aging, 1*, 434–463.

Cantor, M. H. (1983). Strain among caregivers: A study of experience in the United States. *The Gerontologist, 23*, 597–604.

Carstensen, L. (1991). Selectivity theory: Social activity in life-span context. In K. W. Schaie. (Ed.), *Annual review of gerontology and geriatrics*, 11, (195–217). New York: Springer.

Cicirelli, V. G. (1983). Adult children's attachment and helping behavior to elderly parents: A path model. *Journal of Marriage and the Family, 45*, 815–824.

Cicirelli, V. G. (1992). *Family caregiving: Autonomous and paternalistic decision making*. Newbury Park, CA: Sage.

Cohen, S. (1988). Psychosocial models of the role of social support in the etiology of physical disease. *Health Psychology, 7*, 269–297.

Cohen, S., & McKay, G. (1984). Social support, stress and the buffering hypothesis: A theoretical analysis. In A. Baum, S. E. Taylor, & J. E. Singer (Eds.), *Handbook of psychology and health* (pp. 253–267). Hillsdale, NJ: Erlbaum.

Cohen, C., Teresi, J., & Holmes, D. (1985). Social networks, stress, and physical health: A longitudinal study of an inner-city elderly population. *Journal of Gerontology, 40*, 478–486.

Cohen, C., Teresi, J., & Holmes, D. (1988). The physical well-being of old homeless men. *Journal of Gerontology: Social Sciences, 43*, S121–S128.

Cohen, C., Teresi, J., Holmes, D., & Roth, E. (1988). Survival strategies of older homeless men. *The Gerontologist, 28*, 58–65.

Cohen, S., & Wills, T. A. (1985). Stress, social support, and the buffering hypothesis. *Psychological Bulletin, 98*, 310–357.

Connell, C. M., Fisher, E. B. Jr., & Houston, C. A. (1992). Relationships among social support, diabetes outcomes, and morale among older men and women. *Journal of Aging and Health, 4*, 77–100.

Costa, P. T., Zonderman, A. B., & McCrae, R. R. (1985). Longitudinal course of social support among men in the Baltimore Longitudinal Study of Aging. In I. G. Sarason & B. R. Sarason (Eds.), *Social support: Theory, research, and applications* (pp. 136–154). Dordrecht, the Netherlands: Martinus Nijhoff.

Cutrona, C. E., & Russell, D. W. (1987). The provisions of social relationships and adaptation to stress. In W. H. Jones & D. Perlman (Eds.), *Advances in personal relationships* (Vol. 1, pp. 37–67). Greenwich, CT: JAI Press.

Cutrona, C. E., Russell, D. W., & Rose, J. (1986). Social support and adaptation to stress by the elderly. *Psychology and Aging, 1*, 47–54.

Dean, A., Kolody, B., & Wood, P. (1990). Effects of social support from various sources on depression in elderly persons. *Journals of Health and Social Behavior, 31*, 148–161.

Dean, A., Kolody, B., Wood, P., & Ensel, W. (1989). Measuring the communication of social support from adult children. *Journal of Gerontology: Social Sciences, 44*, S71–S79.

Dean, A., Kolody, B., Wood, P., & Matt, G. E. (1992). The influence of living alone on depression in elderly persons. *Journal of Aging and Health, 4*, 3–18.

DeLongis, A., & O'Brien, T. (1990). An interpersonal framework for stress and coping: An application to the families of Alzheimer's patients. In M. A. P. Stephens, J. H. Crowther, S. E. Hobfoll, & D. L. Tennenbaum (Eds.), *Stress and coping in later-life families* (pp. 221–239). New York: Hemisphere.

Depner, C. E., & Ingersoll-Dayton, B. (1988). Supportive relationships in later life. *Psychology and Aging, 3*, 348–357.

Dunkel-Schetter, C., & Bennett, T. L. (1990). Differentiating the cognitive and behavioral aspects of social support. In B. R. Sarason, I. G. Sarason, & G. R. Pierce (Eds.), *Social support: An interactional view* (pp. 267–296). New York: Wiley.

Durkheim, E. (1951). *Suicide: A study in sociology.* (J. Spaulding & G. Simpson, Trans.). New York: Free Press. (Original work published 1897)

Ensel, W. M. (1991). "Important" life events and depression among older adults: The role of psychological and social resources. *Journal of Aging and Health, 3*, 546–566.

Ensel, W. M., & Woelfel, M. (1986). Measuring the instrumental and expressive functions of social support. In N. Lin, A. Dean, & W. M. Ensel (Eds.), *Social support, life events, and depression* (pp. 129–151). Orlando, FL: Academic Press.

Ewart, C. K., Taylor, C. B., Kraemer, H. C., & Agras, W. S. (1991). High blood pressure and marital discord: Not being nasty matters more than being nice. *Health Psychology, 10*, 155–163.

Felton, B. J. & Berry, C. A. (1992). Do the sources of the urban elderly's social support determine its psychological consequences? *Psychology and Aging, 7*, 89–97.

Field, D., & Minkler, M. (1988). Continuity and change in social support between young-old and old-old or very-old age. *Journals of Gerontology: Psychological Sciences, 43*, P100–P106.

Finch, J. F., & Zautra, A. J. (1992). Testing latent longitudinal models of social ties and depression among the elderly: A comparison of distribution-free and maximum likelihood estimates with nonnormal data. *Psychology and Aging, 7*, 107–18.

Finch, J. F., Okun, M. A., Barrera, M. Jr., Zautra, A. J., & Reich, J. W. (1989). Positive and negative social ties among older adults: Measurement models and the prediction of psychological distress and well-being. *American Journal of Community Psychology, 17*, 585–605.

Fiore, J., Becker, J., & Coppel, D. (1983). Social network interactions: A buffer or a stress? *American Journal of Community Psychology, 11*, 423–439.

Fischer, C. S. (1982a). *To dwell among friends: Personal networks in town and city.* Chicago: University of Chicago Press.

Fischer, C. S. (1982b). What do we mean by "friend"? *Social Networks, 3*, 287–306.

Gordon, C., & Gaitz, C. M. (1976). Leisure and lives: Personal expressivity across the life span. In R. H. Binstock & E. Shanas (Eds.), *Handbook of aging and the social sciences* (pp. 310–341). New York: Van Nostrand Reinhold.

Gove, W. (1973). Sex, marital status, and mortality. *American Journal of Sociology, 79*, 45–67.

Gove, W., Hughes, M., & Style, C. B. (1983). Does marriage have positive effects on the psychological well-being of the individual? *Journal of Health and Social Behavior, 24*, 122–131.

Granovetter, M. (1973). The strength of weak ties. *American Journal of Sociology, 78*, 1361–1380.

Haines, V. A., & Hurlbert, J. S. (1992). Network range and health. *Journal of Health and Social Behavior, 33*, 254–266.

Hall, A., & Wellman, B. (1985). Social networks and social support. In S. Cohen & S. L. Syme (Eds.), *Social support and health* (pp. 23–41). Orlando, FL: Academic Press.

Hansson, R. O. (1990). Troubled relationships in later life: Implications for support. *Journal of Social and Personal Relationships, 7*, 451–463.

Hansson, R. O., Jones, W. H., Carpenter, B. N., & Remondet, J. H. (1986–87). Loneliness and adjustment to old age. *International Journal of Aging and Human Development, 24*, 41–53.

Hays, R. B. (1985). A longitudinal study of friendship development. *Journal of Personality and Social Psychology, 48*, 909–924.

Heller, K., & Mansbach, W. E. (1984). The multifaceted nature of social support in a community sample of elderly women. *Journal of Social Issues, 40*, 99–112.

Heller, K., Thompson, M. G., Trueba, P. E., Hogg, J. R., & Vlachos-Weber, I. (1991). Peer support telephone dyads for elderly women: Was this the wrong intervention? *American Journal of Community Psychology, 19*, 53–74.

Heitzmann, C. A., & Kaplan, R. M. (1988). Assessment of methods for measuring social support. *Health Psychology, 7*, 75–109.

Henderson, S., Duncan-Jones, P., Byren, D. G., & Scott, R. (1980). Measuring social relationships: The Interview Schedule for Social Interaction. *Psychological Medicine, 10*, 723–734.

Hirsch, B. J. (1980). Natural support systems and coping with major life changes. *American Journal of Community Psychology, 8*, 159–172.

Hogan, R. (1982). A socioanalytic theory of personality. In M. Page (Ed.), *Nebraska Symposium on Motivation* (pp. 58–89). Lincoln, NE: Univ. of Nebraska.

Holahan, C. K., & Holahan, C. J. (1987). Self-efficacy, social support, and depression in aging: A longitudinal analysis. *Journal of Gerontology, 42*, 65–68.

House, J. S. (1981). *Work stress and social support.* Reading, MA: Addison-Wesley.

House, J. S., & Kahn, R. L. (1985). Measures and concepts of social support. In S. Cohen & S. L. Syme (Eds.), *Social support and health* (pp. 83–108). Orlando, FL: Academic Press.

House, J. S., Umberson, D., & Landis, K. (1988). Structures and processes of social support. *Annual Review of Sociology, 14*, 293–318.

Hughes, M., & Gove, W. R. (1981). Living alone, social integration, and mental health. *American Journal of Sociology, 87*, 48–74.

Jacobson, D. E. (1986). Types and timing of social support. *Journal of Health and Social Behavior, 27*, 250–264.

Johnson, T. P. (1991). Mental health, social relations, and social selection: A longitudinal analysis. *Journal of Health and Social Behavior, 32*, 408–423.

Kahn, R. L., & Antonucci, T. C. (1980). Convoys over the life course: Attachment, roles, and social support. In P. B. Baltes & O. G. Brim (Eds.), *Life-span development and behavior* (pp. 253–286). New York: Academic Press.

Kaniasty, K., & Norris, F. H. (1993). A test of the social support deterioration model in the context of natural disaster. *Journal of Personality and Social Psychology, 64*, 395–408.

Kaplan, R. M., & Toshima, M. T. (1990). The functional effects of social relationships on chronic illness and disability. In B. R. Sarason, I. G. Sarason, & G. R. Pierce (Eds.), *Social support: An interactional view* (pp. 427–453). New York: Wiley.

Kessler, R. (1992). Perceived support and adjustment to stress: Methodological considerations. In H. O. F. Veiel & U. Baumann (Eds.), *The meaning and measurement of social support* (pp. 259–271). Washington, DC: Hemisphere.

Kessler, R. C., McLeod, J. D., & Wethington, E. (1985). The costs of caring: A perspective on the relationship between sex and psychological distress. In I. G. Sarason & B. R. Sarason (Eds.), *Social support: Theory, research and applications* (pp. 491–506). Dordrecht, the Netherlands: Martinus Nijhoff.

Kiecolt-Glaser, J. K., Dyer, C. S., & Shuttleworth, E. C. (1988). Upsetting social interactions and distress among Alzheimer's disease family caregivers: A replication and extension. *American Journal of Community Psychology, 16*, 825–837.

Kiecolt-Glaser, J. K., Glaser, R., Gottman, J., Chee, M. A., & Malarkoy, W. (1992, July). *Immunological consequences of marital discord.* Paper presented at the biennial meeting of the International Society for the Study of Personal Relationships, Orono, ME. Krause, N. (1986). Social support, stress, and well–being among older adults. *Journal of Gerontology, 41*, 512–519.

Krause, N. (1987a). Chronic financial strain, social support, and depressive symptoms among older adults. *Psychology and Aging, 2*, 185–192.

Krause, N. (1987b). Understanding the stress process: Linking social support with locus of control beliefs. *Journal of Gerontology, 42*, 589–593.

Krause, N. (1989). Issues of measurement and analysis in studies of social support, aging, and health. In K. S. Markides & C. L. Cooper (Eds.), *Aging, stress and health* (pp. 43–66). New York: Wiley.

Krause, N., & Jay, G. (1991). Stress, social support, and negative interaction in later life. *Research on Aging, 13*, 333–363.

Krause, N., Liang, J., & Yatomi, N. (1989). Satisfaction with social support and depressive symptoms: A panel analysis. *Psychology and Aging, 4*, 88–97.

Larson, R., Mannell, R., & Zuzanek, J. (1986). Daily well-being of older adults with friends and family. *Psychology and Aging, 1*, 117–126.

Lawton, M. P. (1983). The varieties of well-being. *Experimental Aging Research, 9*, 65–72.

Lawton, M. P., & Moss, M. (1987). The social relationships of older adults. In E. F. Borgatta & R. J. V. Montgomery (Eds.), *Critical issues in aging policy: Linking research and values* (pp. 92–126). Newbury Park, CA: Sage.

Lee, G. R., & Ishii-Kuntz, M. (1987). Social interaction, loneliness, and emotional well-being among the elderly. *Research on Aging, 9*, 459–482.

Levitt, M. J., Weber, R. A., & Guacci, N. (1993). Convoys of social support: An intergenerational analysis. *Psychology and Aging, 8*, 323–326.

Lewis, M. A. (1992). *The influence of social control on health behaviors and psychological distress*. Unpublished doctoral dissertation, University of California, Irvine. (University Microfilm No. 934100).

Lin, N. (1986). Modeling the effects of social support. In N. Lin, A. Dean, & W. M. Ensel (Eds.), *Social support, life events, and depression* (pp. 173–209). Orlando, FL: Academic Press.

Litwak, E. (1985). *Helping the elderly: The complementary roles of informal networks and formal systems*. New York: Guilford.

Litwak, E., & Messeri, P. (1989). Organizational theory, social supports, and mortality rates: A theoretical convergence. *American Journal of Sociology, 54*, 49–67.

Lopata, H. Z. (1979). *Women as widows: Support systems*. New York: Elsevier.

Mancini, J. A., & Blieszner, R. (1992). Social provisions in adulthood: Concept and measurement in close relationships. *Journal of Gerontology: Psychological Sciences, 47*, P14–P20.

Marsden, P. V. (1990). Network data and measurement. *Annual Review of Sociology, 16*, 435–463.

Matt, G. E., & Dean, A. (1993). Social support from friends and psychological distress among elderly persons: Moderator effects of age. *Journal of Health and Social Behavior, 34*, 187–200.

Maton, K. I. (1989). Community settings as buffers of life stress? Highly supportive churches, mutual help groups, and senior centers. *American Journal of Community Psychology, 17*, 203–232.

McAdams, D. P. (1988). Personal needs and personal relationships. In S. Duck (Ed.), *Handbook of personal relationships* (pp. 7–22). Chichester, England: Wiley.

McCallister, L., & Fischer, C. S. (1978). A procedure for surveying personal networks. *Sociological Methods and Research* , *7*, 131–148.

Milardo, R. (1988). Families and social networks: An overview of theory and methodology. In R. Milardo (Ed.), *Families and social networks* (pp. 13–47). Newbury Park, CA: Sage.

Monroe, S. M., & Johnson, S. L. (1992). Social support, depression, and other mental disorders: In retrospect and toward future prospects. In H. O. F. Veiel & U. Baumann (Eds.), *The meaning and measurement of social support* (pp. 93–105). Washington, DC: Hemisphere.

Mullins, L. C., Johnson, D. P., & Anderson, L. (1987). In M. Hojat & R. Crandall (Eds.), *Loneliness: Theory, research, and applications* (pp. 225–238). Newbury Park, CA: Sage.

Murrell, S., Norris, F., & Chipley, Q. (1992). Functional versus structural social support desirable events, and positive affect in older adults. *Psychology and Aging, 7*, 562–570.

Newcomb, M. D. (1990). What structural equation modeling can tell us about social support. In B. R. Sarason, I. G. Sarason, & G. R. Pierce (Eds.), *Social support: An interactional view* (pp. 26–63). New York: Wiley.

Norbeck, J. S., Lindsey, A., & Carerri, V. L. (1981). The development of an instrument to measure social support. *Nursing Research, 30*, 264–269.

Norris, F. H., & Murrell, S. (1987). Transitory impact of life-event stress on psychological symptoms in older adults. *Journal of Health and Social Behavior, 28*, 197–211.

Norris, F. H., & Murrell, S. A. (1990). Social support, life events, and stress as modifiers of adjustment to bereavement by older adults. *Psychology and Aging, 5*, 429–436.

Norris, V. K., Stephens, M. A. P., & Kinney, J. M. (1990). The impact of family interactions on recovery from stroke: Help or hindrance? *The Gerontologist, 30*, 535–542.

Okun, M. A., Melichar, J. F., & Hill, M. D. (1990). Negative daily events, positive and negative social ties, and psychological distress among older adults. *The Gerontologist, 30*, 193–199.

O'Reilly, P. (1988). Methodological issues in social support and social network research. *Social Science and Medicine, 26*, 863–873.

Orth-Gomer, K., & Unden, A. L. (1987). The measurement of social support in population surveys. *Social Science and Medicine, 24*, 83–94.

Oxman, T. E., & Berkman, L. F. (1990). Assessments of social relationships in the elderly. *International Journal of Psychiatry in Medicine, 21*, 65–84.

Pagel, M. D., Erdly, W. W., & Becker, J. (1987). Social networks: We get by with (and in spite of) a little help from our friends. *Journal of Personality and Social Psychology, 53*, 793–804.

Poulshock, S. W., & Deimling, G. T. (1984). Families caring for elders in residence: Issues in the measurement of burden. *Journal of Gerontology, 39*, 230–239.

Procidano, M. E., & Heller, K. (1983). Measures of perceived social support from friends and from family: Three validation studies. *American Journal of Community Psychology, 11*, 1–24.

Revicki, D. A., & Mitchell, J. (1986). Social support factor structure in the elderly. *Research on Aging, 8*, 232–248.

Riley, D., & Eckenrode, J. (1986). Social ties: Costs and benefits within differing subgroups. *Journal of Personality and Social Psychology, 51*, 770–778.

Rivera, P. A., Rose, J. M., Futterman, A., Lovett, S. B., & Gallagher-Thompson, D. (1991). Dimensions of perceived social support in clinically depressed and nondepressed caregivers. *Psychology and Aging, 6*, 232–237.

Roberts, B. L., Dunkle, R., & Haug, M. (1994). Physical, psychological, and social resources as moderators of the relationship of stress to mental health of the very old. *Journals of Gerontology: Social Sciences, 49*, S35–S43.

Rook, K. S. (1984). The negative side of social interaction: Impact on psychological well-being. *Journal of Personality and Social Psychology, 46*, 1097–1108.

Rook, K. S. (1987). Social support versus companionship: Effects on life stress, loneliness, and evaluations by others. *Journal of Personality and Social Psychology, 52*, 1132–1147.

Rook, K. S. (1990a). Stressful aspects of older adults' social relationships: An overview of current theory and research. In M. A. P. Stephens, J. H. Crowther, S. E. Hobfoll, & D. L. Tennenbaum (Eds.), *Stress and coping in later-life families* (pp. 173–192). New York: Hemisphere.

Rook, K. S. (1990b). Social relationships as a source of companionship: Implications for older adults' psychological well-being. In B. R. Sarason, I. G. Sarason, & G. R. Pierce (Eds.), *Social support: An interactional view* (pp. 219–250). New York: Wiley.

Rook, K. S. (1992, April). *Social relationships and emotional health: A reconsideration of positivity and negativity effects.* Paper presented at the annual meeting of the Western Psychological Association, Portland, OR.

Rook, K.S., & Pietromonaco, P. (1987). Close relationships: Ties that help or ties that bind?. In W.H. Jones & D. Perlman (Eds.), *Advances in personal relationships* (Vol. 1, pp. 1–35). Greenwich, CT: JAI Press.

Rook, K. S., Thuras, P. D., & Lewis, M. A. (1990). Social control, health risk taking, and psychological distress among the elderly. *Psychology and Aging, 5*, 327–334.

Ruehlman, L. S., & Karoly, P. (1991). With a little flak from my friends: Development and preliminary validation of the test of negative social exchange. *Journal of Consulting and Clinical Psychology, 3*, 97–104.

Rushing, B., Ritter, C., & Burton, R. P. D. (1992). Race differences in the effects of multiple roles on health: Longitudinal evidence from a national sample of older men. *Journal of Health and Social Behavior, 33*, 126–139.

Russell, D. W., & Cutrona, C. (1991). Social support, stress, and depressive symptoms among the elderly: Test of a process model. *Psychology and Aging, 6*, 190–201.

Russell, D. W., Peplau, L. A., & Cutrona, C. E. (1980). The revised UCLA loneliness scale:

Concurrent and discriminant validity evidence. *Journal of Personality and Social Psychology, 39*, 472–480.

Sarason, B. R., Sarason, I. G., & Pierce, G. R. (1990). Traditional views of social support and their impact on assessment. In B. R. Sarason, I. G. Sarason, & G. R. Pierce (Eds.), *Social support: An interactional view* (pp. 9–25). New York: Wiley.

Sarason, B. R., Shearin, E. N., Pierce, G. R., & Sarason, I. G. (1987). Interrelations of social support measures: Theoretical and practical implications. *Journal of Personality and Social Psychology, 52*, 813–832.

Schoenbach, V. J., Kaplan, B. H., Fredman, L., & Kleinbaum, D. G. (1986). Social ties and mortality in Evans County, Georgia. *American Journal of Epidemiology, 123*, 577–591.

Schulz, R., & Rau, M. T. (1985). Social support through the life course. In S. Cohen & S. L. Syme (Eds.), *Social support and health* (pp. 129–149). Orlando, FL: Academic Press.

Schwarzer, R., & Leppin, A. (1991). Social support and health: A theoretical and empirical overview. *Journal of Social and Personal Relationships, 8*, 99–127.

Seeman, T. E., & Berkman, L. F. (1988). Structural characteristics of social networks and their relationships with social support in the elderly. *Social Science and Medicine, 26*, 737–749.

Shahtamasebi, S., Davis, R., & Wegner, C. (1992). A longitudinal analysis of factors related to survival in old age. *The Gerontologist, 32*, 404–413.

Sherbourne, C. D., & Hays, R. D. (1990). Martial status, social support, and health transitions in chronic disease patients. *Journal of Health and Social Behavior, 31*, 328–343.

Seeman, T. E., Kaplan, G. A., Knudsen, L., Cohen, R., & Guralnik, J. (1987). Social network ties and mortality among the elderly in the Alameda County Study. *American Journal of Epidemiology, 126*, 714–723.

Simmel, G. (1949). The sociology of sociability. *American Journal of Sociology, 55*, 254–261.

Spitze, G., & Logan, J. R. (1992). Helping as a component of parent-adult child relations. *Research on Aging, 14*, 291–312.

Steinbach, U. (1992). Social networks, institutionalization, and mortality among elderly people in the United States. *Journals of Gerontology: Social Sciences, 47*, S183–S190.

Stephens, M. A. P. (1990). Social relationships as coping resources in later-life families. In M. A. P. Stephens, J. H. Crowther, S. E. Hobfoll, & D. L. Tennenbaum (Eds.), *Stress and coping in later-life families* (pp. 1–20). New York: Hemisphere.

Stephens, M. A. P., Kinney, J. M., , & Norris, V. K., Ritchie, S. W. (1987). Social networks as assets and liabilities in recovery from stroke by geriatric patients. *Psychology and Aging, 2*, 125–129.

Stoller, E. P., & Earl, L. L. (1983). Help with activities of everyday life: Sources of support of the noninstitutionalized elderly. *The Gerontologist, 22*, 526–631.

Sugisawa, H., Liang, J., & Liu, X. (1994). Social networks, social support, and mortality among older people in Japan. *Journals of Gerontology: Social Sciences, 49*, S3–S13.

Suitor, J. J., & Pillemer, K. (1993). Support and interpersonal stress in the social networks of married daughters caring for parents with dementia. *Journals of Gerontology: Social Sciences, 48*, S1–S8.

Thompson, E. H., Futterman, A. M., Gallagher-Thompson, D., Rose, J. M., & Lovett, S. B.

(1993). Social support and caregiving burden in family caregivers of frail elders. *Journals of Gerontology: Social Sciences, 48*, S245–S254.

Turner, R. J. (1992). Measuring social support: Issues of concept and method. In H. O. F. Veiel & U. Baumann (Eds.), *The meaning and measurement of social support* (pp. 217–233). New York: Hemisphere.

Umberson, D. (1987). Family status and health behaviors: Social control as a dimension of social integration. *Journal of Health and Social Behavior, 28*, 307–319.

Umberson, D. (1992). Gender, marital status, and the social control of health behavior. *Social Science and Medicine, 34*, 907–917.

Vaux, A. (1992). Assessment of social support. In H. O. F. Veiel & U. Baumann (Eds.), *The meaning and measurement of social support* (pp. 193–216). Washington, DC: Hemisphere.

Vinokur, A. D., & van Ryan, M. (1992). Social support and undermining in close relationships: Their independent effects on the mental health of unemployed persons. *Journal of Personality and Social Psychology, 65*, 350–359.

Vinokur, A. D., & Vinokur-Kaplan, D. (1990). "In sickness and in health": Patterns of social support and undermining in older married couples. *Journal of Aging and Health*, 2, 215–241.

Wan, T. T. (1982). *Stressful life events, social support networks and gerontological health.* Lexington, MA: Lexington Books.

Ward, R. A., Sherman, S. R., & LaGory, M. (1984). Subjective network assessments and subjective well-being. *Journal of Gerontology, 39*, 93–101.

Weinberger, M., Hiner, S. L., & Tierney, W. M. (1987). Assessing social support in elderly adults. *Social Science and Medicine, 25*, 1049–1055.

Weiss, R. S. (1974). The provisions of social relationships. In Z. Rubin (Ed.), *Doing unto others* (pp. 17–26). Englewood Cliffs, NJ: Prentice-Hall.

Wellman, B., & Wortley, S. (1990). Different strokes from different folks: Community ties and social support. *American Journal of Sociology, 96*, 558–588.

Wheaton, B. (1985). Models for the stress-buffering functions of coping resources. *Journal of Health and Social Behavior, 26*, 352–364.

Wills, T. A. (1985). Supportive functions of interpersonal relationships. In S. Cohen & S. L. Syme (Eds.), *Social support and health* (pp. 61–82). Orlando, FL: Academic Press.

Wortman, C., & Lehman, D. R. (1985). Reactions to victims of life crises: Support attempts that fail. In I. G. Sarason & B. R. Sarason (Eds.), *Social support: Theory, research, and application* (pp. 463–489). The Hague, The Netherlands: Martinus Nijhoff.

CHAPTER 9

Aging and Personality Assessment

CAROLYN M. ALDWIN

AND

MICHAEL R. LEVENSON
DEPARTMENT OF APPLIED BEHAVIORAL SCIENCES
UNIVERSITY OF CALIFORNIA, DAVIS

The very existence of a chapter on aging and personality assessment reflects an implicit assumption that there is something inherently different about how personality is or should be assessed in older populations, either in terms of instrument selection or administration. This assumption further presupposes that personality somehow changes in later life—a matter of some controversy in the adult development and gerontology literature.

In contrast to the cognition literature, which includes heated debates over the issues of validity, scoring, and norming of cognitive testing in the elderly (cf. Jarvik, 1988), and the psychopathology literature, which has also questioned the validity of standard depression scales for use in the elderly (cf. Aldwin, Spiro, Levenson, & Bossé, 1989), our review of the literature for this chapter revealed very little research which questioned the validity of either administration or scoring procedures for personality tests for the elderly. To our knowledge, only one study (Butcher, Aldwin, Levenson, Ben-Porath, & Spiro, 1991) even addressed the desirability of simplifying a personality instrument format to accommodate visual and motor impairments common in late life.

Although a few studies specifically addressed item validity of personality instruments for the elderly (Levenson, 1974; Shewchuk, Foelker, Camp, & Blanchard-Fields, 1992), the majority of studies addressing aging and personality are concerned with the basic issue of whether or not personality changes over the lifespan. If personality does not change, then the whole issue of aging and per-

Preparation of this chapter was supported by a FIRST Award from the National Institute on Aging (AG07465) to the first author and a grant from the National Institute for Alcohol Abuse and Alcoholism (AA08941) to the second. We would like to thank Karen Sutton and Kent Kiehl for their aid in preparation of this manuscript and Dr. Avron Spiro III for his helpful comments on earlier drafts.

sonality assessment is moot (with the possible exception of the procedural issues raised by Butcher et al., 1991).[1] However, if personality does change, the issue becomes much more complicated. As Lachman (1989) points out, the more appropriate questions are: What are the changes? Under what circumstances do they occur? and How great are they? From an assessment point of view, the basic questions become: Are we even assessing that which changes? and What theory should we be using to decide what should be assessed?

The answer to these questions devolves in large part on two issues: first, how change is defined and assessed, and second, how personality in late life is defined and assessed. For example, researchers could conclude that personality is stable, either because they used a very liberal definition of what stability is and/or because they used an instrument which is insensitive to change.

There are two contrasting approaches to personality assessment in aging research, which we will call trait and process approaches (a distinction also proposed by Kruse, Lindenberger, & Baltes, in press). Trait measures are constructed without much regard to developmental theory and purport to examine personal characteristics which are believed to be relatively stable over time. In contrast, process measures are theoretically based on phenomena which are hypothesized to change across the life span in a systematic fashion, such as moral or ego development (but see Langer and colleagues, 1990, for a discussion of nonsystematic development). There are a variety of ways of constructing trait and process measures that are more or less independent of the type of format, although trait measures usually consist of closed-ended items and process measures often depend upon the scoring of interviews. Further, one must always remember not to confuse the instrument per se with what the instrument is purported to assess (Kagan, 1988).

This chapter will briefly discuss issues in the measurement of and theoretical approaches to change, and then examine the literature on trait and process measures with respect to whether personality changes are stable in adulthood. Finally, we will propose some criteria for theoretical guidelines for examining personality and aging.

ISSUES IN THE MEASUREMENT OF CHANGE

A number of works have been published recently on the statistical assessment of change (Collins & Horn, 1991; Funder, Parke, Tomlinson-Keasey, & Widaman, 1993); Thus, the relevant issues will be summarized only briefly here. Most personality researchers use cross-sectional designs to examine age differences on a trait, or correlate age with scores on that trait. As is well known, such designs confound age, cohort, and period effects. Longitudinal designs follow individuals over time, examining either correlational (rank order) stability or mean level change (usually using multivariate analysis of variance; MANOVAs). However, longitudinal designs also confound age, cohort, and period effects—even if there is change over time, one does not know if it is specific to that cohort, or if the change is due to period effects. Sequential designs, which follow multiple cohorts across time, can aid in teasing out age, cohort, and period effects (see Schaie & Herzog, 1985). However, sequential designs have been used only rarely in personality research.

Another way of assessing stability and change is through structural variance; simply put, there may be systematic, age-related changes in the meaning of items, which would be reflected in different factor structures, factor loadings of items for different age groups or across time, or differences in the correlations among the factors. For example, many personality scales are developed on college-aged populations, and the items may not be germane to an older person's experience. Some items on Rotter's (1966) locus-of-control scale refer to attitudes about the fairness of teachers' grading practices, a problem which Levenson's (1974) multidimensional locus-of-control scale seeks to avoid. However, using items which are specific to an older population's experience may render generalization across the life span problematic. Even if a researcher is careful to utilize apparently age-neutral items, it is entirely possible that the structure of a scale may nonetheless be age specific, as apparently is the case with Levenson's scale (Shewchuk et al., 1992).

For example, a current conception in general personality theory, for which Goldberg (1993) is the main advocate, is that there are five primary personality factors. Interestingly, Mroczek (1993) found it difficult to replicate the "Big 5" personality factor structure in a large sample of older men without extensive data manipulation, mainly by means of ipsatizing the scores both by column and by row. In other words, items may mean different things to an older population (e.g., physical symptoms on depression scales or hopelessness items among the terminally ill). Further, Spiro (personal communication, 1994) also pointed out that different scales have been normed on different cohorts; in some ways, the vocabulary used in the older scales is more suitable to older people.

Finally, some researchers have argued very strongly for idiographic, idiothetic, or ipsative studies of change and development across the life span (Lamiell, 1981), either by using individual growth curve models (Aldwin, Spiro, et al., 1989; Rogosa, Brandt, & Zimowski, 1982) or through in-depth qualitative analysis (Elms, in press; McAdams, 1985). Individual change may well be obscured or nullified in aggregate studies which, in some ways, constitute the sociology of personality—the examination of traits in groups—rather then the development (or lack thereof) of individual personality.

There are a number of problems with even longitudinal assessments of change. The first is that different methods may easily yield contradictory results. It is perfectly plausible, for example, that the relative distribution of a given trait in a population may remain stable over time, but the mean level may shift. This would give a reasonably large Pearson's *r* (signalling stability) but a statistically significant multivariate F (indicating change). Thus, person x may always be more extraverted than person y, but they both may become more introverted from college to midlife. The converse is also possible. The mean level may be stable over time, but the distribution of the trait within groups may change, yielding a smaller r. Would these patterns indicate stability or change in personality?

The second problem lies in interpreting whether change or stability is seen in any given data set—a classic "Is the glass half empty or half full?" dilemma. Moderate correlations of .4–.6 are routinely touted as demonstrating stability by those researchers with that bias; however, Lamiell (1987) pointed out that an examination of individual change scores in a population with even higher correlations yields evidence of considerable change at the individual (as opposed to group) level. Conversely, Butcher et al. (1991) found statistically significant age group differences on the Minnesota Multiphasic Personality Inventory (MMPI-2), but decided that the magnitude of these differences was so small (generally less than one-half a standard deviation) as to be clinically insignificant, and concluded that special norms for the elderly on the MMPI-2 were unwarranted. What constitutes significant stability or change, statistical significance, or clinical meaning? Given the lack of criteria for indicating change or stability, the same data set could conceivably yield opposite conclusions, depending upon the method of analysis and the predilections of the researchers.

There are other assessment issues, such as whether one can differentiate true change from statistical error due to unreliability in measurement; whether there are individual differences in change, and what the sources of those differences are; and over what time period should individuals be followed and how frequently should they be assessed. Finally, one issue that is seldom addressed in the personality literature is whether demonstrated changes are attributable to developmental, cohort, or period effects? The relative rarity of sequential designs, which attempt to differentiate among these three potential sources of change in longitudinal personality research, is not surprising, given the practical difficulties inherent in following multiple cohorts over sufficient periods of time to assess meaningful change.

Obviously, statistical techniques alone, no matter how elegant, are inadequate to determine the existence of change or stability in personality in adulthood. The need for sound theoretical bases for explaining personality change and stability in adulthood is manifest.

THEORETICAL APPROACHES TO PERSONALITY STABILITY AND CHANGE IN ADULTHOOD

Several possible scenarios of change/stability have been proposed over the years.

1. Personality may remain so stable over the life course that any apparent change can be attributed to error. McCrae and Costa (1990) appear to take

this position and McCrae (1993) goes so far as to suggest that research on change in the adult personality is pointless.

2. Personality traits may change in later life due to age-related physiological changes, especially illness. Alzheimer's disease can result in profound personality change (Strauss, Pasupathi, & Chatterjee, 1993), but more subtle changes can follow transient ischemic attacks and other forms of cardiovascular disease. Indeed, sudden personality change is one of the warning signs of dementia (Raskind & Peskind, 1992). The widely held belief that depression increases in later life will be addressed elsewhere in this volume (Pachana, Gallagher-Thompson, & Thompson, chapter 11; Schulz, O'Brien, & Tompkins, chapter 10).
3. From the viewpoint of the study of interpersonal perception, perceived personality traits may be under considerable situational influence. Different situations may be conducive to different trait attributions in the same person (cf. Jones, 1990). From a contextual viewpoint, observed change need not be permanent to be viewed as change rather than error.
4. A reciprocal relationship may exist between personality and situation which produces sufficient consistency in experience to render personality stable in most cases. Rigidified interpersonal expectancies may render change unlikely even when it would be beneficial (Caspi, Bem, & Elder, 1989).
5. Personality may change as a reflection of changes in social roles (cf. Brim, 1965). This sociological perspective is compatible with the social psychological view of interpersonal perception but further holds that change is built into the social structure. This sociogenic approach holds that apparent traits may change across the life course and from one situation to another at the same life stage. A hypothesis that could be derived from this perspective is that personality stability will be related to the stability of social structure.
6. Personality may be modified by other types of experience throughout the life course, such as trauma (for reviews, see Aldwin, in press; Epstein, 1991). Psychological therapy also attempts to change traitlike characteristics, such as shyness, phobias, and assertiveness, with the appropriate treatment and effort on the part of the client.
7. A maturational approach to change in adult personality suggests such change is more ontogenic than sociogenic (cf. Erikson, 1950). That is, observed changes should reflect like stages more than social roles per se. Some mixture of sociogenic and maturational effects would be anticipated in many cases (Baltes, Reese, & Lipsitt, 1980).
8. Personality may be intentionally changed, or it may be changed as a product of efforts to develop qualities and capacities, e.g., wisdom or the ideal self (Brandtstädter, Wentura, & Greve, 1993). Alternatively, traits such as introversion may remain relatively stable while other dimensions emerge (e.g., Eriksonian generativity).

The empirical studies reviewed below do not address each of these possibilities equally. The approach featured in a given study depends on the assumptions and measures employed by the investigators. However, the reader should keep these issues in mind because clues concerning the degree and sources of change in personality in adulthood appear when the studies are compared.

Stability and Change in Trait Assessments of Personality

Table 9.1 summarizes information from 12 longitudinal studies. These were selected on several criteria: recency (publication since 1984); use of a standardized personality instrument (preferably one assessing multiple dimensions), the use of the same instrument (or assessment techniques) at all time points, a follow-up period of at least 5 years, follow-up at least until midlife and preferably later life, and publication in refereed journals. For the most part, we followed the format adopted by McCrae and Costa (1990) in their review of earlier studies, which provided information about the sample size, length of follow-up, and some indication of the findings. While this table cannot be considered exhaustive, it does summarize the most recent literature on longitudinal change and stability in personality traits.

The creation of Table 9.1 was surprisingly difficult due to the extreme variation in the type, quality, and amount of information presented. We presented the initial *N*, because it was often difficult to determine what the *N* was at follow-up, or because the follow-up *N* was allowed to vary as a function of missing data, differences in follow-up times for different samples, etc.[2] Most studies reported the ages of the respondents, but in two studies estimation was required (indicated by a ~). Some studies used more than one cohort, which were indicated by C1, C2, etc. Unless otherwise noted, most studies had only two intervals. However, the interval often varied as a function of logistic requirements. Often, several years were required to do both the initial testing and the follow-up testing, so we computed the longest possible interval.

Finally, we had hoped to duplicate McCrae and Costa's (1990) column on the median stability correlation, but this was not always possible, because some researchers only provided ranges of correlations, whereas others presented changes in mean levels, and so forth. Indeed, there were marked differences in how researchers reported change and stability, which made summarization in the results column on Table 9.1 somewhat awkward. When the studies examined mean level differences across time, the findings are presented either in terms of increases, decreases, or no mean differences. If many subscales were used, we indicated the proportion which changed significantly (e.g., 5/23). For those studies which used correlational techniques, we divided the correlations into three categories. High (H) stability indicated those correlations greater than or equal to .70 (although caveats concerning mean level and ipsative stability should be kept

TABLE 9.1 Summary Information from Recent Longitudinal Studies of Personality Traits

Study	*Initial N*	*Initial Age*	*Measure*	*Longest Retest Interval (yrs)*	*Results*
Costa et al. (1987)	3,089 (F) 1,853 (M)	25–74	GWB[a]	9	No mean diffs. (3 scales)
Costa & McCrae (1988)	Varies	21–96	NEO (+AC)[b]	6	Decreased N, A, C; Stable E, O
Dudek & Hall (1991)	124 (M)	37–63	ACL,[c] CPI[d]	25	ACL[b]: 9H, 26M, 2L[e] CPI[c]: 3H 13M, 2L[e]
Field & Millsap (1991)	51 (F) 21 (M)	~27	Interview	14	Primary: 0H, 3M, 18L[e] 2nd Order: 0H, 4M, 1L[e]
Field, Schaie, & Leino (1991)	41 (F) 16 (M)	C1: 74–84 C2: 85–93	Interview	14	All five subscales changed: age x sex variations
Finn (1986)	281 (M) 178 (M)	C1: 43–53 C2: 17–25	MMPI[f]	30	C1: 9H, 5M, 3L; C2: 2H, 12M, 3L[e] 11 of 17 sig. diffs. betw. C1 & C2
Haan et al. (1986)	138 (F) 136 (M)	5–67	California Q-sort	47	Early—Mid adult: 0H, 5M, 1L[e] Mid—Late adult: 0H, 6M, 0L[e]
Helson & Moane (1987)	81 (F)	21	CPI[d]	22	0H, 4M, 16L
Helson & Wink (1992)	101 (F)	43	CPI[d] ACL[c]	9	CPI[d]: Med r = .73; 5/23 sig. diff. ACL[c] Med r = .73; 6/37 sig. diff. Coping: Med r = .50; 4/10 sig. diff.
Lachman & Leff (1989)	42 (F) 21 (M)	~73	LMC[g] PIC[h]	5	0H, 2M, 1L; no mean diff. 0H, 3M, 0L; 1 mean change
Schaie & Willis (1991)	1,814 (F) 1,628 (M)	22–84	TBR[i]	28	Mean stable through midlife; 2/3 subscales decreased after age 60
Stevens & Truss (1985)	66 (F) 114 (M)	18–20	EPPS[j]	20	Cohort 1 (to age 30): 0H, 17M, 15L[e] Cohort 2 (to age 40): 3H, 21M, 5L

[a]GWB: General Well Being
[b]NEO (+AC): Neuroticism, Extraversion Openness, Agreeableness, & Conscientiousness
[c]ACL: Adjective Checklist
[d]CPI: California Personality Inventory
[e]H M L: High ($r > .70$), Medium (.4–.69), Low (<.40)
[f]MMPI: Minnesota Multiphasic Personality Inventory
[g]LMC: Levenson Multidimensional Control
[h]PIC: Personality in Intellectual Contexts
[f]TBR: Test of Behavioral Rigidity
[j]EPPS: Edwards Personality Preference Schedule

in mind); moderate (M) coefficients were those between .40 and .69; and low (L) coefficients were those less than .40. Thus, 9H, 26M, 2L indicates that 9 of the correlations were high, 26 were moderate and 2 were low.

We had planned to perform a metanalysis to examine factors affecting stability and change but, as is obvious from Table 9.1, the range of measures utilized by the different laboratories precluded this possibility. Thus, we will only address highlights from the table, supplemented by cross-sectional, behavioral genetic or other studies which did not meet the criteria for inclusion in the table, but nonetheless provide interesting additional information.

First, it is obvious that there is considerable variability in the stability of different traits, both within and across studies. While McCrae (1993) stated that the average correlation across time for personality traits is .70, indicating little change, an examination of both a stability coefficient table compiled by McCrae and Costa (1990, p. 87) and Table 9.1 reveals moderate stability, at best. In McCrae and Costa's table, the median stability coefficients range from .34 to .71, with a computed average of .48; in Table 9.1, the modal correlation is clearly moderate, between .40 and .69. Thus, the available longitudinal studies clearly indicate both change and stability. The next task is to examine the possible sources of the variance.

Duration of Study. Length of follow-up is clearly a factor in the degree of stability of personality traits in a study. In Table 9.1, the three studies which evidenced the most stability had a follow-up interval of less than 10 years. Not surprisingly, the longer the follow-up time, the less the stability.

Heritability. Differences in the types of traits examined may also account for some of the variance. Lachman (1989) suggested that traits which are more heritable are more stable. If some traits are based on a biological substrate, it is sensible to suppose that they would be more stable than patterns based on socialization. Emotionality and extraversion appear to be good candidates for genetic determination (Eysenck, 1987; Buss & Plomin, 1975, 1984; Kagan, Reznik, & Snidman, 1988; Kagan, 1989). Indeed, some of the scales with high consistency in the two studies that also demonstrated high stability in Table 9.1 (Dudek & Hall, 1991; Helson & Wink, 1992) included some approximations of sociability. Unfortunately, only one of the longitudinal studies in Table 9.1 utilized specific measures of neuroticism and extraversion.

Costa and McCrae (1988) found that older age groups reported lower scores on five of the six neuroticism subscales on the NEO Personality Inventory. Following up the respondents over a period of 6 years, overall self-reported neuroticism declined slightly. Similarly, substantial differences in extraversion were also seen in cross-section, but little change over the 6-year period, although the warmth subscale appeared to increase in the cross-sequential analysis. While the authors claim that this demonstrates that personality is stable, a more parsimonious conclusion is that the time period was simply too short to assess change.

In a 45-year longitudinal study with data collection at three points in time, Conley (1985) examined consistency over time, for neuroticism and social introversion derived from the Bernreuter Personality Inventory (Times 1 and 2) and the Cornell Medical Index (Time 3). Correlations between Times 1 and 2 were fairly high (.60 for neuroticism; .70 for extraversion) but lowered substantially when a different measure was used at Time 3. T1–T3 correlations were .31 and .27 and T2–T3 received .34 and .29, for neuroticism and extraversion, respectively. These results highlight the importance of consistency of assessments (however outdated) in longitudinal research. In a cross-sectional study, Eysenck (1987) found that successively older cohorts evidenced lower scores on neuroticism and extraversion, suggesting that even if correlational stability is high, mean level change may nonetheless occur.

In a 13-year longitudinal study, Spiro, Levenson, and Aldwin (1992) conducted 2-point longitudinal analyses employing a short form of the Eysenck Personality Inventory (EPI–Q; Floderus, 1974). They found mean level stability for emotionality and an increase for extraversion but also found that 10% of the respondents changed by more than 3 points on one or both of the scales. Correlation coefficients over time for the two trait measures were high: the correlations were .66 for extraversion and .57 for emotionality (disattenuated stability coefficients were .92 and .76, respectively). Nonetheless, scores for approximately one quarter of the respondents changed more than one quartile. Of these, a large majority decreased on each of the two scales. This finding is similar to that reported by McCrae (1993), who found considerable ipsative change for various components of neuroticism on the NEO. Thus, even in these most stable of characteristics, some individual-level change can be seen.

In other studies, the question of genetic influence was addressed explicitly. In a behavior genetic study of the second half of the life span, Plomin, Pedersen, McClearn, Nesselroade, and Bergeman (1988) examined heritabilities for the traits of emotionality, activity level, and sociability (approximately equivalent to Eysenck's extraversion). Using the Emotionality, Activity, and Sociability Temperament Survey for adults (Buss & Plomin, 1984), they found significant genetic influence but they also found that half of the variance on this measure was due to unshared environment. Also, heritability estimates were lower than in younger samples.

In a metanalysis of twin studies, McCartney, Bernieri, and Harris (1990) found that correlations between both monozygotic and dizygotic twins declined significantly with age on such measures as activity/impulsivity and masculinity/femininity while monozygotic twins alone evidenced significantly declining correlations on dominance, anxiety, and task orientation. Several studies using MMPI scale scores have found that some scales, such as Depression (D), Psychopathic Deviate (Pd), Schizophrenia (Sc), and Social Introversion (Si), which evidence significant genetic influence in adolescence (Gottesman, 1963, 1966), show no significant genetic influence in early-to-mid adulthood (Dworkin,

Burke, Maher, & Gottesman, 1976; Reznikoff & Honeyman, 1967). Pogue-Geile and Rose (1985) found significant genetic variance on four scales (Wiggin's Social Maladjustment; Sc; Welsh Anxiety and Welsh Depression 30) both at ages 20 and 25 but for Pd and Wiggin's Religiosity, genetic variance was significant at age 20 only.

These studies suggest that genetic effects on personality may be most notable in early life, and dissipate in later life. However, an examination of Table 9.1 suggests that younger age groups are less stable than older groups (see also McCrae & Costa, 1990), which presents a bit of a conundrum. If it is assumed that heritability means stability, how is it that the personality of young adults, in whom the heritability effects are presumably strongest, are less stable?

Age/Cohort Differences in Stability. In a longitudinal study with an older and a younger cohort, Finn (1986) observed significantly higher 30-year correlation consistencies on 9 of 15 MMPI factor scales and one of two higher order factors for the older cohort. The younger cohort was significantly more consistent on only one factor scale (denial of somatic problems). These findings suggest maturational change toward greater stability.

However, age and cohort effects may have been confounded in Finn's study. Using the Edwards Personal Preference Schedule, Stevens and Truss (1985) examined longitudinal stability in 15 traits in two college graduate samples, one of which (30-year-olds) was assessed at a 12-year interval and the other (40-year-olds) at a 20-year interval. These authors measured change and stability by combining cross-time correlation and mean level change. They found evidence for both maturational (ontogenic) and generational (sociogenic) change. The 40-year-olds (who were first tested in the 1950s) evidenced much more correlational consistency than the 30-year-olds (who were first tested in the 1960s), even though their follow-up time was longer than the 1960s cohort. This suggests that the age effect on overall personality consistency is sociogenic rather than maturational. However, the combined analyses indicated that there were maturational (i.e., shared by both cohorts) increases in need for dominance, autonomy, and achievement and decreases in need for affiliation and abasement. The order, deference, succorance, exhibition, and endurance scales showed longitudinal stability. Comparing the initial scores of the male and female 40- and 30-year-olds with those of a group of 20-year-olds at the time of final testing, Stevens and Truss found that the 40-year-old men and women had initially differed on eight scales, the 30-year-olds on four, while the 20-year-olds differed on none.

In connection with the argument advanced by McCrae (1993) that longitudinal change in trait scores is due to error, the changes shown in this study are rationally interpretable in light of recent changes in gender roles. It would have been interesting to look at individual change scores in the two longitudinal cohorts to determine whether the number of respondents exhibiting large change scores was greater in the 30-year-old sample than among the 40-year-olds.

Thus, while older adults are generally more consistent in their self-reported personality traits, there may be interesting cohort differences in personality stability, which may also account for some of the cross-study differences in Table 9.1.

Maturational/Volitional Sources of Change. Perhaps the conundrum posed above by the heritability and age differences in consistency controversy can be explained by a maturational model. From this viewpoint, young adulthood is a time in which individuals assess their personalities and shape them, suppressing undesirable characteristics (even if genetically based) and enhancing desirable ones; by midlife one has developed a personality that one can "live with," as it were, and thus it becomes more stable. (The role of the selection of situational contexts in this regard is obvious. With luck, the individual finds a mate and a work role or other social contexts which support or reinforce the desired characteristics; see Caspi et al., 1989.)

This hypothesis is supported by Haan, Hartka, and Millsap (1986), who found that positive characteristics uniformly increased from young adulthood to midlife. However, each personality component had its own unique developmental signature exhibiting different patterns of stability and change, with some showing far more change in adulthood than others. Also, significant sex × time differences were found for the cognitive commitment and warm versus hostile traits. In both cases, women went from a lower level than men in adolescence to a higher level in adulthood. There was significant decline in only one component after midlife: women's assertiveness.

A study by Helson and Wink (1992) suggests that positive change can continue into midlife, even in the midst of relative rank-order stability. In a longitudinal study of women (Mills College graduates) in their early forties and, again, in their early fifties, Helson and Wink found fairly high stability coefficients of .56 or greater for subscales of the California Personality Inventory (CPI; median r = .73) and of .53 or greater for subscales of the Adjective Checklist (ACL; median r = .73) but significant mean level change on five of the CPI scales and six of the ACL scales. The women increased on CPI Responsibility, Self-Control, Good Impression, and Norm Favoring and decreased on Femininity. They increased on ACL Dominance, Self-Confidence, Favorableness of Adjectives Checked and Congruence between Self and Ideal Self and decreased in Abasement and Succorance. The Haan Coping scale, which was derived from the CPI, had lower stability coefficients than the other two scales (.40 or greater with median r = .50). Significant mean level change occurred in 4 of the 10 scales, including Intellectuality, Logical Analysis, Tolerance of Ambiguity, and Substitution (a measure of cognitive flexibility). Helson and Wink found no relationships between life events (menopause, empty nest, and involvement in the daughter role) and personality change. The authors interpret their findings as indicating normative changes in the adult personalities of women including increased self-assurance, dominance, self-control, and identification with social norms.

On the other hand, it may be that these well-educated and presumably affluent women have had opportunities to develop these qualities that are not available to women in general. Their circumstances may also bear on the failure to find effects of life events. Many persons are not so well insulated against unpleasant and unexpected life events, a fact that may have long-term consequences on some aspects of personality. Further, less fortunate individuals may well refuse to participate in a longitudinal study. A study of the influence of social class on personality change would help resolve the controversy between advocates of ontogenic explanations of adult development and those who favor a sociogenic model. Vaillant (1993) recently compared three different longitudinal studies, which included upper class men (the Grant Study), highly intelligent women (from the Terman Study), and lower class men (a comparison group for a study of inner city delinquents). All of these groups showed maturational effects in defense mechanisms, suggesting that development is not limited to upper middle class samples. These studies clearly suggest the existence of maturational change in personality from early to middle adulthood, even if all adults do not exhibit that change.

Social Roles as a Source of Change. There is a fairly large literature on social roles and personality which can only be briefly mentioned here. Although most studies are cross sectional and deal primarily with early adulthood, there is some longitudinal evidence for systematic personality change with changes in social roles from early adulthood to midlife. Although Helson and Wink (1992) found little impact of social roles on general personality, Wink and Helson (1993) found such effects by examining personality traits which are more closely linked with specific roles. They examined both the cross-sectional and longitudinal effects of parenting on ACL measures of succorance and competence. They found that women decreased in succorance from the early parental to the postparental period, whereas both sexes increased in competence over the same time period. A sequential study by Parker (1993) also showed systematic changes in gender role identity in early adulthood which was consistent across cohorts, but was nonetheless moderated by the timing of parenthood.

Change and Stability in Late Life

Less is known about personality change in late life, but at first glance it would appear to be less positive than the changes from young adulthood to midlife. Schaie and Willis (1991) report decreases in three indices of behavioral flexibility after age 60, although Fiske and Chiriboga, using the ACL, (1990) report no change in flexibility. Costa and McCraw (1988) found decline in some of the openness to experience subscales on the NEO, but no change in intellectual openness. This finding was echoed by Giambra, Camp, and Grodsky (1992), who found decreasing susceptibility to boredom with age, but no change in intellectual curiosity. Locus-of-control measures appear relatively stable, except for increases in the perception of powerful others (Lachman & Leff, 1989). Although Costa and McCrae (1988) found a decrease in agreeableness over 6 years, they also found an increase in warmth, suggesting some individual differences in the direction of change.

In the one study which focused on very old individuals, Field, Schaie, and Leino (1991) found different patterns of personality change between the old-old (75–84) and the very-old (85–93). For example, while the old-old were stable or decreased slightly in agreeableness, the very-old appeared to increase slightly. Field et al. also analyzed the distribution of individual change scores and found that about half of the sample remained stable on the five personality measures, and the rest showed varying patterns of increase or decrease. A 5-year study of the MMPI–2 among the Normative Aging Study men, who ranged in age from 45 to 90 at follow-up, also found considerable aggregate stability, but the change scores were normally distributed. About 20% of the men changed at least one standard deviation on various scales. This suggests that personality continues to be somewhat malleable in late life. It would be very interesting to examine the sources of that change, which might include the social context, health status, and perhaps even maturational processes in late life.

Summary of Stability and Change Data

The longitudinal literature on personality change provides evidence for some of the eight positions on change in adult personality summarized at the beginning of this section. First, there is clear evidence of change in adulthood, even among studies which utilize measures of purportedly stable personality traits. The majority of studies showed moderate correlations; the studies with high stability coefficients generally had the shortest follow-up periods. The moderate stability across adulthood supports Caspi et al.'s (1989) suggestion that person–situation interactions may act to support stability. Nonetheless, there is also substantial evidence for change. Further, contrary to McCrae (1993), not all of the change can be viewed as error. Although some is undoubtedly due to unreliability in measures, the change found in many of the studies makes good maturational sense. There appears to be a decrease in levels of neuroticism and increases in those personality traits reflecting competence from early adulthood to midlife, which supports a maturational viewpoint. The nature of the maturational changes, in light of their generally positive emphasis, implies that some of the changes may be volitional, supporting the position of Brandtstädter et al. (1993).

Genetic influence on personality traits appears to be most prominent in early life, dissipating in midlife. This suggests that social roles may play a larger role in personality in midlife. Note, however, that social roles may influence very specific personality characteristics rather than the overall constellation of personality traits. In general, cross-sectional differences between cohorts were much larger than longitudinal change (Costa & McCrae, 1988; Schaie & Willis, 1991), and there were suggestions of cohort differences in personality stability. This presents intriguing evidence for powerful cohort—and therefore social—effects on personality.

In other words, change and stability in personality in adulthood is highly complex. Support was found for at least half of the theoretical approaches to change and stability in personality listed above. Although genetics and cohort effects may be strong influences on personality in early adulthood, maturational and volitional forces may provide impetus for personality change through midlife, with the selection of social contexts reinforcing that change (or lack thereof, as the case may be). Studies in late life show that change can continue, although the nature of that change may not be as strongly positive. Clearly, research on adult development is far from pointless. If trait measures can show this degree of change, what do process measures reveal?

Process Approaches to Personality Change

Surprisingly, studies of ego development processes in late life are generally rare. For purposes of this study, these are termed *process approaches*, as they are generally based on assumptions of systematic teleological personality change in adulthood. Process theories may be cast in the form of stages or dialectical processes, including theories of ego development (Loevinger, 1977), ego integrity and generativity (Erikson, 1950), as well as moral development (Kohlberg, 1984) and wisdom (cf. Sternberg, 1990). Process measures are usually based on the coding of interview material, although some scales assess various aspects of Erikson's (1950) theory. Research on personality development, especially in later life, is still in its infancy, and those studies which do exist are mainly cross-sectional rather than longitudinal.

Ego Development. A review of the literature revealed that the vast majority of studies of ego development using the Sentence Completion Test (SCT; Loevinger, 1966) have been done on adolescents; only a handful have reported on middle-aged and older samples. Although McCrae and Costa (1980) found no association with age and level of ego development in men, White (1985) found that middle-aged women were higher in ego development than younger women. Vaillant and McCullough (1987) compared ego levels in the Grant Study men to levels reported in studies of young individuals, and found their respondents to be consistently higher than college students. The one study of ego development in late life that we located unfortunately did not report on associations with age (Beaton, 1991).

Moral Development. Most studies of moral development are also conducted on adolescent samples. However, there is some suggestion that moral development increases from young adulthood to midlife, in both cross-sectional (Bakken &

Ellsworth, 1990) and longitudinal studies (Colby, Kohlberg, Gibbs, & Lieberman, 1983; Walker, 1989), especially among the educated (White, 1988). In later life, however, the issue may become more complicated. Pratt, Golding, and Hunter (1991) compared younger (35–55) and older (65–85) adults on several measures that are relevant to wisdom, Kohlberg's (1984) Moral Judgment Interview (MJI), personal dilemmas scored for ego development, moral orientation, and integrative complexity, and found no age group differences. However, in an earlier study, Pratt, Diessner, Hunsberger, Pancer, and Savoy (1991) compared moral reasoning (in the MJI) with preferred stage of moral thinking (in the Defining Issues Test; Rest 1979) and found them to be completely uncorrelated in young adults, moderately correlated in mature adults, and strongly correlated (.70) in older adults. The authors interpret the strikingly greater moral consistency of older people as supporting Kohlberg's (1973) hypothesis that moral reflectiveness increases with age.

Generativity and Integrity. Some empirical work has been done testing various aspects of Erikson's (1950) theory, but again, studies in older adults are relatively rare, and longitudinal studies even scarcer. Cross-sectional studies generally find modest increases in generativity and integrity with age (Darling-Fisher & Leidy, 1988; Domino & Affonso, 1990), even in cross-cultural samples (Ochse & Plug, 1986; Viney, 1987). Interestingly, generativity scores appear to peak in midlife (Ryff & Heincke, 1983), although this may vary by type of generativity (McAdams, de St. Aubin, & Logan, 1993). Vaillant and Milofsky (1980) did conduct a longitudinal study of Erikson's model of the life cycle using two 40-year prospective studies of men. Although the study found some evidence for sequentiality of stages, there were individual differences in the age at which the men mastered the various stages, which might account for the generally rather weak correlations with age found in other studies.

Wisdom. Finally, wisdom is a construct to which gerontologists are just beginning to devote attention. While often thought of primarily as a cognitive construct (Smith & Baltes, 1990), it clearly includes both affective (Labouvie-Vief, 1990) and characterological components (Chandler & Holliday, 1990), and thus falls under the rubric of personality assessment. Assessing wisdom is an extremely complex task because it is a multidimensional construct that includes complexity in processing and perspicacity in integrating both information and emotions, a certain level of practical knowledge, cogency in the provision of advice to others, ego strength in the ability to set goals and persevere, and as yet poorly specified virtues such as generosity, honesty, and so forth. Thus, it is not surprising that preliminary work has often relied upon analysis of interview data.

Baltes and his colleagues (Smith & Baltes, 1990; Staudinger, Smith, & Baltes, 1992) assessed wisdom by rating along several dimensions the advice older and younger respondents would give concerning specific life problems. They found that the quality of advice respondents provided received higher ratings when the person in the life problem was similar in age to the respondent. In other words, wisdom did not necessarily increase with age, but rather was highly context-specific. However, using a similar format but a different scoring scheme, Kitchener, King, Wood, and Davison (1989) found increases in reflective judgment, at least in early adulthood. Further, Labouvie-Vief and her colleagues found that older respondents were more complex than younger respondents in both cognitive (Adams, Labouvie-Vief, Hobart, & Dorosz, 1990) and emotional processing (Labouvie-Vief, DeVoe, & Bulka, 1989; Labouvie-Vief, Hakim-Larson, DeVoe, & Schoeberlein, 1989).

Others study wisdom by asking respondents to describe in their own language the characteristics of individuals they think are wise (Clayton & Birren, 1980; Holliday & Chandler, 1986; Sternberg, 1986). Although wisdom is commonly associated with older individuals, the link between age and wisdom decreases when self-ratings are examined (Sternberg, 1986).

Wisdom is not a personality trait per se, but rather a process, or a way of looking at the world, which is developed as a function of both experience and volition. As such, it has connections to several literatures, including cognition, values, and coping research, but transcends all of these. Therefore, wisdom has special problems vis-à-vis assessment, but the development of this construct and its measurement is crucial for understanding aging and positive mental health.

Comparison of Personality Measures

There is no "gold standard" in personality assessment. Which measure to use depends upon both the research question and the characteristics of the sample, e.g., high functioning or impaired elders. If one wishes to assess basic personality traits in a young-old (65–74) or high-functioning group, then most standard measures of personality traits would be appropriate, depending on the research question. When using more specialized scales, however, the item content should be evaluated. Many scales were developed using college students, and the item content may not be appropriate for an older population. For example, the Rotter (1966) Locus of Control scale contains several items relevant primarily to student populations; the Levenson Multidimensional Control Scale (Levenson, 1974) is much more appropriate for use in older populations.

Scale choice may be critical in dealing with old-old or impaired elders, especially those with cognitive impairments. Shorter versions of personality scales should be used, if possible with a simplified response format. Visual and hearing impairments also mitigate against the use of longer instruments. Shorter versions of scales should also be used when doing community surveys to try to enhance response rates.

Although it is not possible to review all possible personality assessments in the space available, we will try to discuss the most widely used general trait measures and those of special interest for adult development. However, the reader should be aware that, although there is a literature on whether or not standard deviations of various measures goes up with age, almost no work has been done comparing the reliability and validity of personality measures in older versus younger populations. This is undoubtedly due to the fact that much work on scale development and validation takes place using captive college populations who will tolerate filling out multiple versions of the same construct. Such research in an older population would be much more expensive and would require fairly tolerant respondents.

Our subjective experience in working with older people suggests that there may be validity issues, especially in old-old populations. Our observation is that older adults are often intolerant of redundancy in questionnaires. Further, those over age 70 or with less formal education are often uncomfortable with assigning numbers to their experience, as rating scales require. Those with even mild cognitive impairment may quickly forget what the appropriate response format is, or fall quickly into response sets. When conducting interviews, we find cue cards with the rating scales printed on them in large print to be very helpful. When doing surveys, we repeat the response formats frequently to try to reduce response set bias. This is especially important when the formats change from scale to scale. To the extent possible, we group scales with the same formats together, and use visual cues to make it very clear when the response format changes. There may also be cohort difference in language use that make validity issues vital. For example, young and middle-aged adults have no problem whatsoever in talking about stress in their life and their coping strategies; older adults often do not respond as quickly, and may prefer not to characterize their lives in terms of "problems" or "stresses" (Aldwin, 1992). Thus, although many studies have examined correlations or mean level change with age, almost no one has examined systematically how the validity and reliability issues in the instruments themselves might change with age.

Minnesota Multiphasic Personality Inventory (MMPI). The MMPI or its revised version, the MMPI–2 (Butcher, Dahlstrom, Graham, Tellegen, & Kaemmer, 1989) is the instrument of choice for investigating pathological personality traits, or traits which may be conducive to pathology whether mental or physical. It has the advantage of a long track record and has received considerable use in older samples. Further, it is the instrument most often used by health psychologists in examining the relationship between personality and health (Piotrowski & Lubin, 1990). As noted above (Butcher et al., 1991), it does not appear that a special or separate version is needed for elderly samples—except for the impaired elderly, for which the brief MMPI (Kincannon, 1968) would be preferable, although Butcher (1991, personal communication) believes that it is not as reliable as the long version. The principal disadvantage of the MMPI is that its scales are unidirectional. That is, it is scored in the direction of more or less pathology, and the scale dimensions do not have explicitly "healthy" ends. To our knowledge, explicit studies of the reliability and validity of the MMPI or the MMPI–2 in the elderly have not been conducted, although the Butcher et al. (1991) study suggested a fair amount of similarity in item endorsement rates across age groups (with some obvious exceptions, such as whether a respondent used marijuana). However, several of the clinical scales include items which assess physical symptoms; thus, older respondents may appear depressed, hypomanic, or hypochondriacal when actually they have legitimate health complaints. Confirmatory factor analytic studies of the MMPI–2 have not been published.

California Personality Inventory (CPI). The CPI (Gough, 1960) is similar in appearance to the MMPI, but its emphases are rather different. The principle difference is the emphasis of the CPI on socialization and social maturity. Because of this, the CPI is not very appropriate for aging research in late life, although some of the subscales, such as Responsibility, Self-Control, and Tolerance of Ambiguity may be useful indices of development in young adulthood to midlife (Helson & Moane, 1987; Helson & Wink, 1992).

The 16 Personality Factor Scale (16PF). The 16PF scales (Cattell, 1973; Cattell, Eber, & Tatsuoka, 1980) based on factor analysis (rather than item analysis, as with the MMPI). 16PF is designed to be a taxonomy of personality traits rather than an assessment of pathology or pathology risk per se. It is designed to be bipolar, without regard to whether one end of the pole should be considered "healthy" or not. There are three forms, A, B, and the combination form, C. The 16PF is rather lengthy, but a shorter form (A or B) can be used. While at least 50 factor analyses have been conducted on the 16PF to try to determine what exactly the taxonomy of personality is (Cattell & Krug, 1986), none of them were apparently conducted with reference to older populations.

NEO Personality Inventory. The NEO Personality Inventory (Costa & McCrae, 1985) includes five dimensions, neuroticism, extraversion, openness to experience, agreeableness, and conscientiousness. Although the NEO has been used extensively with the Baltimore Longitudinal Study of Aging (BLSA) population (see McCrae & Costa, 1990 for a review), no work to our knowledge has been published indicating whether age differentials exist in the reliability or validity of the NEO. However, the NEO has both a self-rated and an observer-rated version, which is very useful in studies of personality change. Although Costa and McCrae (1988) found little correlation between self- and spouse-rated change using the NEO, Strauss et al. (1993) did find fairly good concordance when assessing personality change consequent upon Alzheimer's disease. Although both the patients and their spouses agreed that the patient's personality had changed, the spouses' ratings actually suggested greater change than that reported by the patients. Thus, the NEO can apparently be used successfully with even somewhat impaired populations.

Eysenck Personality Inventory (EPI). The EPI (Eysenck & Eysenck, 1968) is a two-dimensional scale which assesses introversion/extraversion and neuroticism, sometimes called emotionality. It is an extremely widely used instrument. A short form exists, the EPI–Q (Floderus, 1974), which is very useful for the elderly, since it only contains 18 dichotomous items. The EPI–Q predicts both mental health and stress ratings in older populations (Aldwin, Levenson, Spiro, & Bossé, 1989; Levenson, Aldwin, Bossé, & Spiro, 1988). The three-dimensional Eysenck Personality Questionnaire (EPQ; Eysenck & Eysenck, 1976) was developed later, which adds a psychoticism dimension to the original two. The interpretation of the psychoticism dimension is much more controversial (Block, 1977). Again, little information exists on age differences in reliability and validity on this measure.

Adjective Checklist (ACL). The ACL (Gough & Heilbrun, 1983) may be especially suited for aging research, as it covers a broad array of personality traits and has a very simple format—lists of adjectives which the respondent rates as like self or not like self. Again, no information exists on its validity or reliability in older people, although it appears reasonably sensitive to change (Helson & Moane, 1987; Helson & Wink, 1992).

California Q Sort. The California Q Sort (Block, 1978) is often very useful in longitudinal research, as it is a system for rating interview data and thus is not dependent upon instruments which are older and perhaps outdated. The research group from the Institute for Human Development has published extensively using this method with data from the Oakland Growth and Berkeley Guidance studies (Block, 1971; Eichorn, Clausen, Haan, Hanzika, & Mussen, 1981). In this procedure, raters read the interviews and sort cards into rank-ordered categories, based upon which characteristics are more or less dominant in each individual. Thus, the reference point is the rank order of characteristics within persons, rather than across persons, as with self-report inventories. In other words, most self-report inventories have the explicit or implicit instruction that, compared to other people, how much is some trait characteristic of the respondent. Thus, two people could be primarily characterized by introversion on a Q-sort, but one person could be much more introverted than the other. It could be argued that aggregating Q-sort ratings across individuals may be partly misleading; however, Q-sorts may be particularly useful for ipsative analyses. It would be interesting to see if age bias on the part of raters might exist in the use of this procedure.

Measures of Adult Development. A number of efforts have been made to psychometrically assess Erikson's life stages. Unfortunately, most of the instruments that have been developed have included only the first six stages, to the neglect of generativity and integrity, which are of greater interest to adult developmentalists. The most widely used one is the Erikson Psychosocial Stage Inventory (Rosenthal, Gurney, & Moore, 1981). Darling-Fisher and Leidy (1988) modified this instrument to include the last two stages and found good reliabilities for each of the subscales, .75 for generativity and .80 for ego integrity. Domino and Affonso (1990) developed the Inventory of Psychosocial Balance (IPB) to assess Erikson's stages. They found an eight-factor solution that paralleled the eight stages, which accounted for 72% of the total variance. Six of the IPB scales were significantly correlated with the CPI Social Maturity Index (Gough, 1966).

Some of the most extensive work on scales relevant to adult development has been done by Ryff and colleagues (Ryff, 1989a; Ryff & Essex, 1991; Ryff & Heincke, 1983). The Developmental Personality Scales (Ryff & Heincke, 1983) include measures of complexity, generativity, integrity, and interiority. The reliabilities for these scales range from .70 to .82. The Scales of Psychological Well-Being (Ryff, 1989a) consist of six subscales assessing Self-Acceptance, Positive Relations with Others, Autonomy, Environmental Mastery, Purpose in Life, and Personal Growth. Their reliabilities range from .83 to .91. These factor into three dimensions assessing Well-Being, Personal Growth, and Autonomy (Ryff & Essex, 1991). These scales are relatively short and have item content that is appropriate to older populations. Although cross-sectional age differences and studies of projected change (Ryff, 1989b) suggest that these scales are sensitive to developmental processes, as of yet no longitudinal data have been published.

Summary: Selecting an Instrument

Researchers and clinicians interested in conducting personality assessment in older adults should be aware of procedural and validity issues in such testing. While special forms of tests may not be needed with young-old or high-functioning elders, researchers should try to avoid tests which have been developed primarily with younger populations in mind. In general, simpler, briefer versions of personality instruments should be used in dealing with old-old or impaired elders.

WHITHER AGING AND PERSONALITY ASSESSMENT?

In some ways, the scattered nature of the literature on personality and aging is reminiscent of unconstrained chickens in a farmyard. They wander off in all directions, without much concern for what the others are doing. Thus, the various research groups that have longitudinal data generally use different instruments. In all fairness, the diversity reflects the very early stage of personality assessment at the time many of these studies were started. Unfortunately, it leads to many unanswered questions in aging and personality assessment.

A key and relatively unexplored issue is whether personality instruments as they currently exist are appropriate for older populations. Basic questions exist as to whether reliability, validity, and factor structures for the most widely used personality instruments are similar in late life to those found in younger samples. The dearth of studies utilizing confirmatory factor analysis for personality structure across age groups is surprising. Second, many major personality instruments are very long and often use scantron sheets. The old-old in particular may have difficulty with lengthy instruments with complex formats; motor tremors and poor eyesight may make the use of scantron sheets problematic. Whether personality instruments should be shortened and simplified for use in late life is an open question, but a particularly important one when conducting research with the cognitively impaired elderly.

A question which no longer needs to be addressed is whether personality changes or is stable across the life span. The studies of personality traits reviewed here clearly demonstrate moderate stability, coupled with maturational changes as well as cohort differences in the distribution of personality traits. However, most work has been done examining change from young to middle adulthood; longitudinal studies into late life are still rare. However, there are intriguing hints in the literature that change occurs even in very late life, and more research is needed to examine the nature of that change. Studies which examine both the trajectory and predictors of positive change, stability, and negative change in personality structure across the life span are also needed.

The relative rarity of studies of ego processes in late life was also surprising. From the few studies that do exist, it would appear that most development occurs from the early years to midlife, with the possibility of some further consolidation of ego processes within a single stage throughout life. Much more work is clearly needed in the conceptualization and assessment of wisdom. Integrating wisdom research with work in moral and ego development might simplify that task.

Finally, cohort effects on personality structure were surprisingly strong, which raises issues concerning the effect of social structure on personality. Unfortunately, secular trends appear to be negative. Schaie and Willis (1991) found decreases in social responsibility across cohorts, while Helson (personal communication, 1992) has documented increasing levels of narcissism in her samples. Thus, the sociology of personality approach has raised an interesting possibility. If successive cohorts are changing in some undesirable ways, it is equally likely that future cohorts could change in desirable ways. This possibility renders research into both how social structure affects personality and the factors which promote the development of wisdom a potentially critical contribution of geropsychology to societal well-being.

NOTES

1. Validity issues in the elderly, of necessity, speak to change, either within a person or across cohorts. If an instrument is deemed valid in a younger sample but not in an older one, obviously there is something different about the elderly and their experience. Reliability issues, on the other hand, may be a function of validity or they may be a function of physiological problems, such as impaired memory or visual acuity. In the latter case these issues would be subsumed under procedural issues rather than any question of personality change per se.
2. With longitudinal data, the issue of missing data is always difficult. Listwise deletion, in which all respondents must have data on all measures at all points, often re-

sults in losing a large portion of the population. This, in turn, results in problems of generalizability—respondents who are especially compliant may well differ systematically from those who are less dependable. In smaller samples, listwise deletion may mean that too much power may be lost for any meaningful results. On the other hand, maximizing the sample size by using pairwise deletion results in the *N* varying across samples results in interpretation problems. Surprisingly, none of the studies reported here either presented alternative analyses based upon pairwise versus listwise deletion or attempted to use missing data estimation techniques. Most simply allowed the *N* to vary across analyses, which is why we reported only the initial *N*.

REFERENCES

Adams, C., Labouvie-Vief, G., Hobart, C. j., & Dorosz, M. (1990). Adult age group differences in story recall style. *Journals of Gerontology: Psychological Sciences, 45*, P17–P27.

Aldwin, C. M. (in press). *Stress, coping, and development across the lifespan: A transactional approach.* New York: Guilford.

Aldwin, C. M. (1992). Aging, coping, and efficacy: Theoretical framework for examining coping in life-span developmental context. In M. L. Wykle, E. Kahana, & J. Kowal, (Eds.), *Stress and health among the elderly* (pp. 96–113). New York: Springer.

Aldwin, C. M., Levenson, M. R., Spiro, A. III, & Bossé, R. (1989). Does emotionality predict stress? Findings from the Normative Aging Study. *Journal of Personality and Social Psychology, 56*, 618–624.

Aldwin, C. M., Spiro, A. III, Levenson, M. R., & Bossé, R. (1989). Longitudinal findings from the Normative Aging Study. I. Does mental health change with age? *Psychology and Aging, 4*, 295–306.

Bakken, L., & Ellsworth, R. (1990). Moral development in adulthood: Its relationship to age, sex, and education. *Education Research Quarterly, 14*, 2–9.

Baltes, P. B., Reese, H. W., & Lipsitt, L. P. (1980). Lifespan developmental psychology. *Annual Review of Psychology, 31*, 65–110.

Baltes, P. B., & Smith, J. (1990). Toward a psychology of wisdom and its ontogenesis. In R. Sternberg (Ed.), *Wisdom: Its nature, origins, and development* (pp. 87–120). New York: Cambridge University Press.

Beaton, S. R. (1991). Styles of reminiscence and ego development of older women residing in long-term care settings. *International Journal of Aging and Human Development, 32*, 53–63.

Block, J. (1971). *Lives through time.* Berkeley: Bancroft Books.

Block, J. (1977). The Eysencks and psychoticism. *Journal of Abnormal Psychology, 86*, 653–654.

Block, J. (1978). *The Q–sort method in personality assessment and psychiatric research.* Palo Alto, CA: Consulting Psychologists Press.

Brandtstädter, J., Wentura, D., & Greve, W. (1993). Adaptive resources of the aging self: Outlines of an emergent perspective. *International Journal of Behavioral Development, 16*, 323–349.

Brim, O. C. (1965). Adult socialization. In J. A. Clausen (Ed.), *Socialization and society* (pp. 182–226). Boston: Little Brown.

Buss, A. H., & Plomin, R. (1975). *A temperament theory of personality development.* New York: Wiley–Interscience.

Buss, A. H., & Plomin, R. (1984). *Temperament: Early development of personality traits.* Hillsdale, NJ: Erlbaum.

Butcher, J. N., Aldwin, C. M., Levenson, M. R., Ben-Porath, Y. S., & Spiro, A. (1991). Personality and aging: A study of the MMPI–2 among older men. *Psychology and Aging, 6*, 361–370.

Butcher, J. N., Dahlstrom, W. G., Graham, J. R., Tellegen, A., & Kaemmer, B. (1989). *MMPI–2: Minnesota Multiphasic Personality Inventory–2. Manual for administration and scoring.* Minneapolis: University of Minnesota Press.

Caspi, A., Bem, D. J., & Elder, G. H. (1989). Continuities and consequences of interactional styles across the life course. *Journal of Personality, 57*, 375–406.

Cattell, R. B. (1973). *Personality and mood by questionnaire.* San Francisco: Jossey-Bass.

Cattell, R. B., Eber, H. W., & Tatsuoka, M. M. (1980). *Handbook for the Sixteen Personality Factor Questionnaire (16PF).* Champaign, Ill.: Institute for Personality and Ability Testing.

Cattell, R. B., & Krug, S. E. (1986). The number of factors in the 16PF: A review of the evidence with special emphasis on methodological problems. *Educational & Psychological Measurement, 46*, 509–522.

Chandler, M. J., & Holliday, S. G. (1990). Wisdom in a postapocalyptic age. In R. Sternberg (Ed.), *Wisdom: Its nature, origins, and development* (pp. 121–141). New York: Cambridge University Press.

Clayton, V., & Birren, J. E. (1980). The development of wisdom across the life span: A reexamination of an ancient topic. In P. B. Baltes and O. R. Brim (Eds.), *Life span development and behavior* (pp. 103–135). New York: Academic Press.

Colby, A., Kohlberg, L., Gibbs, J., & Lieberman, M. (1983). A longitudinal study of moral judgment. *Monographs of the Society for Research in Child Development, 48* (1–2, Serial No. 200).

Collins, L. M., & Horn, J. L. (1991). *Best methods for the analysis of change: Recent advances, unanswered questions, future directions.* Washington, DC: American Psychological Association.

Conley, J. J. (1985). Longitudinal consistency of adult personality: Self-reported psychological characteristics across 45 years. *Journal of Personality and Social Psychology, 47*, 1325–1333.

Costa, P. T., Jr., & McCrae, R. R. (1985). *The NEO personality inventory manual.* Odessa, FL: Psychological Assessment Resources.

Costa, P. T., Jr., & McCrae, R. R. (1988). Personality in adulthood: A six-year longitudinal study of self-reports and spouse ratings on the NEO Personality Inventory. *Journal of Personality and Social Psychology, 54*, 853–863.

Costa, P. T., Zonderman, A. B., McCrae, R. R., Cornoni-Huntley, J., Locke, B. Z., & Barbano, H. E. (1987). Longitudinal analyses of psychological well-being in a national sample: Stability of mean levels. *Journal of Gerontology, 42*, 50–55.

Darling-Fisher, C. S., & Leidy, N. K. (1988). Measuring Eriksonian development in the adult: The Modified Erikson Psychosocial Stage Inventory. *Psychological Reports, 62*, 747–754.

Domino, G., & Affonso, D. D. (1990). A personality measure of Erikson's life stages: The Inventory of Psychosocial Balance. *Psychological Assessment, 54*, 576–588.

Dudek, S. Z., & Hall, W. B. (1991). Personality consistency: Eminent architects 25 years later. *Creativity Research Journal, 4*, 213–231.

Dworkin, R. H., Burke, B. W., Maher, B. A., & Gottesman, I. I. (1976). A longitudinal study of the genetics of personality. *Journal of Personality and Social Psychology, 34*, 510–518.

Eichorn, D. H., Clausen, J. A., Haan, N., Honzik, M., & Mussen, P. (Eds.) (1981). *Present and past in middle life*. New York: Academic Press.

Elms, A. (in press). *One life at a time*. Oxford University Press.

Epstein, S. (1991). The self-concept, the traumatic neurosis, and the structure of personality. In D. Ozer, J. H. Healy, & A. J. Stewart (Eds.), *Perspective in Personality, 3*, 63–98.

Erikson, E. H. (1950). *Childhood and society*. New York: Norton.

Eysenck, H. J. (1987). Personality and ageing: An exploratory analysis. *Journal of Social Behavior and Personality, 3*, 11–21.

Eysenck, H. J., & Eysenck, S. B. G. (1976). *Psychoticism as a dimension of personality*. London: Hodder and Stoughton.

Eysenck, H. J., & Eysenck, S. B. (1968). *Manual of the Eysenck Personality Inventory*. San Diego: Educational and Industrial Testing Service.

Field, D., & Millsap, R. (1991). Personality in advanced old age: Continuity or change? *Journals of Gerontology: Psychological Sciences, 46*, P299–P308.

Field, D., Schaie, K. W., Leino, E. V. (1991). Continuity in intellectual functioning: The role of personality. *Mensa Research Journal, 30*, 6–19.

Finn, S. E. (1986). Stability of personality self-ratings over 30 years: Evidence for an age/cohort interaction. *Journal of Personality and Social Psychology, 50*, 813–818.

Fiske, M., & Chiriboga, D. A. (1990). *Change and continuity in adult life*. San Francisco: Jossey-Bass.

Floderus, B. (1974). Psychosocial factors in relation to coronary heart disease and associated risk factors [Monograph]. *Nordisk Hygienisk Tidskrift [Supplementum 6]*, 1–48.

Funder, D. C., Parke, R. D., Tomlinson-Keasey, C., & Widaman, K. (1993). *Studying lives through time*. Washington, DC: American Psychological Association.

Giambra, L. M., Camp, C. J., & Grodsky, A. (1992). Curiosity and stimulation seeking across the adult life span: Cross-sectional and 6- to 8-year longitudinal findings. *Psychology and Aging, 7*, 150–157.

Goldberg, L. R. (1993). The structure of phenotypic personality traits. *American Psychologist, 48*, 26–34.

Gottesman, I. I. (1963). Heritability of personality: A demonstration. *Psychological Monographs, 77* (Whole No. 572).

Gottesman, I. I. (1966). Genetic variance in adaptive personality traits. *Journal of Child Psychology and Psychiatry, 7*, 199–208.

Gough, H. G. (1960). *Manual for the California Psychological Inventory* (rev. ed.). Palo Alto, CA: Consulting Psychologists Press.

Gough, H. G. (1966). Appraisal of social maturity by means of the CPI. *Journal of Abnormal Psychology, 71*, 189–195.

Gough, H. G., & Heilbrun, A. B. Jr. (1983). *The adjective check list manual*. Palo Alto, CA: Consulting Psychologist Press.

Haan, N., Hartka, E., & Millsap, R. (1986). As time goes by: Change and stability in personality over fifty years. *Psychology and Aging, 1*, 220–232.

Helson, R., & Moane, G. (1987). Personality change in women from college to midlife. *Journal of Personality and Social Psychology, 53*, 176–186.

Helson, R., & Wink, P. (1992). Personality change in women from the early 40's to the early 50's. *Psychology and Aging, 7*, 46–55.

Holliday, S. G., & Chandler, M. J. (1986). *Wisdom: Explorations in adult competence*. Basel, Switzerland: Karger.

Jarvik, L. (1988). Aging of the brain: How can we prevent it? *The Gerontologist, 28*, 739–747.

Jones, E. E. (1990). *Interpersonal perception*. New York: Freeman.

Kagan, J. (1988). The meanings of personality predicates. *American Psychologist, 43*, 614–620.

Kagan, J. (1989). *Unstable ideas*. Cambridge, MA: Harvard University Press.

Kagan, J., Reznik, J. S., & Snidman, N. (1988). Biological bases of childhood shyness. *Science, 240*, 167–171.

Kincannon, J. C. (1968). Prediction of the standard MMP II scale scores from 71 items: The Mini-Mult. *Journal of Consulting and Clinical Psychology, 32*, 319–325.

Kitchener, K. S., King, P. M., Wood, P. K., & Davison, M. L. (1989). Consistency and sequentiality in the development of reflective judgment: A six year longitudinal study. *Journal of Applied Developmental Psychology, 10*, 73–95.

Kohlberg, L. (1973). Stages and aging in moral development: Some speculations. *The Gerontologist, 13*, 497–502.

Kohlberg, L. (1984). *The psychology of moral development*. San Francisco: Harper and Row.

Kruse, A., Lindenberger, U., & Baltes, P. B. (in press). Longitudinal research on human aging: The power of combining real-time, microgenetic, and simulation approaches. In D. Magnusson (Ed.), *Methodological and research strategical issues in longitudinal research*. Cambridge, England: Cambridge University Press.

Labouvie-Vief, G. (1990). Wisdom as integrated thought: historical and developmental perspectives. In R. Sternberg (Ed.), *Wisdom: Its nature, origin, and development* (pp. 52–86). New York: Cambridge University Press.

Labouvie-Vief, G., DeVoe, M., & Bulka, D. (1989). Speaking about feelings: Conceptions of emotion across the life span. *Psychology and Aging, 4*, 425–437.

Labouvie-Vief, G., Hakim-Larson, J., DeVoe, M., & Schoeberlein, S. (1989). Emotions and self-regulation: A life span review. *Human Development, 32*, 279–299.

Lachman, M. E. (1989). Personality and aging at the crossroads: Beyond stability versus change. In K. W. Schaie & C. Schooler (eds.), *Social structure and aging: Psychological processes*. Hillsdale, NJ: Erlbaum.

Lachman, M. E., & Leff, R. (1989). Perceived control and intellectual functioning in the elderly: A 5-year longitudinal study. *Developmental Psychology, 25*, 722–738.

Lamiell, J. T. (1987). *The psychology of personality: An epistemological inquiry*. New York: Columbia University Press.

Lamiell, J. T. (1981). Toward an idiothetic psychology of personality. *American Psychologist, 36*, 276–289.

Langer, E. J., Chanowitz, B., Palmerino, M., Jacobs, S., Rhodes, M., & Thayer, P. (1990). Nonsequential development and aging. In C. N. Alexander & E. J. Langer (Eds.),

Higher stages of human development (pp. 114–136). New York: Oxford University Press.

Levenson, H. (1974). Activism and powerful others: Distinctions within the concept of internal-external control. *Journal of Personality Assessment, 38*, 377–383.

Levenson, M. R., Aldwin, C. M., Bossé, R., & Spiro, A., III. (1988). Emotionality and mental health: Longitudinal findings from the Normative Aging Study. *Journal of Abnormal Psychology, 97*, 94–96.

Loevinger, J. (1966). The meaning and measurement of ego development. *American Psychologist, 21, 195–206.*

Loevinger, J. (1977). *Ego development: Conceptions and theories.* San Francisco: Jossey-Bass.

McAdams, D. P. (1985). *Power, intimacy and the life story: Personological inquiries into identity.* Homewood, Ill: Dorsey Press.

McAdams, D. P., de St. Aubin, E., & Logan, R. L. (1993). Generativity among young, midlife, and older adults. *Psychology and Aging, 8*, 221–230.

McCartney, K., Bernieri, F., & Harris, M. J. (1990). Growing up and growing apart: A developmental meta-analysis of twin studies. *Psychological Bulletin, 107*, 226–237.

McCrae, R. R. (1993). Moderated analyses of longitudinal personality stability. *Journal of Personality and Social Psychology, 65*, 577–585.

McCrae, R. R., & Costa, P. T. (1980). Openness to experience and ego level in Loevinger's Sentence Completion Test: Dispositional contributions to developmental models of personality. *Journal of Personality and Social Psychology, 39*, 1179–1190.

McCrae, R. R., & Costa, P. T. (1990). *Personality in adulthood.* New York: Guilford Press.

Mroczek, D. K. (1993). *Personality and psychopathology in older men: The five factor model and the MMPI–2.* Unpublished doctoral thesis, Boston University. *Dissertation Abstracts International,* 1992, Oct., *53*(n-4-B):2095.

Ochse, R., & Plug, C. (1986). Cross-cultural investigation of the validity of Erikson's theory of personality development. *Journal of Personality and Social Psychology, 50*, 1240–1252.

Parker, R. (1993). *The effect of social roles on sex role identity development in early and middle adulthood.* Unpublished doctoral thesis, University of California, Davis.

Piotrowski, C., & Lubin, B. (1990). Assessment practices of health psychologists: Survey of APA Division 38 clinicians. *Professional Psychology Research and Practice, 21*, 99–106.

Plomin, R., Pedersen, N. L., McClearn, G. E., Nesselroade, J. R., & Bergeman, C. S. (1988). EAS temperaments during the last half of the life span: Twins reared apart and twins reared together. *Psychology and Aging, 3*, 43–50.

Pogue-Geile, M. F., & Rose, R. J. (1985). Developmental genetic studies of adult personality. *Developmental Psychology, 21*, 547–557.

Pratt, M. W., Diessner, R., Hunsberger, B., Pancer, S. M., & Savoy, K. (1991). Four pathways in the analysis of adult development and aging: Comparing analyses of reasoning about personal-life dilemmas. *Psychology and Aging, 6*, 666–675.

Pratt, M. W., Golding, G., & Hunter, W. (1991). Age as ripening: Character and consistency of moral judgment in young, mature, and older adults. *Human Development, 26*, 277–288.

Raskind, M. A., & Peskind, E. R. (1992). Alzheimer's disease and other dementing disorders. In J. E. Birren, R. B. Sloane, & G. D. Cohen (Eds.), *Handbook of mental health and aging* (pp. 487–515). San Diego, CA: Academic Press.

Rest, J. (1979). *Development in judging moral issues.* Minneapolis: University of Minnesota Press.

Reznikoff, M., & Honeyman, M. A. (1967). MMPI profiles of monozygotic and dizygotic twins. *Journal of Consulting Psychology, 31*, 100–104.

Rogosa, D. R., Brandt, D., & Zimowsky, M. (1982). A growth curve approach to the measurement of change. *Psychological Bulletin, 90*, 726–748.

Rosenthal, D. A., Gurney, R. M., & Moore, S. M. (1981). From trust to intimacy: A new inventory for examining Erikson's stages of psychosocial development. *Journal of Youth and Adolescence, 10*, 525–537.

Rotter, J. B. (1966). Generalized expectancies of internal versus external control of reinforcement. *Psychological Monographs, 80* (Whole No. 609).

Ryff, C. D. (1989a). Happiness is everything, or is it? Explorations on the meaning of psychological well-being. *Journal of Personality and Social Psychology, 57*, 1069–1081.

Ryff, C. D. (1989b). In the eye of the beholder: Views of psychological well-being among middle-aged and older adults. *Psychology and Aging, 4*, 195–210.

Ryff, C. D., & Essex, M. J. (1991). Psychological well-being in adulthood and old age: Descriptive markers and explanatory processes. In K. W. Schaie (Ed.), *Annual Review of Gerontology and Geriatrics, 11*, 144–171. New York: Springer.

Ryff, C. D., & Heincke, S. G. (1983). Subjective organization of personality in adulthood and aging. *Journal of Personality and Social Psychology, 44*, 807–816.

Schaie, K. W., & Herzog, C. (1985). Measurement in the psychology of adulthood and aging. In J. E. Birren & K. W. Schaie (Eds.), *Handbook on the psychology of aging* (2nd ed., pp. 65–90). New York: Van Nostrand Reinhold.

Schaie, K. W., & Willis, S. (1991). Adult personality and psychomotor performance: Cross-sectional and longitudinal analyses. *Journals of Gerontology: Psychological Sciences, 46*, P275–P285.

Shewchuk, R. M., Foelker, G. A., Camp, C. J., Blanchard-Fields, F. (1992). Factorial invariance issues in the study of adult personality: An example using Levenson's locus of control scale. *Experimental Aging Research, 18*, 15–24.

Smith, J., & Baltes, P. B. (1990). Wisdom-related knowledge: Age/cohort differences in response to life-planning problems. *Developmental Psychology, 26*, 494–505.

Spiro, A., III, Butcher, J. N., Levenson, M. R., Aldwin, C. M., & Bossé, R. (in press). Personality change and stability over five years: The MMPI–2 in older men. *Journal of Personality.*

Spiro, A., III, Levenson, M. R., & Aldwin, C. (August, 1992). *How stable is personality?* Paper presented at the annual meeting of the American Psychological Association, Washington, DC.

Staudinger, U. M., Smith, J., & Baltes, P. B. (1992). Wisdom-related knowledge in a life review task: Age differences and the role of professional specialization. *Psychology and Aging, 7*, 271–281.

Sternberg, R. (1986). Implicit theories of intelligence, creativity, and wisdom. *Journal of Personality and Social Psychology, 49*, 607–627.

Sternberg, R. (1990). Wisdom and its relations to intelligence and creativity. In R. Sternberg (Ed.), *Wisdom: Its nature, origins, and development* (pp. 142–159). New York: Cambridge University Press.

Stevens, D. P., & Truss, C. V. (1985). Stability and change in adult personality over 12 and 20 years. *Developmental Psychology, 21*, 568–584.

Strauss, M. E., Pasupathi, M., & Chatterjee, A. (1993). Concordance between observers in descriptions of personality change in Alzheimer's disease. *Psychology and Aging, 8*, 475–480.

Vaillant, G. (1993). *The wisdom of the ego.* Cambridge, MA: Harvard University Press.

Vaillant, G., & McCullough, L. (1987). The Washington University Sentence Completion Test compared with other measures of adult ego development. *American Journal of Psychiatry, 144*, 1189–1194.

Vaillant, G. E., & Milofsky, E. (1980). Natural history of male psychological health: IX. Empirical evidence for Erikson's model of the life cycle. *American Journal of Psychiatry, 137*, 1348–1359.

Viney, L. L. (1987). A sociophenomenological approach to life-span development complementing Erikson's sociodynamic approach. *Human Development, 30*, 125–136.

Walker, L. (1989). A longitudinal study of moral reasoning. *Child Development, 60*, 157–166.

White, C. (1988). Age, education, and sex effects on adult moral reasoning. *International Journal of Aging and Human Development, 27*, 271–281.

White, M. S. (1985). Ego development in adult women. *Journal of Personality, 53*, 561–574.

Wink, P., & Helson, R. (1993). Personality change in women and their partners. *Journal of Personality and Social Psychology, 65*, 597–605.

CHAPTER 10

The Measurement of Affect in the Elderly

RICHARD SCHULZ

AND

ALISON T. O'BRIEN
DEPARTMENT OF PSYCHIATRY
AND UNIVERSITY CENTER FOR SOCIAL RESEARCH
UNIVERSITY OF PITTSBURGH

AND

CONNIE A. TOMPKINS
DEPARTMENT OF COMMUNICATION DISORDERS
UNIVERSITY OF PITTSBURGH

The experience and expression of affect are central features of human existence. Affect is a pervasive element of everyday life and helps to characterize the quality of life for most individuals. For more than a century, the centrality and ubiquity of emotional phenomena have secured the status of affect among behavioral scientists as a major focus for theory development and empirical investigation. The range of phenomena encompassed by this topic is so vast and the accompanying literature so extensive, it would be impossible to adequately cover it in one chapter. In keeping with the goals of this volume, we have limited our discussion to the following issues: conceptual issues regarding the definition and components of affect, rationales for studying affect, and methods of assessing affect.

CONCEPTUAL ISSUES: WHAT DO WE MEAN BY AFFECT?

Terms such as affect, emotion, and mood commonly occur in everyday discourse, and their meanings are generally well understood. These terms are often used interchangeably because they describe underlying phenomena that have much in common. Despite the unclear boundaries between the states these terms represent, there are some common variations in their use. Affect is a general term referring to the continuum of states comprised of *emotions*, *moods*, and *feeling states* (Clark & Isen, 1982). The term emotion describes a heightened state of arousal, usually elicited by an environmental stimulus. Emotions are likely to interrupt ongoing behavior, and redirect it toward a specific target in the external environment (Schulz, 1985). Emotions tend to be transient and intense experiences. In contrast, moods are more pervasive states that do not interrupt behavior and lack specific behavioral targets and consequences (Clark & Isen, 1982). Moods affect behaviors in a more subtle manner by influencing perception and cognition.

One of the ways scientists have enhanced our understanding of this area is by showing that affect refers to a very broad range of phenomena that includes behavioral, cognitive, physiological, and subjective feeling components (Stone, in press). Thus, encountering a bear while hiking in the woods is likely to elicit behaviors such as running away, cognitions about what bears can do to people, a racing heart and sweaty palms, along with subjective feelings of fear. Researchers interested in theories of emotion and affect have focused their attention on issues such as the essential elements necessary for the experience of a particular emotion and the temporal order in which these elements appear.

Dimensions that characterize affect states quantitatively include *intensity, frequency, and duration* (Schulz, 1985). Some researchers argue that the intensity of emotions can be described by the concurrent level of autonomic nervous system (ANS) arousal (Mackay, 1980). Thus, intense emotions such as rage occupy the extreme end of the ANS arousal continuum, whereas milder states such as sadness are characterized by more moderate degrees of physiological arousal. Affective states can also vary in the frequency with which they occur, and some researchers have suggested that intensity and frequency are discrete, independent components of affect (Diener, Larsen, Levine, & Emmons, 1985). Finally, emotional states vary in their duration. A given episode of affect may last for only seconds, as in the case of rage, or it may persist for weeks or even years, as is often true of depressed affect. In addition to studying *states*, or isolated instances of mood or emotion, investigators have also examined affect over extended periods of time to yield aggregate descriptions of emotional experience. These cumulative assessments are referred to as *traits* and provide information about affect commonly experienced by individuals (Anderson, 1989).

Thus far we have focused on components or elements of affect without defining the many specific, qualitatively different types of emotions commonly experienced. How to characterize different emotional states qualitatively remains a contentious issue, with two distinct camps advocating two different views of the structure of affect. The *specific affects approach* supports the existence of 6 to 12 independent monopolar factors, each with unique characteristics and response patterns (Izard, 1977; Plutchik, 1980; Tomkins, 1963). For example, Izard (1977) describes 10 basic emotions: joy, surprise, interest, sadness, anger, disgust, contempt, fear, shame/shyness, and guilt. An underlying assumption of the specific affects approach is that each distinct affect can be measured as a unique entity and a specific psychophysiological response is associated with each particular affective state (Stone, in press). Some of the research conducted by such theorists is concerned with developing and applying methods to identify these distinct emotions, and clarifying the functions of basic emotions in an evolutionary context. Universal facial expressions that reflect the basic emotions of anger, disgust, enjoyment, fear, sadness, and surprise have been identified in both Western and non-Western cultures, including preliterate societies (Ekman, 1992). Less consistent evidence also exists for universal facial expressions of contempt, guilt, interest and shame. Differences in ANS activity for five basic emotions have been isolated, and research in this area continues in an effort to determine the distinct physiological responses associated with each emotion (Levenson, 1992).

The *dimensional approach* claims that affects do not exist as discrete entities, but instead are related to each other in a highly systematic fashion, and are best characterized in terms of a few basic dimensions. Russell (1980) suggests that emotions are organized in accordance with two orthogonal dimensions, pleasure/displeasure and high/low activation, and that distinct affects can be arranged in a circumplex which reflects their relationship to each other. Thus, within this conceptual framework, anger would be represented by displeasure and high activation. Watson and Tellegen (1985) argue for negative affect and positive affect as the two basic dimensions, and arrange distinct affects in a similar circumplex. Anger would be described as loading positively and highly on negative affect and minimally on positive affect in this factor structure. The different dimensions obtained by these researchers can be accounted for by different factor analytic procedures. Although the dimensional approach appears to be dominant among researchers at this time, it has been criticized for failing to capture the richness of human emotional experience.

A final issue to consider in conceptualizing affect concerns the distinction between the *experience, expression* or display, and *perception* of affect. The large majority of the literature on affect and emotion in aging focuses on how and why individuals experience affect. Relatively little attention has been paid to age-related changes in the expression or display of affect, or to age-related changes in our ability to perceive affect in others (Malatesta, 1981; Malatesta, Izard, Culver, & Nicolich, 1987). We would encourage the development of research focused on the way in which age-related physical changes may influence the expression of affect through voice and face, and the perception of emotion through sensory modalities. For example, negative emotions such as grief and sadness may be perceived more often in the elderly because of age-related changes in vocal characteristics such as slow rates of speaking, diminished amounts of vocal inflection or emphasis, and lower pitch (Schulz & Tompkins, 1989). Extremes of either positive or negative affect may be less well communicated due to reduced vocal modulation. Similar arguments could be made for tissue and musculature changes in the face leading to more frequent perceptions of minimized or blended emotions among the elderly

(Malatesta & Izard, 1984). In addition, individuals without their glasses or dentures have facial characteristics (e.g., squinting or slack jaw) which may lead others to perceive negative affect more frequently. Perceiving affect in others may be influenced by age-related hearing and vision changes, possibly reducing the ability of older persons to detect subtle changes associated with communication of emotion .

To summarize this section, one can identify many factors that are used to characterize affect and have implications for measurement. One can measure any of a number of different components of affect that may vary in intensity, duration, and frequency. Divergent perspectives on the structure of affect also suggest different measurement strategies. Finally, even though most work (including this chapter) focuses on ways to measure the experience of affect in aging, it is important to recognize that one can also assess how individuals express affect, or detect it in others (e.g., Buck, 1984).

Distinguishing Between Affect and Conceptually Related Constructs

Given the importance of affect in human experience, it is not surprising that a number of constructs are conceptually related to emotion. For instance, affect is an important dimension of most well-being and life satisfaction measures. Some individual difference constructs are related to the quality or intensity of emotion people are likely to experience, and many psychiatric disorders have affective features. Assessments of these domains include dimensions in addition to affect, indicating that they are distinct from measures designed to assess affect exclusively. As the definition of any construct is critical to its measurement, a discussion of how affect differs from related concepts follows in an effort to further clarify our definition of this construct.

Life Satisfaction. Life satisfaction represents a cognitive evaluation of an individual's life in general, and implies a comparison between actual and ideal situations. (George, 1981). The extent to which a person's life situation is congruent with a desired or ideal life reflects the degree of life satisfaction or dissatisfaction. While affect may be related to life satisfaction, the predominant feature of this construct is a cognitive, rather than affective, assessment of one's life circumstance.

Subjective Well-Being. Subjective well-being is a multidimensional construct which includes both affective and cognitive components. Although there is disagreement as to the specific dimensions which constitute well-being, some investigators suggest the existence of three higher order factors: cognitive evaluation (similar to life satisfaction), positive affect, and negative affect (Kercher, 1992). Thus, the inclusion of a cognitive assessment dimension in subjective well-being distinguishes this construct from affect.

Demoralization. Jerome Frank (1974, 1985) describes a state he terms demoralization, which consists of two requisite components. One feature characterizing demoralization is negative affect, commonly experienced as depression, guilt, anxiety, or shame. In addition to these feelings, a demoralized individual is overwhelmed by a profound sense of incompetence and hopelessness. A perceived inability to cope with one's life situation and the accompanying emotional distress together comprise demoralization.

Psychopathology. Features of many psychiatric disorders are described as the excess or absence of particular emotions. For example, a predominant feature of major depression is the persistence of intense negative affect, particularly sadness, and a concurrent lack of positive affect. Accompanying these affective features in major depression are somatic symptoms. Eating, sleeping, and concentration are disturbed. Psychomotor agitation or retardation may be present. These neurovegetative symptoms differentiate major depression from sadness (American Psychiatric Association [APA], 1987). Other disorders have less obvious affective components. Conduct disorder is considered a behavioral disorder; however, individuals with this disorder display a great deal of aggression, and very little guilt (APA 1987). It is the constellation of affective, behavioral, and somatic symptoms that lead to the description of psychopathology. Another way in which psychopathology differs from affect is that an implicit requirement for diagnosis is the impairment of normal functioning by the presence of psychiatric symptoms.

Personality and Individual Differences. Personality refers to the stable and enduring characteristics of an individual. In contrast, emotions or moods are considered transient states, and may change quickly. Some conceptual approaches to personality do include components which are relevant to affect. For instance, the neuroticism and extraversion dimensions proposed by McCrae and Costa (1984) incorporate proneness to experience negative affect and positive affect, respectively. Larsen and Diener (1987) propose an individual difference variable, affect intensity, which refers to the intensity of emotion a person typically experiences. Both of these concepts describe dispositional characteristics rather than specific instances of affect.

Why Measure Affect? Affect has long been recognized as an important outcome for characterizing the status of older people. In many gerontological studies, it is used as an outcome measure in its own right, or as a mediator or moderator of outcomes thought to be associated with affective states. For example, virtually all instruments assessing subjective well-being contain items or scales assessing affective functioning (Birren, Lubben, Rowe, & Deutchman, 1991; Lawton, 1991; Spilker, Molinek, Johnston, & Simpson, 1990; Ware & Sherbourne, 1992). A good example is the widely used SF-36 Health Survey (McHorney, Ware, & Raczek, 1993; Ware and Sherbourne, 1992) which includes a separate scale for mental health with items such as "felt downhearted and blue," "been a happy person," "felt calm and peaceful." Although distilling the essence of life into a few dimensions can be a risky proposition, there exists strong consensus that negative and positive affect as well as energy and vitality are essential metrics for characterizing quality of life (Arnold, 1991).

Investigators interested in understanding age-related differences in the experience of affect also typically view measures of affect as outcomes. Early theoretical work on affective experience in late life predicted increasing negative affect with age, accompanied by blunting and constriction of affective states, (Tomkins, 1963). However, some recent work challenges this view (Malatesta & Kalnok, 1984). Empirical research addressing theoretical issues in this area is still relatively rare (Lawton, Kleban, Rajagopal, & Dean, 1992; Malatesta et al., 1987; Malatesta & Kalnok, 1984), but much descriptive work has been conducted which does characterize individuals on one or more affective dimensions. A good example can be found in the extensive research efforts using screening instruments such as the Center for Epidemiologic Studies Depression Scale (CES-D; Radloff, 1977). This instrument was designed as a screening tool for a clinical condition, but it can also be viewed as a means for describing the affective status of an individual on one or possibly two dimensions: depression/sadness and vitality.

A third common use of measures of affect is predicated on the role of affect in many stress-coping models as a predictor of other important outcomes such as morbidity and mortality. The model of Cohen, Kessler, and Gordon (in press) serves as a good example of how affect is viewed in the stress-coping context. According to this model, once a stressor is appraised as demanding and the individual is unable to cope with it, an affective response is elicited. This response in turn elicits a physiological and/or behavioral reaction. Although one might take exception to the details of this model, it nevertheless shows how affective response can be viewed as a mediator or moderator of antecedent conditions and subsequent outcomes. In keeping with the stress-coping paradigm, investigators have also suggested that specific enduring affective states, such as anger and hostility, may be linked to important health outcomes such as mortality (Barefoot, Dodge, Peterson, & Dahlstrom, 1989; Barefoot, Siegler, Nowlin, & Peterson, 1987).

Many scientists study the association between affective experience and diverse motivational, social and communicative behaviors (Frijda, 1986; Izard, 1977; Malatesta, 1981). Emotions interrupt ongoing behavior and redirect attention to factors in the external environment which may be threatening to the individual (Clark & Isen, 1982). In the context of ongoing intimate relationships, the experience of emotion often indicates that the pursuit of shared goals has been impeded (Berscheid, 1983). Affect can also serve as an indicator as to whether or not progress is being made toward goals and may influence the way in which certain goals are pursued (Emmons & Diener, 1986). Social behavior or interactions may be influenced by affect, and may, in turn, influence impact feeling states. For example, moods influence whether or not people engage in prosocial behavior (Carlson, Charlin, & Miller, 1988), which may be followed by an increase in positive affect

(Williamson & Clark, 1989). Social comparison processes often result in affective outcomes (Buunk, Collins, Taylor, Van Yperen, & Dakof, 1990), which in turn influence self-evaluations (Sedikides, 1992). Finally, individuals may communicate their needs to others through emotional expression, particularly in the context of close relationships (Clark, 1983; Clark & Taraban, 1991).

The interaction between feeling states and cognition provides another domain in which affect is a variable of interest. Affect is a pervasive contextual factor that influences sensory, perceptual, learning, and memory processes. For example, Tompkins and colleagues (Tompkins, Spencer, & Boada, in press) have demonstrated that different affective contexts can alter the interpretation of ambiguous vocal expressions. Similarly, Russell and Fehr (1987) have shown that the same facial expression can be perceived as conveying different types and degrees of emotion, depending on what other faces are seen before it. Mood influences on learning and memory have been reported by researchers examining mood-congruent memory effects (e.g., Blaney, 1986; Gilligan & Bower, 1984). This research indicates that individuals are generally better able to recall information when mood states are the same during learning and retrieval.

In sum, the ubiquity of affect in daily life has its counterpart in the world of research. Hundreds and perhaps thousands of studies are reported each year in which the measurement of affect is a primary focus. Although the work on affect in the gerontological domain is less extensive, there are many rationales for examining the role of affect in cognitive, behavioral and social aspects of late life. This leads to us to ask, What measures are available to assess emotion, and how and when should they be used?

MEASURES OF AFFECT

An extensive range of measures has been developed to assess affect. Our focus here is on self-report measures, but it is important to keep in mind that the literature offers many additional options, including measures of facial musculature (Ekman & Friesen, 1978) and facial expression (Buck, 1984; Ekman, 1982), blood flow to the brain (Zajonc & McIntosh, 1992; Zajonc, Murphy, & Inglehart, 1989), and other physiological indicators such as skin conductance (Levenson, Ekman, & Friesen, 1990).

Self-report measures of affect are summarized in Table 10.1. Our intent is not to be exhaustive, but rather to provide a representative sample of instruments currently available, with special emphasis on scales used with elderly individuals. Not included in this list are the many global quality of life measures, such as the Life Satisfaction Index (Neugarten, Havighurst, & Tobin, 1961), or psychiatric screening instruments, such as the CES-D, even though measures of affect are frequently a key element in these measures.

Affect Measures Used Extensively with the Elderly

The Affect Balance Scale. The measures of affect most commonly used to assess emotion in the elderly are the Bradburn Affect Balance Scale (Bradburn, 1969) and the Profile of Mood States (POMS; McNair, Lorr, & Droppleman, 1971). The Affect Balance Scale is a 10-item instrument consisting of a 5-item positive affect scale (PAS) and a 5-item negative affect scale (NAS). Respondents indicate whether or not they have experienced different affective states over some period of time, usually the past few weeks. Scores on the PAS and NAS are summed to provide information on positive and negative affect separately, and an affect balance score is obtained by taking the difference between PAS and NAS (i.e., affect balance = PAS–NAS). Although the relatively small number of items and the simple response format contribute to the ease with which the scale can be administered to elderly samples, several properties of the scale have been criticized (Diener & Emmons, 1985; Watson, 1988). Most of the items on the positive subscale refer to specific instances when affect is experienced (e.g., "pleased about having accomplished something"), and items on the negative subscale tend to refer to more general feeling states (e.g., "depressed or very unhappy"), indicating that the items presented on this scale may not reflect an adequate range of affective experiences. In addition, the dichotomous response format does not capture the frequency and intensity of feeling states, and artificially biases factor structures against intercorrelation (see Russell, 1979). Finally, the positive and negative subscales are consistently found to have low reliability (Watson, 1988). A modified 9-item version of this scale with a 4-point response format (Warr, Barter, & Brownbridge, 1983) demonstrates somewhat better reliability than the original scale (Watson, 1988).

The Profile of Mood States (POMS). POMS consists of 65 emotion adjectives that respondents rate on a 4-point scale for the extent to which they felt that way during the past week (McNair et al., 1971). Originally titled the Psychiatric Outpatient Mood Scale, this instrument was designed to measure mood changes in psychiatric outpatients. Consequently, the POMS assesses clinical aspects of affect more than most measures, a fact reflected by the factor structure of the scale. The six factors identified include Tension-Anxiety, Depression-Dejection, Anger-Hostility, Vigor-Activity, Fatigue-Inertia, and Confusion-Bewilderment. Since its development, the instrument has been widely used with a variety of samples including elderly respondents. Administering the POMS to nursing home patients has proven quite difficult, however, as few are able to complete the scale (Kaye et al., 1988). The primary difficulty in using this measure with the elderly is the length of the scale, which may fatigue more impaired elders. Further, some investigators have raised the concern that the instruction to report mood over a 1-week period may measure trait aspects of affect, rather than current affective state (Howarth & Schokman-Gates, 1981). A 40-item version of the POMS exists with instructions

TABLE 10.1 Measures of Affect

Scale	*Number of items*	*Item style response categories*	*No. of factors or dimensions*	*Use with elderly*	*Comments*
Affect Balance Scale (Bradburn, 1969)	10	phrases describing feeling states (5 positive, 5 negative) rated yes or no	2	Extensively used with the elderly	Low reliability consistently demonstrated, heavily critiqued
Profile of Mood States (McNair, Lorr, & Droppleman, 1971)	65	adjectives rated on 4- or 5-point scales	6	Extensively used with the elderly	Widely used, but difficult to administer to nursing home residents
Multiple Affect Adjective Checklist (Zuckerman & Lubin, 1965, 1985)	132	adjectives that are checked or not checked	3	Some use with the elderly	Subscales demonstrate high reliability but high intercorrelation
Eight State Questionnaire (Curran & Cattell, 1976)	96	descriptions of feelings rated on 4-point scales	8	No recent use with the elderly	Widely used
Clyde Mood Scale (Clyde, 1963)	44	adjectives rated on 4-point scales	6	No recent use with the elderly	Scale is most appropriate for use in drug studies
Nowlis Mood Adjective Checklist (Nowlis, 1965)	36	adjectives rated on 4-point scales	12	No recent use with the elderly	A shorter, 12-item version of the MACL, which excludes the "cannot decide" response, has been used by Stone (1981)
Differential Emotions Scale (Izard, Dougherty, Bloxom & Kotsch, 1974)	36	descriptions of feelings rated on 5-point scales	10–12	Some use with the elderly	High intercorrelation between subscales measuring negative affective states
Semantic Differential Mood Scale (Lorr & Wunderlich, 1988)	35	pairs of bipolar adjectives rated on 5-point scales	5	Not used with the elderly	Internal consistency adequate

Positive and Negative Affect Schedule (Watson, Clark, & Tellegen, 1988)	20	adjectives rated on 5-point scales	2	Some use with the elderly	High reliability reported in both student and nonstudent adult samples
Diener & Emmons (1985)	9 or 12	4 or 6 positive and 5 or 6 negative affect terms rated on 7-point scales	2	Part of sample elderly	Fairly high reliability in both student and community samples
PGC Positive and Negative Affect Scales (Lawton, Kleban, Dean, Rajagopal, & Parmelee, 1992)	10	5 positive and 5 negative affect terms rated on 5-point scales	2	Some use with the elderly	Different factor structures appeared in different age groups
Positive States of Mind Scale (Horowitz, Adler, & Kegeles, 1988)	6	descriptions of feelings rated on 4-point scales	1	Not used with the elderly	Adequate reliability and some convergent validity established in an undergraduate sample
Neutral Word Ratings (Kuykendall, Keating, & Wagaman, 1988)	6	neutral words rated on 7-point scales for pleasantness	1	Not used with the elderly	Discriminates between subjects induced to be in positive, neutral, or negative moods
Visual Analogue Scale (numerous investigators)	1	respondent marks mood on a 100 mm line with descriptive terms at ends	1	Some use with the elderly	Difficult to evaluate reliability; face validity good for a global measure of mood
Circular Mood Scale (Jacob et al., 1989)	1	circle outlined with adjectives and marked for current mood	2	Not used with the elderly	Useful for assessing general affect; must use angular statistics
Affect Grid (Russell, Weiss, & Mendelsohn, 1989)	1	adjectives around a 9 x 9 matrix that is marked for cell best describing mood	2	Not used with the elderly	Responses change with mood induction as expected; further evaluation necessary

to report current mood, but the reliability and validity of this scale need further evaluation (Grove & Prapavessis, 1992).

In short, the two measures most commonly employed to assess affect in elderly samples may not be the most appropriate instruments for use with some older samples. An overview follows of other measures of affect that have been used less extensively with the elderly. The progression of this presentation is approximately chronological; earlier instruments are considered separately from those developed more recently.

Early Measures of Affect: The Multidimensional Approach

The earliest developed affect instruments[1] consist of a number of dimensions, ranging from 3 to 12 (see Table 10.1). Their multidimensional structure is consistent with the *specific affects*, or *differential emotions*, conceptualization of emotion. These multidimensional instruments contain a relatively large number of items (between 35 and 132) and have been used much more extensively than the recently developed measures, reviewed subsequently. Advantages to using older measures are that, generally, they have been administered to a diverse range of samples in the context of a variety of research designs, and have well-established psychometric properties. Despite their advantages, these older, multidimensional measures of affect raise several concerns for use with the elderly. For instance, the length of these scales can fatigue all but the healthiest of elderly individuals. In addition, some scales include emotion terms that may lie beyond the scope of the average respondent's vocabulary, particularly when English is not the native language.

The Multiple Affect Adjective Checklist (MAACL). Developed by Zuckerman and Lubin (1965, 1985), the MAACL consists of 132 adjectives that respondents check if they have felt that way during some period of time, usually the past week. The MAACL has been used in hundreds of studies, including studies of the elderly (Lubin et al., 1988; Salzman, Kochansky, Shader, & Cronin, 1972). This instrument was specifically designed to measure anxiety, depression and hostility, and like the POMS, the MAACL emphasizes clinical aspects of these emotions more than most scales. The Anxiety, Depression, and Hostility subscales demonstrate high reliability, but there is a great deal of intercorrelation between the three subscales. Consequently, there is some dispute as to whether the three subscales should be treated as separate measures, rather than summed to yield an overall measure of negative affect (Howarth & Schokman-Gates, 1981). In addition, factor analyses have yielded between one and five factors, with no consistent explanations for the observed variations in factor structure. The large number of scale items limits the usefulness of this instrument for gerontological research (Salzman et al., 1972); however, the trait form has been used recently with the elderly (Lubin et al., 1988).

The Eight State Questionnaire (8SQ). This is a widely used instrument containing 96 items designed to assess eight different affective states (Curran & Cattell,

1976). The items are grouped into eight subscales, Anxiety, Stress, Depression, Regression, Fatigue, Guilt, Extraversion, and Arousal, each containing 12 items rated on 4-point scales for current feelings. Investigators commonly use only those subscales that are relevant to their research questions. Some analyses have demonstrated high intercorrelations between the subscales of the 8SQ (Boyle, 1985), whereas others have not (Boyle & Katz, 1991). Two advantages of this measure are, first, items are descriptions of affective states rather than adjectives, which may minimize vocabulary difficulties, and, second, it has been clearly established as a state instrument. The length of the scale may pose difficulty for some older persons (e.g., the frail elderly) and certain protocols (e.g., those including many assessments). The 8SQ has not been used in recent years with the elderly.

The Clyde Mood Scale. This scale (Clyde, 1963) consists of 48 adjectives that respondents rate on 4-point scales, indicating the extent to which the words describe their current feelings. The scale was initially developed to assess mood changes in psychiatric patients and designed for use in drug studies (Clyde, 1963). Factor analyses have identified six dimensions labelled Friendly, Aggressive, Clear-Thinking, Sleepy, Unhappy and Dizzy, indicating that the instrument assesses arousal and clarity of consciousness in addition to affect. An advantage of this scale is that it does not include a *cannot decide* category in the response options; such a category has been found to bias factor analyses towards a unidimensional structure (Russell, 1979). Little research involving elderly individuals has been conducted using this scale.

The Nowlis Mood Adjective Checklist (MACL). Originally created with 130 adjectives, the most commonly used form of the MACL consists of 36 adjectives that respondents rate on 4-point scales to describe current mood (Nowlis, 1965). The Nowlis MACL has been well validated and continues to be used frequently in social science research. A 12-factor structure has been identified for the MACL, and on this basis, Stone (1981) developed a 12-item version of the scale that has been used in a number of studies (e.g., Kennedy-Moore, Greenberg, Newman, & Stone, 1992). Stone's (1981) 12-item MACL is brief, excludes the *cannot decide* category from the original set of response options, and factors into positive and negative engagement scales.

The Differential Emotions Scale-IV (DES-IV). The DES consists of 36 descriptions of feelings that are rated on 5-point scales for how often the respondent has felt that way over a specified period of time (Kotsch, Gerbing, & Schwartz, 1982). It was originally designed to assess the 10 basic emotions identified by differential emotions theorists (Izard, Dougherty, Bloxom, & Kotsch, 1974), but has been slightly modified to include 12 subscales (Interest, Enjoyment, Surprise, Sadness, Anger, Disgust, Contempt, Fear, Guilt, Shame, Shyness, and Inward Hostility). The reliability of many of the subscales is quite high, but a few, such as the Disgust and Shame subscales, demonstrate slightly less impressive psychometric properties (Kotsch et al., 1982). Earlier versions of the DES have been used with elderly individuals, but there is no recent research using the DES-IV with the elderly.

The Semantic Differential Mood Scale (SDMS). Respondents rate 35 pairs of mood antonyms on 5-point scales for which descriptor better indicates their current mood (Lorr & Wunderlich, 1988). The SDMS was created as a bipolar instrument based on the assumption that every mood state has a bipolar opposite. The scale was designed to be used with nonpsychiatric samples, and to include a wide range of positive affect items. Recently developed with high school respondents, the scale needs to be further evaluated with a variety of samples and research designs.

Recent Assessments of Affect: The Basic Dimensions Approach

Recent research on the measurement of affect has led to the development of instruments that assess one or two fundamental dimensions, and consequently, are more consistent with the *basic dimensions* view of affect than the previously discussed multidimensional instruments. As shown in Table 10.1, the newer measures, containing 6 to 20 items, are typically shorter than multidimensional assessments. Three of the following six measures have been used minimally with elderly samples, but all merit further exploration in gerontological research, given the potential advantages of using shorter assessments with the elderly. These instruments take less time to complete, and may prove less fatiguing to frail elders, than the preceding scales. In addition, they can be included easily in studies assessing a number of constructs, and some are short enough for frequent assessments over time. The primary problem with using these recently developed measures of affect is the paucity of available information on their reliability and validity, particularly with older respondents.

The Positive and Negative Affect Schedule (PANAS). Respondents rate 10 positive and 10 negative affect adjectives on 5-point scales to reflect the extent to which they have felt that way during a specific period of time (Watson, Clark, & Tellegen, 1988). The PANAS was developed to maintain independence of the Positive Affect (PA) and Negative Affect (NA) scales, and the intercorrelation between the two is consistently low, independent of the time frame over which respondents report. Both subscales exhibit high reliability in student and nonstudent adult samples (Watson, Clark, & Tellegen, 1988). Older adults have completed a 10-item version of the PANAS, and the factor structure obtained in this sample is quite consistent with other age groups (Kercher, 1992).

Diener and Emmons Affect Scales. Diener and Emmons (1985) used affect of several types in a series of studies designed to clarify the association between positive and negative affect. Two of these scales were later evaluated by Watson (1988) and found to be highly internally consistent. One scale is composed of 9 affect items, 4 positive (enjoyment/fun, happy, joyful, and pleased) and 5 negative (angry/hostile, depressed/blue, frustrated, unhappy, and worried/anxious). The other consists of

12 adjectives, 6 positive (content, delighted, glad, happy, pleased, and satisfied), and 6 negative (annoyed, depressed, frustrated, gloomy, miserable, and sad). The second scale was found to be somewhat more reliable than the first. Both measures employ the common procedure of having respondents rate the extent to which they have felt each emotion over a specified time frame, using 7-point scales. Some community dwelling elderly individuals were included in Diener and Emmons' fifth study (1985), but these measures have not been applied with more extensive samples of older adults.

The Philadelphia Geriatric Center (PGC) Positive and Negative Affect Scales. These scales were recently designed to provide a brief assessment of emotion that includes a wider range of affective states than other short instruments (Lawton, Kleban, Dean, Rajagopal, & Parmelee, 1992). Both the Positive and Negative Affect Scales consist of five adjectives that are rated on 5-point scales for how often the feelings were experienced over a particular time period. Although this instrument was developed primarily for use with elderly samples, it has also been completed by young and middle-aged adults. Differences in factor loadings between age groups dictate caution when making age comparisons. Two important advantages of Lawton and colleagues' measure are its brevity and demonstrated utility with both frail and healthy elders (Lawton et al., 1992). Given the recent development of this instrument, further evaluation of its psychometric properties is recommended.

The Positive States of Mind Scale (PSOM). Horowitz, Adler, & Kegeles (1988) developed the PSOM to provide an assessment of several positive mood states, an area that has received less attention than the evaluation of negative states. The PSOM consists of six descriptions of distinct positive feeling states that are rated on 4-point scales for the degree to which they were experienced over the preceding week. The instrument demonstrates adequate internal reliability, and some convergent validity has been established. The PSOM has only been used with undergraduate students, so it will be important to evaluate this scale with diverse individuals and research designs.

Neutral Word Ratings. A relatively nonreactive method of assessing affect, neutral word ratings require respondents to rate the pleasantness of neutral word stimuli. The method is based on the premise that moods will influence perception of affectively neutral objects (Kuykendall, Keating, & Wagaman, 1988). Respondents are given six words purported to be emotionally neutral (rock, solitude, coffee, bear, weight, down), to be rated on 7-point scales for pleasantness-unpleasantness. It is unclear whether this method can be used in the same way as other self-report measures of affect, but it does discriminate, albeit imperfectly, between subjects induced to be in positive, neutral, or negative moods. This approach to affect measurement was developed with undergraduate students, and has not been extended to other age groups. It might be particularly appropriate for use in situations where demand characteristics or reactivity are expected to exert significant influences on subjective reports of affect.

Single-Item Assessments of Affect

Several available measures of affect consist of one item. If retest reliability and validity are adequate, these measures may be useful when assessing affect in the frail elderly, when a research question requires only a global measure of affect, or when repeated assessments of affect must be completed over an extended period of time.

Visual Analogue Scales (VAS). VAS have been used in a variety of research areas to provide subjective, global information on psychological and physiological states. Visual analogue scales can be used to measure a wide range of constructs, and they are easy for subjects to complete. Respondents are presented with a 100-mm line with descriptors at each end and are asked to indicate their current state by placing a mark on the line. Often, one VAS is presented to assess general mood, but some investigators use more items with greater specificity. For example, Monk (1989) describes an 8-item VAS that includes a general vigor and a general affect dimension. A VAS is particularly useful when global affect must be assessed frequently but may not be appropriate for measuring distinct feeling states (Cella & Perry, 1986). It is difficult to evaluate the psychometric properties of a single VAS, but the face validity is good for a general assessment of affect. These instruments have been used occasionally with the elderly.

The Circular Mood Scale (CMS). Recently designed to provide a quick, easily completed assessment of current mood (Jacob et al., 1989), the CMS is based on the assumption that affect is bipolar in nature, and can be represented as a circle reflecting varying degrees of arousal and positive or negative affect. Respondents are presented with mood adjectives placed around a circle at 45-degree intervals and are asked to mark their current mood along the circle. Intensity of mood can also be assessed by instructing subjects to vary the distance of their rating from the center of the circle. In addition, respondents check any of 10 specific moods that they may currently feel. Scores on the CMS are determined trigonometrically, and data analysis requires the use of angular statistics. The scale seems useful for capturing current mood, and appears to have adequate reliability with a college sample. Further evaluation of its psychometric properties is needed with other subject groups.

The Affect Grid. Similar to the CMS in that it is also a one-item assessment that presents respondents with a graphical representation of bipolar affective space, the Affect Grid is a 9 × 9 matrix with mood descriptors reflecting varying levels of pleasantness and arousal, placed at eight points around the matrix (Russell, Weiss, & Mendelsohn, 1989). Respondents mark the cell that best describes their current mood. This is also a new measure that has not been tested extensively or used with elderly subjects. An advantage of this measure over the similar CMS is that the Affect Grid does not require the use of angular statistics.

Trait Measures of Affect

The measures discussed above are generally considered state measures in that their intent is to capture current emotional status. However, many researchers may be interested in obtaining information on dispositional or trait aspects of affect in the elderly. Assessing trait affect provides us with an understanding of emotion typically experienced by individuals, which may be crucial to characterizing affective experience in a given population. A few measures exist that were developed specifically to assess trait affect, in addition to state affect. Among these are the State-Trait Anxiety Inventory (Spielberger, 1983) and the State-Trait Anger Expression Inventory (Spielberger, 1988), both of which include questions on affect as well as clinical symptoms. Another common method of assessing trait affect involves asking respondents either to report mood over a long period of time (e.g., the past month or year), or to indicate how they usually feel, on a measure that is typically used as a state measure. A number of scales discussed in the previous sections (e.g., MAACL, Nowlis MACL, and PANAS) have been used in this manner. Thomas and Diener (1990) do report that people underestimate the frequency with which they experience positive affect relative to negative affect and overestimate the intensity of experienced emotions in retrospective reports, indicating that single assessments encompassing long periods of time are generally inaccurate. However, retrospective measures provide researchers with valuable information on how individuals perceive their own emotional experiences, despite the potential inaccuracy of those perceptions.

Potential Biases in the Assessment of Affect

In general, the rules that apply to gathering any type of reliable self-report data from elderly respondents apply as well to the collection of mood data (see Carp, 1989). For example, researchers need to ensure that they establish good rapport with respondents, that their tasks and procedures are clearly explained and well understood, and that their instruments are appropriate to the respondents' functional abilities and stamina. In addition to these broad prescriptions, collecting reliable mood data requires sensitivity to a number of social and cognitive factors that can potentially influence self-report results. These factors, described below, include (a) positivity and social desirability, (b) perceived demand characteristics, (c) display rules, (d) cultural factors, and (e) contextual effects (e.g. trait characteristics, location in the life course).

Positivity and Social Desirability. It has been suggested that elderly respondents are reluctant to complain or to report negative feelings, particularly in reference to themselves (Carp, 1989; Schulz & Fritz, 1988). This positivity or social desirability bias may contribute to exaggerated reports of positive affect and underestimation of negative affect. Positivity is most likely to emerge in response to global questions, such as one-item ratings of overall mood (Carp, 1989), or measures of affect with dichotomous response formats (Lorr, 1989).

Perceived Demand Characteristics. Assessments with high reactivity or obvious demand characteristics may bias self-report data as well. Elderly respondents, in a variation of a social desirability effect, may unknowingly try to be "good subjects" by reporting what they have deduced that the examiner wants or expects to hear. Each of these problems can be minimized by encouraging respondents to be candid and by implementing procedures to assure both their anonymity and the confidentiality of results.

Display Rules. A similar pitfall is related to socially conditioned display rules that specify appropriate emotional expressions in the presence of others (Hochschild, 1979). For example, the presence of a male investigator has been shown to inhibit expressions of tenderness in males, but not in females (Buck, 1984), suggesting that gender specific display rules can influence reports of affect. Some research indicates that older adults endorse display rules against expressing certain emotions more often than other age groups, but these rules may have less actual impact on the expressive behavior of older adults (Malatesta & Kalnok, 1984).

Cultural Factors. Cultural factors will also influence emotional expressiveness and displays, particularly with interviewers from cultures other than the respondents'. It is difficult to assess these kinds of effects procedurally without large research samples. With large samples, the potentially systematic influences of variables like gender or culture can be evaluated analytically. Other, less obvious, individual differences should not exert significant influence on the data when samples are randomly selected. When selection is not random, the potential effects of such factors can still be anticipated and acknowledged. In research with smaller samples, it is useful to characterize gender and cultural status and interviewer/respondent relationships for purposes of generalizability.

Contextual Effects. Individual contextual effects on affective interpretation and experience are ubiquitous. Affective experiences stored in memory are likely to provide individuals with a context to evaluate new emotion-related events (Schulz, 1985). As a consequence, affective responses to similar events may become less intense over time. These hypothesized contextual effects are likely to be most pronounced in late life; however, they have not been examined through empirical investigation. A variety of other individual difference factors, such as personality characteristics and self-monitoring ability, have been associated with variations in affective expressiveness and experience (see Buck, 1984) and may similarly mediate subjective reports of emotion. These effects can also be systematically examined with large, randomly selected samples.

Choosing a Measure

The choice of measurement tools is first and foremost determined by the question to be addressed. For example, if the goal of a study is to characterize momentary fluctuations in mood over time, a trait measure of mood would be inappropriate. On the other hand, researchers who inquire about the role of dispositional affective states and their influence on other outcomes would need a trait measure of mood. Investigators interested in documenting qualitatively different moods should select a measure that will yield information about discrete moods rather than general dimensions of affect. In sum, the hypotheses or questions guiding a study will immediately constrain the number of relevant alternatives.

Another consideration in selecting measures involves achieving a balance between the logistics of data collection and psychometric adequacy of the instrument. A lengthy affect inventory may be impossible to administer in a study in which other types of data have a higher priority and would also be inappropriate for studies in which multiple ratings are collected over short time intervals. In such cases, a brief inventory is more appropriate; however, the inventory should not be so brief that measurement reliability is compromised. As a general rule, we would recommend against single item assessments of mood because of the inherent instability of such measures. If these scales are used, retest reliability could be estimated through multiple administrations, repeated in close succession. More generally, the ideal assessment would have established reliability and validity data, derived from a sample of the population to which the measure is to be applied. With this in mind, we encourage investigators to report available reliability and validity information on affect measures; this information is particularly lacking for samples of older adults. Further investigation is needed to achieve the most desirable balance between psychometric adequacy and practical concerns.

Protocols involving the assessment of qualitatively distinct emotions will require the use of a multidimensional scale. Of the instruments discussed earlier, we would strongly recommend the Differential Emotions Scale (Izard et al., 1974), which is founded on a strong theoretical background and designed specifically to measure discrete emotions. In addition, we recommend the Profile of Mood States (McNair et al., 1971) for research with healthy older adults because of the diverse and extensive gerontological literature concerning this measure. If a research question does not require the amount of detail provided by a multidimensional assessment, shorter instruments consistent with the basic dimensions approach should be considered. We particularly encourage further use of the PGC Positive and Negative Affect Scales (Lawton et al., 1992) and the PANAS (Watson et al., 1988) for this purpose. The PANAS seems to be the best instrument for making age comparisons because the factor structure appears consistent across age groups (Kercher, 1992). We caution against using scales with asymmetric (e.g., Nowlis MACL) or dichotomous response categories (e.g., Affect Balance Scale) as these formats are known to bias factor structures (Russell, 1979), and elderly respondents have reported that dichotomous formats are too restrictive (Carp, 1989). On the other hand, a great number of response options may be confusing to frail elderly persons.

FUTURE DIRECTIONS

Given the wide range of affect measures available, the creation of new ones should receive low priority unless there are good reasons for their development. More pressing is the need for research aimed at addressing both general and focused questions regarding affect and aging. For example, a number of important physical changes should be relevant to understanding differences in the experience, display, and perception of emotions over the life course. Among these are functional changes in the central nervous system, a general systems decline including reduced sensory abilities and increased chronic disabling conditions, and changes in the vocal tract, facial musculature and skin. To date, little research investigating age-related changes in these areas and their relation to affect has been carried out. Preliminary research in this area suggests that some age-related differences in the expression and perception of affect may exist (Malatesta et al., 1987), and that the physiological responses of older adults to emotional stimuli are smaller in magnitude than those of younger adults (Levenson, Carstensen, Friesen, & Ekman, 1991).

Aging can also be characterized in terms of the accumulation of experience over time. It is likely that events associated with high-intensity affect become particularly salient elements in the long—term memory networks of individuals, and that such experiences provide a context for the evaluation of new experiences. This leads to the question, How do such experiences and associated expectations affect the experience of emotion as one ages?

Some emotion researchers propose that emotion-related concepts are represented in a memory network that is analogous to the lexical-semantic network in which non-emotional concepts are stored. In a such a network, activation spreads from one node, be it lexical or emotional, to others that are associated through past experience. The quality and quantity of related information brought to the interpretation of an event or feeling depends on both the time course and extent of spreading activation, both of which are neurophysiologically determined. Some evidence indicates that activation spreads more slowly in the lexicon with age (Howard, Shaw, & Heisey, 1987). If we pursue the analogy, we can speculate that the time course and/or extent of spreading activation through an emotional network may change with age. One potential result would be a less rich, or less complete framework with which to interpret events or feelings. Another would be a delayed reaction to emotional stimuli or situations. These age-related changes are likely to have implications for how we measure affect, although the exact nature of their impact will require future research.

These are just a few of the questions that might be pursued in future research, and they all require that we pay close attention to issues regarding the measurement of affect. Advancing knowledge in these and other areas rests on a careful choice of measures and an appreciation of their limitations.

NOTE

1. One recent measure, the Semantic Differential Mood Scale (Lorr & Wunderlich, 1988), has been included in the discussion of early instruments because its design and factor structure is more consistent with the differential emotions approach than the basic dimensions approach.

REFERENCES

American Psychiatric Association. (1987). *Diagnostic and statistical manual of mental disorders* (rev., 3rd ed.). Washington, DC: Author.

Anderson, N. H. (1989). Information integration approach to emotions and their measurement. In R. Plutchik & H. Kellerman (Eds.), *Emotion: Theory, research, and experience: Vol. 4. The measurement of emotions* (pp.133–186). San Diego: Academic Press.

Arnold, M. B. (1991). Measurement of quality of life in the frail elderly. In J. E. Birren, J. E. Lubben, J. C., Rowe, & D. E. Deutchman (Eds.), *The concept and measurement of quality of life in the frail elderly* (pp. 50–73). San Diego: Academic Press.

Barefoot, J. C., Dodge, K. A., Peterson, B. L., & Dahlstrom, W. G. (1989). The Cook-Medley Hostility Scale: Item content and ability to predict survival. *Psychosomatic Medicine*, *51*, 46–57.

Barefoot, J. C., Siegler, I. C., Nowlin, J. B., & Peterson, B. L. (1987). Suspiciousness, health, and mortality: A follow-up study of 500 older adults. *Psychosomatic Medicine*, *49*, 450–457.

Berscheid, E. (1983). Emotion. In H. H. Kelley, E. Berscheid, A. Christensen, J. Harvey, T. Huston, G. Levinger, E. McClintock, L. A. Peplan, & D. Peterson (Eds.), *Close relationships* (pp. 110–168). San Francisco: Freeman.

Birren, J. E., Lubben, J. E., Rowe, J. C., & Deutchman, D. E. (Eds.). (1991). *The concept and measurement of quality of life in the frail elderly.* San Diego: Academic Press.

Blaney, P. (1986). Affect and memory: A review. *Psychological Bulletin*, *99*, 229–246.

Boyle, G. J. (1985). Self-report measures of depression: Some psychometric considerations. *British Journal of Clinical Psychology*, *24*, 45–59.

Boyle, G. J., & Katz, I. (1991). Multidimensional scaling of the Eight State Questionnaire and the Differential Emotions Scale. *Personality and Individual Differences*, *12*, 565–574.

Bradburn, N. (1969). *The structure of psychological well-being*. Chicago: Aldine.

Buck, R. (1984). *The communication of emotion*. New York: Guilford Press.

Buunk, B. P., Collins, R. L., Taylor, S. E., Van Yperen, N. W., & Dakof, G. A. (1990). The affective consequences of social comparison: Either direction has its ups and downs. *Journal of Personality and Social Psychology*, *59*, 1238–1249.

Carlson, M., Charlin, V., & Miller, N. (1988). Positive mood and helping behavior: A test of six hypotheses. *Journal of Personality and Social Psychology*, *55*, 211–229.

Carp, F. (1989). Maximizing data quality in community studies of older people. In M. P.

Lawton & A. R. Herzog (Eds.), *Special research methods for gerontology* (pp. 93–122). Amityville, N.Y.: Baywood.

Cella, D. F., & Perry, S. W. (1986). Reliability and concurrent validity of three visual-analogue scales. *Psychological Reports, 59*, 827–833.

Clark, M. S. (1983). Some implications of close social bonds for help seeking. In B. M. DePaulo, A. Nadler, & J. D. Fisher (Eds.), *New directions in helping. Vol. 2: Help seeking*. New York: Academic Press.

Clark, M. S., & Isen, A. M. (1982). Toward understanding the relationship between feeling states and social behavior. In A. H. Hastorf & A. M. Isen (Eds.), *Cognitive and social psychology* (pp. 73–108). The Netherlands: Elsevier.

Clark, M. S., & Taraban, C. (1991). Reactions to and willingness to express emotion in communal and exchange relationships. *Journal of Experimental Social Psychology, 27*, 324–336.

Clyde, D. (1963). *Manual for the Clyde Mood Scale*. Coral Gables, FL: University of Miami.

Cohen, S. & Kessler, R. C., & Gordon, L. G. (in press). Strategies for measuring stress in studies of psychiatric and physical disorders. In S. Cohen, R. C. Kessler, & L.G. Gordon (Eds.), *Measuring stress: A guide for health and social scientists*. New York: Oxford.

Curran, J. P. & Cattell, R. B. (1976). *Manual for the Eight State Questionnaire*. Champaign, IL: Institute for Personality and Ability Testing.

Diener, E., & Emmons, R. A. (1985). The independence of positive and negative affect. *Journal of Personality and Social Psychology, 47*, 1105–1117.

Diener, E., Larsen, R. J., Levine, S., & Emmons, R. A. (1985). Intensity and frequency: Dimensions underlying positive and negative affect. *Journal of Personality and Social Psychology, 48*, 1253–1265.

Ekman, P. (1982). *Emotion in the human face* (2nd ed.). Cambridge, England: Cambridge University Press.

Ekman, P. (1992). Facial expressions of emotion: New findings, new questions. *Psychological Science, 3*, 34–38.

Ekman, P., & Friesen, W. V. (1978). *Facial action coding system*. Palo Alto, CA: Consulting Psychologists Press.

Emmons, R. A., and Diener, E. (1986). A goal-affect analysis of everyday situational choices. *Journal of Research in Personality, 20*, 309–326.

Frank, J. D. (1974). *Persuasion and healing*. New York: Schocken Books.

Frank, J. D. (1985). Further thoughts on the anti-demoralization hypothesis of psychotherapeutic effectiveness. *Integrative Psychiatry, 3*, 17–26.

Frijda, N. H. (1986). *The emotions*. Cambridge, England: Cambridge University Press.

George, L. K. (1981). Subjective well-being: Conceptual and methodological issues. In C. Eisdorfer (Ed.) *Annual review of geriatrics and gerontology, 2*, 345–382. New York: Springer.

Gilligan, S. G. & Bower, G. H. (1984). Cognitive consequences of emotional arousal. In C. E. Izard, J. Kagan, & R. B. Zajonc (Eds.), *Emotions, cognition and behavior* (pp. 547–588). New York: Cambridge University Press.

Grove, J. R. & Prapavessis, H. (1992). Preliminary evidence for the reliability and validity of an abbreviated Profile of Mood States. *International Journal of Sports Psychology, 23*, 93–109.

Hochschild, A. R. (1979). Emotion work, feeling rules, and social structure. *American Journal of Sociology, 85*, 551–575.

Horowitz, M., Adler, N., & Kegeles, S. (1988). A scale for measuring the occurrence of positive states of mind: A preliminary report. *Psychosomatic Medicine*, *50*, 477–483.

Howard, C. V., Shaw, R. J., & Heisey, J. C. (1987). Aging and the time course of semantic activation. *Journal of Gerontology, 41,* 195–203.

Howarth, E., & Schokman-Gates, K. (1981). Self–report multiple mood measures. *British Journal of Psychology, 72,* 421–441.

Izard, C. E. (1977). *Human emotions*. New York: Plenum.

Izard, C. E., Dougherty, F., Bloxom, B., & Kotsch, W. (1974). The differential emotions scale: A method of measuring subjective experience of discrete emotions. Unpublished manuscript. Department of Psychology, Vanderbuilt University.

Jacob, R. G., Simons, A. D., Manuck, S. B., Rohay, J. M., Waldstein, S., & Gatsonis, C. (1989). The circular mood scale: A new technique of measuring ambulatory mood. *Journal of Psychopathology and Behavioral Assessment*, *11*, 153–173.

Kaye, J. M., Lawton, M. P., Gitlin, L. N., Kleban, M. H., Windsor, L. A., & Kaye, D. (1988). Older people's performance on the Profile of Mood States (POMS). *Clinical Gerontologist,* 7, 35–56.

Kennedy-Moore, E., Greenberg, M. A., Newman, M. G., & Stone, A. A. (1992). The relationship between daily events and mood: The mood measure may matter. *Motivation and Emotion*, *16*, 143–155.

Kercher, K. (1992). Assessing subjective well-being in the old-old. *Research on Aging,* 14, 131–168.

Kotsch, W. E., Gerbing, D. W., & Schwartz, L. E. (1982). The construct validity of the Differential Emotions Scale as adapted for children and adolescents. In C. E. Izard (Ed.), *Measuring emotions in infants and children* (Vol. 1, pp. 251–278). Cambridge, England: Cambridge University Press.

Kuykendall, D., Keating, J. P., & Wagaman, J. (1988). Assessing affective states: A new methodology for some old problems. *Cognitive Therapy and Research*, *12*, 279–294.

Larsen, R. J., & Diener, E. (1987). Affect intensity as an individual difference characteristic: A review. *Journal of Research in Personality, 21*, 1–39.

Lawton, M. P. (1991). A multidimensional view of quality of life in frail elders. In J. E. Birren, J. E. Lubben, J. C. Rowe, & D. E. Deutchman (Eds.), *The concept and measurement of quality of life in the frail elderly* (pp. 3–27). San Diego: Academic Press.

Lawton, M. P., Kleban, M. H., Dean, J., Rajagopal, D., & Parmelee, P. A. (1992). The factorial generality of brief positive and negative affect measures. *Journals of Gerontology: Psychological Sciences, 47*, P228–P237.

Lawton, M. P., Kleban, M. H., Rajagopal, D., & Dean, J. (1992). Dimensions of affective experience in three age groups. *Psychology and Aging*, *7*, 171–184.

Levenson, R. W. (1992). Autonomic nervous system differences among emotions. *Psychological Science, 3*, 23–27.

Levenson, R. W., Carstensen, L. L., Friesen, W. V., & Ekman, P. (1991). Emotion, physiology, and expression in old age. *Psychology and Aging, 6*, 28–35.

Levenson, R. W., Ekman, P., & Friesen, W. V. (1990). Voluntary facial action generates emotion-specific autonomic system activity. *Psychophysiology*, *27*, 363–384.

Lorr, M. (1989). Model and methods for measurement of mood. In R. Plutchik & H. Kellerman (Eds.), *Emotion: Theory, research and experience. Vol. 4. The measurement of emotions* (pp. 37–53). New York: Academic Press.

Lorr, M., & Wunderlich, R. A. (1988). A semantic differential mood scale. *Journal of Clinical Psychology*, *44*, 33–36.

Lubin, B., Zuckerman, M., Breytspraak, L. M., Bull, N. C., Gumbhir, A. K. & Rinck, C. M.

(1988). Affects, demographic variables and health. *Journal of Clinical Psychology, 44*, 131–141.

Mackay, C. J. (1980). The measurement of mood and psychophysiological activity using self-report techniques. In I. Martin & P. H. Venables (Eds.), *Techniques in psychophysiology* (pp. 501–562). Chichester, New York: Wiley.

Malatesta, C. Z. (1981). Affective development over the lifespan: Involution or growth? *Merrill-Palmer Quarterly, 27*, 145–173.

Malatesta, C. Z., & Izard, C. E. (1984). The facial expression of emotion: Young, middle-aged and older adult expressions. In C.Z. Malatesta & C. E. Izard (Eds.), *Emotion in adult development* (pp. 253–273). Beverly Hills, CA: Sage.

Malatesta, C. Z., Izard, C. E., Culver, C., & Nicolich, M. (1987). Emotion communication skills in young, middle-aged, and older women. *Psychology and Aging, 2*, 193–203.

Malatesta, C. Z., & Kalnok, M. (1984). Emotional experience in younger and older adults. *Journal of Gerontology, 39*, 301–308.

McCrae, R. R., & Costa, P. T., Jr. (1984). *Emerging lives, enduring dispositions*. Boston: Little, Brown.

McHorney, C. A., Ware, J. E., & Raczek, A. E. (1993). The MOS 36-Item Short-Form Health Survey (SF-36): II. Psychometric and clinical tests of validity in measuring physical and mental health constructs. *Medical Care, 31*, 247–263.

McNair, D., Lorr, M., & Droppleman, L. (1971). *Manual for the Profile of Mood States*. San Diego: Educational and Industrial Testing Service.

Monk, T. H. (1989). A visual analogue scale technique to measure global vigor and affect. *Psychiatry Research, 27*, 89–99.

Neugarten, B. L., Havighurst, R. J., & Tobin, S. S. (1961). The measurement of life satisfaction. *Journal of Gerontology, 16*, 134–143.

Nowlis, V. (1965). Research with the Mood Adjective Checklist. In S. S. Tomkins & C. E. Izard (Eds.), *Affect, cognition, and personality* (pp. 352–389). New York: Springer.

Plutchik, R. (1980). Emotion: *A psychoevolutionary synthesis*. New York: Harper and Row.

Radloff, L. S. (1977). The CES-D scale: A self-report depression scale for research in the general population. *Journal of Applied Psychological Measurement, 1*, 387–393.

Russell, J. A. (1979). Affective space is bipolar. *Journal of Personality and Social Psychology, 37*, 345–356.

Russell, J. A. (1980). A circumplex model of emotion. *Journal of Personality and Social Psychology, 39*, 1161–1178.

Russell, J. A. & Fehr, B. (1987). Relativity in the perception of emotion in facial expressions. *Journal of Experimental Psychology: General, 116*, 223–237.

Russell, J. A., Weiss, A., & Mendelsohn, G. (1989). Affect grid: A single-item scale of pleasure and arousal. *Journal of Personality and Social Psychology, 57*, 493–502.

Salzman, C., Kochansky, G. E., Shader, R. I., & Cronin, D. M. (1972). Rating scales for psychotropic drug research with geriatric patients. II: Mood ratings. *Journal of the American Geriatrics Society, 20*, 215–221.

Schulz, R. (1985). Emotion and affect. In J. E. Birren & K. W. Schaie (Eds.), *Handbook of the psychology of aging* (2nd ed., pp. 531–543). New York: Van Nostrand Reinhold.

Schulz, R., & Fritz, S. (1988). Origins of stereotypes of the elderly: An experimental study of the self-other discrepancy. *Experimental Aging Research, 13*, 189–200.

Schulz, R., & Tompkins, C. A. (1989, August). Emotion, affect, and aging: Developments and future directions. Symposium on *Affect in adult development and aging*; Symposium conducted at the meeting of the American Psychological Association, New Orleans.

Sedikides, C. (1992). Changes in the valence of the self as a function of mood. In M. S. Clark (Ed.), *Review of personality and social psychology. Vol. 14: Emotion and social behavior* (pp. 271–311). Newbury Park, CA: Sage.

Spielberger, C. D. (1983). *Manual for the State-Trait Anxiety Inventory.* Palo Alto, CA: Consulting Psychologists Press.

Spielberger, C. D. (1988). *State-Trait Anger Expression Inventory: Research edition professional manual.* Odessa, FL: Psychological Assessment Resources.

Spilker, B., Molinek, F. R., Johnston, K. A., & Simpson, R. L. (1990). Quality of life bibliography and indexes. *Medical Care, 28,* DS1-DS77.

Stone, A. A. (1981). The association between perception of daily experience and self- and spouse-related mood. *Journal of Research in Personality, 15,* 510–522.

Stone, A. A. (in press). Measures of affective response. In S. Cohen, R. C. Kessler, & L.G. Gordon (Eds.), *Measuring stress: A guide for health and social scientists.* New York: Oxford University Press.

Thomas, D. L., & Diener, E. (1990). Memory accuracy in the recall of emotions. *Journal of Personality and Social Psychology, 59,* 291–297.

Tomkins, S. (1963). *Affect, imagery, and consciousness. Vol. 2. The negative affects.* New York: Springer.

Tompkins, C. A., Spencer, K. A., & Boada, R. (in press). Contextual influences on judgments of emotionally ambiguous stimuli by brain-damaged and normally aging adults. *Clinical Aphasiology.*

Ware, J. E., & Sherbourne, C. D. (1992). The MOS 36-Item Short-Form Health Survey (SF-36): I. Conceptual framework and item selection. *Medical Care, 30,* 473–483.

Warr, P., Barter, J., & Brownbridge, G. (1983). On the independence of positive and negative affect. *Journal of Personality and Social Psychology, 44,* 644–651.

Watson, D. (1988). The vicissitudes of mood measurement: Effects of varying descriptors, time frames, and response formats on measures of positive and negative affect. *Journal of Personality and Social Psychology, 55,* 128–141.

Watson, D., Clark, L. A., & Tellegen, A. (1988). Development and validation of brief measures of positive and negative affect: The PANAS scales. *Journal of Personality and Social Psychology, 54,* 1063–1070.

Watson, D., & Tellegen, A. (1985). Towards a consensual structure of mood. *Psychological Bulletin, 98,* 219–235.

Williamson, G. M., & Clark, M. S. (1989). Providing help and desired relationship type as determinants of changes in moods and self-evaluations. *Journal of Personality and Social Psychology, 56,* 722–734.

Zajonc, R. B. & McIntosh, D. N. (1992). Emotions research: Some promising questions and some questionable promises. *Psychological Science, 3,* 70–74.

Zajonc, R. B., Murphy, S. T., & Inglehart, M. (1989). Feeling and facial efference: Implications of the vascular theory of emotion. *Psychological Review, 96,* 395–416.

Zuckerman, M., & Lubin, B. (1965). *Manual for the Multiple Affect Adjective Checklist.* San Diego: Educational and Industrial Testing Service.

Zuckerman, M., & Lubin, B. (1985). *Manual for the Multiple Affect Adjective Checklist-revised.* San Diego: Educational and Industrial Testing Service.

CHAPTER 11

Assessment of Depression

NANCY A. PACHANA
HARBOR MEDICAL CENTER
UNIVERSITY OF CALIFORNIA, LOS ANGELES

AND

DOLORES GALLAGHER-THOMPSON

AND

LARRY W. THOMPSON
STANFORD UNIVERSITY SCHOOL OF MEDICINE AND
VETERANS AFFAIRS MEDICAL CENTER, PALO ALTO

INTRODUCTION AND CONCEPTUAL FRAMEWORK

When one considers the issues surrounding assessment of depression in the elderly, one needs to first distinguish between depression as a negative affect and depression as a clinical syndrome. We raise this issue at the outset because we wish to convey to the reader a sense of the inadequacy of current nosological systems in capturing, both qualitatively and quantitatively, the full aspects of late-life depression. On the one hand, according to recent epidemiological studies conducted in five sites across the United States, the prevalence of major depressive disorder (or the clinical syndrome of depression) in the 5,700 elderly persons who were interviewed was less than 1% (0.4% in men and 1.4% in women); this rate is only about a quarter of that reported in adults aged 18 to 44 (Koenig & Blazer, 1992). On the other hand, when depressive symptoms (rather than disorders) have been examined in a variety of studies, their prevalence in older adults was substantially increased; one report, using the same epidemiological data set noted above, found

This project was supported in part by the National Institute of Mental Health Grants MH37196 and MH40041.

that depressive symptoms (such as dysphoria and other indices of negative mood) were present in about 30% of the sample (Blazer, Hughes, & George, 1987). Estimates vary still further when self-report measures are used with community samples (averaging about 20% in several studies; see Koenig & Blazer, 1992) or when special subgroups, such as the medically ill or institutionalized elderly, are studied (e.g., from a low of about 10% to a high of just under 50%; see Koenig & Blazer, 1992), or when family caregivers are assessed, where rates close to 50% have been reported (Gallagher, Rose, Rivera, Lovett, & Thompson, 1989). Other subgroups that are at risk for higher levels of both depression as a clinical syndrome and depressive symptoms, include the recently bereaved and those with other psychiatric diagnoses, such as substance abuse (see Bliwise, McCall, & Swan, 1987, for a very informative presentation of sociodemographic and other factors influencing rates of depression in the elderly). In their thorough and thoughtful recent review of this literature, Koenig and Blazer (1992) present about 50 studies showing widely varying prevalence rates for depression in the elderly. At least two explanations for the considerable differences involve the different definitions of depression that are used—whether the researchers were looking for evidence of a full-blown syndrome versus reports of dysphoric mood—and whether the information was collected in an interview or in a self-report format. Given the current confusion about how to define and how to measure what is loosely called depression in the field overall, it is not surprising that similar confusion exists in the geriatric literature.

The diagnostic criteria of depression as a clinical syndrome are set forth in the Diagnostic and Statistical Manual for Mental Disorders (DSM-III-R), the current standard for definition of terms for professionals in the mental health field (American Psychiatric Association, 1987). Although major depression as a syndrome is clearly delineated there, its unique manifestation in varying populations, especially the elderly, is inadequately described. For example, older men tend to deny or refuse to acknowledge feelings of depression when asked directly about them, but they may acknowledge "depression equivalents" such as feelings of emptiness or other negative affects including frustration or worry. Do these feelings qualify to meet the first diagnostic criteria of depressed affect, or not? Also, there are currently no categories to capture the situationally determined dysphoric reactions that many elders experience following the loss of a loved one, or in prolonged situations of family caregiving. The use of strict criteria for a clinical level of depression has resulted not only in a low prevalence rate of depressive disorders among elders but has led to confusion in the field with regard to the development and refinement of our assessment instruments and strategies. The inadequate nomenclature of depression in elders is a conceptual problem, one of whose consequences is assessment instruments that fail to fully survey specific depressive symptomatology in the elderly. In our opinion, there are no currently existing measures that are truly sensitive to the nuances of late-life depression (see Futterman, Gallagher-Thompson, Thompson, & Moak, in press, for a fuller discussion of this point). Having acknowledged this dilemma, we attempt in this chapter to provide useful information concerning the psychometric properties of instruments currently in use, as well as those under development. We will also suggest additional research to improve the diagnostic process.

COMMENTS AND RECOMMENDATIONS REGARDING SPECIFIC ASSESSMENT INSTRUMENTS

Due to space limitations, a summary of current depression assessment instruments used with geriatric populations has been provided in table form (see Tables 11.1 and 11.2). These tables provide information on the format, target population, reliability, validity, sensitivity and specificity, and purpose, of the various instruments covered, along with key references. Both interview and observer-rated as well as self-rated report scales are included.

Interviewer-Administered or Observer-Rated Instruments

In terms of interviewer scales for use with an elderly population, the Schedule for Affective Disorders and Schizophrenia (SADS) holds an advantage over some others in that published studies are available documenting the validity of the SADS with geriatric patients (Dessonville, Gallagher, Thompson, Finnell & Lewinsohn, 1982). In addition, a shorter form of the SADS (Spitzer & Endicott, 1977) is available specifically to assess change in diagnosis or specific symptoms. Gurland and his colleagues (1977–78) also have spent numerous years refining their instrument, the Comprehensive Assessment and Referral Evaluation (CARE), a lengthy interview measure covering a wide range of psychiatric, medical, and social problems of older adults. The CARE has been modified and shortened twice, with the aim of continuing to refine items that maximize discrimination of depressed elders from nondepressed and other clinical populations. The CORE–CARE (Golden, Teresi, & Gurland, 1984), although shorter than the original CARE, still has a lengthy interview time and may be fatiguing for elderly patients. The SHORT-CARE (Gurland, Golden, Teresi, & Challop, 1984) is a simpler, shorter instrument that places emphasis on identifying dementia, depression, and physical impairment. The CARE interview includes the Geriatric Mental State (GMS, Copeland et al., 1976), without the psychotic items. The GMS, developed by the United States–United Kingdom Diagnostic Project (Copeland et al., 1976; Gurland et al., 1976), was specifically designed for use with the elderly. It is an omnibus symptom inventory which recently has been used with a new computerized diagnostic system, Automated Geriatric Examination for Computer Assisted Taxonomy (AGECAT) (Copeland, Dewey, & Griffiths-Jones, 1986; Copeland et al., 1988) to provide a consistent and reliable diagnostic method for epidemiological studies.

A widely used diagnostic interview which fails to take into account both the unique qualities of a geriatric population and the increased skill and sensitivity

TABLE 11.1 Depression Measures: Interview and Observer-Rated

	Instrument Name	*Primary References*	*Length (No. of items)*	*Time to Administer*	*Target Population*
1a	Comprehensive Assessment & Referral Evaluation (CARE)	Gurland et al., 1977–78; Golden et al., 1983, 1984; Teresi, Golden, & Gurland, 1984; Teresi, Golden, Gurland, Wilder, & Bennett, 1984	314 items; 22 indicator scales; (depression subscale has 29 items)	90 minutes; requires skilled interviewer	Elderly patients and nonpatients; designed for use in community surveys
1b	SHORT-CARE	Gurland, Golden, Teresi, & Challop, 1984	6 indicator scales and 2 diagnostic scales (for depression and dementia)	30–45minutes	Elderly patients and nonpatients
2.	Diagnostic Interview Schedule (DIS)	Robins, Helzer, Croughan, & Ratcliff, 1981; Malgady et al., 1992	254 questions (branch system)	45–75 minutes; requires trained interviewer technician rather than clin. professional	Inpatient and outpatient psychiatric; also in community surveys
3.	Geriatric Depression Rating Scale (GDRS)	Jamison & Scogin, 1992	35 items	35 minutes; requires trained interviewer (detailed manual available)	Inpatient and outpatient psychiatric; community volunteers
4.	Hamilton Rating Scale for Depression (HRSD)	Hamilton, 1960, 1967; Williams, 1988	21 items (17 on depression, 4 on other syndromes)	20–30 minutes; requires trained interviewer	Inpatient and outpatient psychiatric patients already diagnosed as depressed
5.	Minnesota Multiphasic Personality Inventory–Depression Scale (MMPI-D)	Hathaway & McKinley, 1951	Depression scale has 60 items; complete MMPI is 250 to 550 items, depending on version used	15–20 minutes for depression subscale	Inpatient and outpatient psychiatric and medical patients

TABLE 11.2 Self-Report Questionnaires

	Instrument Name	*Primary References*	*Length (No. of items)*	*Time to Administer*	*Target Population*
1a	Beck Depression Inventory (BDI)	Beck, Ward, Mendelson, Mock, & Erbaugh, 1961; Beck, Steer & Garbin, 1988; Gallagher, Nies & Thompson, 1982; Gallagher, Breckenridge, Steinmetz, & Thompson, 1983	21 items of graded intensity; time frame = past week, including today	5–10 minutes	Psychiatric patients, medical patients, normals, community volunteers
1b	Beck Depression Inventory – Short Form	Beck & Beck, 1972; Beck et al., 1988	13 items (subset of original BDI)	5 minutes	Psychiatric patients, medical patients, normals, community volunteers
2.	Bradburn Affect Balance Scale (ABS)	Bradburn, 1969	10 items in a yes/no format; 5 positive and 5 negative, yielding 2 subscores as well as an affect/balance score	5 minutes	General population; suitable for elders
3.	Brief Symptom Inventory (BSI)	Derogatis & Spencer, 1982; Hale, Cochran, & Hedgepeth, 1984; Pearson & Gatz, 1982	53 items; respond for intensity of discomfort; 9 symptom dimensions, including depression (6 items) and a global severity index	15–20 minutes for total scale	Psychiatirc or medical patients and normals; norms for elderly for each subscale (by gender)

needed to assess their concerns is the Diagnostic Interview Schedule (DIS) (Robins, Helzer, Croughan, & Ratcliff, 1981). Despite these limitations, the DIS has been used with elderly patients in several major epidemiological studies, such as the NIMH Epidemiological Catchment Area study on the prevalence of psychiatric disorders in the community (cf. Myers, Weissman, & Tischler, 1984; Blazer et al., 1987). Now we are discovering that the DIS may have significantly underreported the incidence of depression in the community in general, leaving questions regarding the true prevalence and incidence of depression among elders. Recent studies have begun to document the lack of empirical research linking DIS diagnoses to external criterion-related standards, bringing the psychometric validity of this instrument into question (Malgady, Rogler, & Tryon, 1992). Although this instrument may have utility in exploring a broad range of psychopathology and obtaining a history of past mental illness, its specific validity in the diagnosis of depression in geriatric populations remains dubious.

Issues of the validity and reliability of the Hamilton Rating Scale for Depression (HRSD; Hamilton, 1960, 1967) with elderly patients are also noteworthy. The HRSD has been considered by many in the psychiatric field as representing the "gold standard" for determining the level of depression at any point in time; however, there is a problem of wide interrater variability in how each question on the scale is asked. It is left to the interviewer's judgment to decide how to actually phrase questions and follow-up probes; only very general guidelines were provided by Hamilton in the original version of this scale. More recently, Williams (1988) developed a Structured Interview Guide for the HRSD (SIGH-D) in order to address this issue. This guide provides specific wording for all questions, thus increasing the likelihood of a standardized administration of the instrument. A test-retest reliability study by Williams demonstrated a substantially improved level of agreement on most HRSD items. Nevertheless, Williams reported that even with use of the SIGH-D, item reliabilities for half of the items still ranged from fair to poor. With regard to the elderly, Lichtenberg, Marcopulos, Steiner, and Tabscott (1992) pointed out some additional problems. For example, in interviewing frail elders with mild cognitive impairment, an unsophisticated interviewer may fail to record the presence of some depressive symptomatology owing to unresponsiveness on the part of the patient, thus underestimating the presence of depression in that individual. These and other concerns (e.g., the fact that over half the items on the HRSD are somatic in nature) are further discussed in Thompson, Futterman, and Gallagher (1988).

In dealing with older persons or patients who may be experiencing a number of complex problems (such as poor health and possibly mild cognitive decline) along with their affective distress, it can be anticipated that fewer problems with reliability and validity will occur if a structured interview is available that was specifically designed for use with the elderly. One such measure is a new interviewer-based rating scale called the Geriatric Depression Rating Scale (GDRS), developed by Jamison and Scogin and first published in 1992. The authors used some items from the widely used self-report Geriatric Depression Scale (GDS) as topic areas to assess in a structured clinical interview format similar to that of the HRDS. They added items of particular relevance to the elderly, such as questions on life satisfaction, morning mood, hopefulness, and several on cognitive function including memory complaints and mental clarity. The authors also developed a detailed manual for administration of the scale. For these reasons, they assert that less rater training and less discretionary decision making on the part of the rater are involved in using the GDRS with the elderly (Jamison & Scogin, 1992). In presenting their initial findings about this instrument, however, Jamison and Scogin gave no breakdown of the data by gender, and the overall size of their sample (68 subjects) was relatively small. Nevertheless, such a scale responds to a long-felt need for an instrument which takes at least some of the specific characteristics of depression in the elderly into account in assessing depression level.

The Minnesota Multiphasic Personality Inventory (MMPI) and MMPI–2, which were not normed on elders, are problematic when used with this population, as Brink (1980) and Gallagher (1987) point out. In a recent study, Harper, Kotik-Harper and Kirby (1990) compared assessment of geriatric medical patients using the MMPI Depression scale, the Brief Symptom Inventory and the Geriatric Depression Scale. False negative rates up to 53% for major depression and 100% for minor depression were found. Misrecognition was unrelated to degree of dementia or education, but was related to age on the MMPI. In an Australian sample, Strassberg, Clutton and Korboot (1991) found the new content scale for depression on the MMPI–2 to have good concurrent validity for male and female subjects. More work needs to be done in looking at the new MMPI–2 and its content scales with a geriatric population. Nevertheless, since the scale is virtually unchanged from the older version, age corrections in interpreting T-scores will continue to have to be made (Graham, 1990).

A relatively new interview scale, which was developed to bridge the gap between research and clinical utility and which has been widely accepted in the psychiatric community at large, is the Structured Clinical Interview for DSM–III-R (SCID). This is a semistructured diagnostic interview developed by Spitzer, Williams, Gibbon and First (1992) that can be used to diagnose major Axis I syndromes as well as Axis II personality disorders. The SCID records the presence or absence of each disorder for both current episodes as well as for lifetime occurrence. Information regarding levels of agreement on the test/retest reliability of diagnostic formulations based on SCID data can be found in Williams et al. (1992). In length of time of administration, the SCID offers an advantage over other interviews, such as the SADS, in that it was designed in a modular format so that sections can be omitted if they are thought to be irrelevant in a given diagnostic situation (for example, the interviewer may omit the section on abuse of street drugs with elders having no history of substance abuse). Another advantage to the SCID is that it (unlike other similar interviews) contains the full criteria for DSM–III-R disorders embedded within the instrument itself; this can be a major convenience for interviewers, who can diagnose as they go along, without having to wait until the interview is completed to check the diagnostic criteria.

Unfortunately, despite its several advantages, the SCID has rarely been used with elders, either in clinical settings or in research investigations. One of the only published studies on the use of the SCID with elders, by Stukenberg, Dura, and Kiecolt-Glaser (1990), found that it worked quite well in terms of assessing depression; in fact, they used it as a gold standard against which to validate other self-report screening scales, and did not report significant problems with its use. They did indicate that all three instruments used (SCID, Beck Depression Inventory, and the Depression subscale of the Brief Symptom Inventory) were able to successfully identify major depression (the clinical syndrome) but none were consistently sensitive to cases of dysthymia or chronic depression. Our preliminary experience has been different: our use of the SCID as a diagnostic instrument with geriatric populations in several studies has not supported its use as such a standard. The SCID appeared less sensitive than we had anticipated for identifying either depressive or anxiety disorders, for which symptoms were noted both clinically and on responses to other measures, such as the Geriatric Depression Scale and/or the Beck Depression Inventory. However, since there appears to be so little experience with the SCID with elders, it is not possible at this point in time to either strongly recommend it, or strongly caution against its use. It is possible that the lack of sensitivity found in our group's use of the SCID may have been due to a lack of sophistication in raters' use of the measure; alternatively, there may truly be a lack of validity in the instrument itself when used with older adults. This remains an open question at present.

Finally, the Older Americans Resources and Services methodology (OARS; Duke University Center for the Study of Aging and Human Development, 1978), like the CARE is a multidimensional assessment tool which includes an index of depression. It has often been used for survey research of geriatric populations (see George & Fillenbaum, 1985, for a review of this research). The mental health scale from the OARS, the Short Psychiatric Evaluation Schedule (SPES) was developed by Pfeiffer (1979) and cited in Gatz, Pedersen, and Harris, (1987) as a simple self-report index of psychopathology. However, Gatz, Pedersen, and Harris (1987) found that because the SPES combines different types of symptoms, especially somatic symptoms, using the total score could obscure age-related patterns. Also, it should be noted that in their review of how the OARS has been used in over a decade of research, George and Fillenbaum (1985) make the point that it is not recommended as a screening device for detection of depression in elders.

In summary, this review of interview-based measures of depression leads to the following recommendations:

1. The SADS interview is recommended over the SCID or DIS to assess the clinical syndromes of depression in older adults because more experience has been reported with it than with the other two, and there are some pub-

lished validity and reliability data on its use with elders. Information of this type is either not currently available and/or less than affirming of the adequacy of the other two.

2. The SHORT–CARE is highly appropriate for use in screening, particularly when the aim is to assess both depression and dementia and/or rule them out, in the elderly.
3. The GDRS is preferred over the HRSD to assess levels of depression in persons already diagnosed, although more research is needed with larger samples so that this recommendation can be made more strongly.

Self-Report Measures

Despite evidence of adequate validity and reliability when used as a screening measure to detect depression in the elderly (see Gallagher, 1986, for review), there are some limitations to consider regarding the widely used Beck Depression Inventory (BDI) (Beck, Ward, Mendelson, Mock, & Erbaugh, 1961). First, like most other self-report depression measures that were not specifically designed with the elderly in mind, it does not include criteria characteristic of depression in the elderly, such as emptiness, feelings of envy, helplessness and a history of depressive feelings (Weiss, Nagel, & Aronson, 1986). Second, the BDI uses a response format based on gradations of intensity for each symptom inquired about; this format requires the respondent to remember and choose from among four levels of severity for each item. Clearly, this manner of responding places greater demands on working memory and attention than the simpler yes/no format used, for example, on the Geriatric Depression Scale (GDS), discussed below. Finally, the number of questions assessing somatic symptoms may also limit the BDI's utility with the elderly in that there is no way for the clinician to ascertain whether symptoms endorsed are secondary to depression or secondary to physical illness (Norris, Gallagher, Wilson, & Winograd, 1987).

The Geriatric Depression Scale (GDS) was developed with many of these very issues in mind. Currently, it is the sole self-rating depression instrument specifically designed for and standardized with an elderly population (Yesavage, Brink, & Rose, 1983). Features of the GDS which facilitate its use with elders include its simplified yes/no response format and a lack of items inquiring about somatic complaints (Brink et al., 1982). Several studies report better validity of the GDS in distinguishing between depressed and nondepressed elders than other rating scales. For example, Brink et al. (1982) found greater sensitivity and specificity for the GDS in comparison with Zung's (1965) Self-Rating Depression Scale and the HRDS. Similarly, Hyer and Blount (1984) reported that the GDS was a better discriminator between depressed and nondepressed elders than the BDI. In a comparison of patient scores on the GDS and the BDI in a nursing home setting, the GDS was more sensitive to depressive symptoms; the BDI appeared to underestimate levels of depression in this population (Kiernan et al., 1986). A short form has also been developed, with adequate reliability compared to the original scale (Sheikh & Yesavage, 1986).

The data have not been so clear-cut with regard to the validity of using the GDS with cognitively impaired populations. One study used the GDS to screen for depression in a nursing home and reported that it was not sensitive enough to be adequate (Kafonek et al., 1989); in contrast, other studies have reported successful use of the GDS as a screening measure in long-term care settings (see, for example, Parmelee, Katz, & Lawton, 1989; Parmelee, Katz, & Lawton, 1992a). In general, the greater the severity of cognitive impairment, the more limited the validity of the GDS (Burke, Houston, Boust, & Roccaforte, 1989). As stated by Feher, Larrabee, and Crook (1992) the GDS does appear to be a valid measure of mild to moderate depressive symptoms in Alzheimer patients with mild to moderate dementia. However, those with more severe dementia tend to deny both their cognitive deficits and their affective distress; the GDS may not be appropriate with such individuals. On the other hand, Parmelee and her associates (Parmelee, Lawton, & Katz, 1989) found that there were no differences in reliability or validity for cognitively impaired and nonimpaired groups in an extended care setting.

Another factor to consider is how the scale is administered: Clinicians working with geriatric populations, especially patients with cognitive impairment, often read the questions aloud to their patients (rater-administered format) rather than use a self-administered format. At least one research team (O'Neill, Rice, Blake, Walsh, & Coakley, 1992) has found a significant difference in GDS scores derived from patients depending on the mode of presentation of the instrument. In their original paper, Yesavage et al. (1983) described a mixed mode of application; the absence of strict administration guidelines for the GDS may contribute to discrepancies in published data on the GDS relative to the demented (O'Neill et al., 1992), and possibly other diagnostic and age groups, such as the old-old or the medically frail. Despite the limitations noted here, it seems to us that the GDS may well be the best all-around self-report depression scale available at present with utility across a broad range of geriatric populations.

The Zung Self-Rating Depression Scale (SDS) was one of the first self-report measures used widely with elderly populations. In their review paper on its use and limitations, Zung and Zung (1986) point out that it has good reliability and validity with the elderly. However, recent comparison studies have documented shortcomings in this instrument. For example, Toner, Gurland, and Teresi (1988) found this scale to be less satisfactory as a screening tool than the SHORT–CARE because the Zung scale has a lower response rate and poorer convergent validity. It is important to note that this measure has a higher false-positive rate for older adults than for younger adults (Zung, 1975), and that depression masked as somatic illness may be missed (Raft, Spencer, Toomey, & Brogan, 1977).

Finally, the Center for Epidemiological Studies–Depression Scale (CES–D) was specifically designed for epidemiological studies of depression in a general population (DeForge & Sobal, 1988) and, like the HRSD and the BDI, has remained a popular assessment instrument for depression in a wide variety of populations. It has also been used to assess the prevalence of depressive symptomatology in the elderly (Murrell, Himmelfarb, & Wright, 1983; O'Hara, Kohout, & Wallace, 1985; Phifer & Murell, 1986). Himmelfarb & Murrell (1983), based on a large representative sample, provide data approaching true norms for the CES–D. A large-scale study conducted by Hertzog and colleagues (Hertzog, Van Alstine, Usala, & Hultsch, 1990), using techniques of confirmatory factor analysis, found that the factor structure of this measure was invariant across two cross-sectional samples of adults and across the various age groups studied. They concluded that the data supported the measurement validity of the CES–D for depression screening in older adult populations. However, some have criticized the CES–D's response format, which asks for frequency ratings of how often the specific symptoms occurred in the past week, suggesting that for older adults (particularly those with cognitive impairments), such distinctions may be very difficult to make with reliability (Gallagher, 1987).

Other scales included in Table 11.2 of this review, such as the Profile of Mood States (POMS), Depression Adjective Checklist (DACL), Multiple Affect Adjective Checklist (MAACL), and Brief Symptom Inventory (BSI), have not been extensively used with the elderly. Considerably more research is needed to ascertain their more appropriate uses.

In summary, this review of self-report measures of depression leads to the following recommendations:

1. At present, the GDS is recommended as the most sensitive and widely accepted self-report scale, though more research is needed on its utility with cognitively impaired elders.
2. The BDI and CES–D are appropriate for more highly educated elders who can understand their more complex response formats.

SPECIAL TOPICS CONCERNING DEPRESSION IN A GERIATRIC POPULATION

Depression in the Physically Ill Elderly

Depression is quite common yet often unrecognized and untreated in physically ill elders (Berkman et al., 1986). A recent study cites the frequency of a depressive disorder among medically ill geriatric inpatients as ranging from 25%–50% (Small & Fawzy, 1988). Similarly, among a community sample of 890 elders, 28.4% of the total sample reported one or more serious physical health problems, which in turn were associated with cognitive impairment, depression, generalized anxiety and agoraphobia (Lindesay, 1990). While the precise frequency of depression secondary to medical illness is not known, commonly cited causes include endocrine and metabolic disorders, structural brain lesions, medication side effects

(Small & Fawzy, 1988) and chronic pain (Parmelee, Katz, & Lawton, 1992b; for reviews, see Romano & Turner, 1985, and Roy, Thomas, & Matas, 1984), particularly if it impacts negatively on functional abilities (Williamson & Schulz, 1992a, 1992b).

It is extremely important to determine the possible contribution that illness, pain, and/or medication might be making to specific depressive symptoms or syndromes when completing an assessment for depression. This is particularly critical when dealing with elderly patient samples, who are at risk for medical complications, such as the old-old for whom no specific depression scale has been validated (Weiss et al., 1986). Unfortunately, there are no depression or other adjunct clinical measures specifically designed to make these distinctions, and therefore it is often necessary to make clinical judgments about the relative significance of physical and psychological factors when attempting to describe a diagnostic type and level of depression. In attempting to do this, it is helpful first to obtain detailed information concerning past and previous illnesses, along with prescribed and over-the-counter medications, and then to consult with appropriate medical specialists concerning their potential importance for the development of specific symptoms associated with depression.

Depression in the Demented Elderly

Dementia is yet another organic illness that frequently coexists with depression. The prevalence of depression in dementia patients has ranged higher than two-thirds in some samples, with a modal response of slightly less than one-third (Teri & Wagner, 1992). The cognitive impairments associated with depression and the impaired self-report capacity of demented patients contribute to the difficulty in teasing apart these two conditions. The reported frequency of the mislabelling of depression as dementia is in the 10%–15% range (Small & Fawzy, 1988) with depressive symptoms being more common than depressive syndromes (Small, 1989).

The assessment of depression in demented populations thus poses a unique challenge. Of the instruments reviewed here, the GDS would seem most aptly suited for screening purposes with this population because of its simplistic format and its low weighting of somatic features. However, as noted previously, research results are mixed regarding its reliability and validity with this population, particularly with the more demented elderly.

In contrast to the physically ill elderly, some progress has been made in the development of depression rating scales specifically for use with dementia patients. For example, the Cornell Scale for Depression in Dementia (Alexopoulos, Abrams, Young, & Shamoian, 1988) uses information from interviews with both the patient and staff members. Preliminary work with 83 elderly demented nursing home patients demonstrated that it has high interrater reliability, internal consistency, and sensitivity. The total scores on the Cornell correlated with depressive subtypes classified according to research diagnostic criteria. A second instrument, the Dementia Mood Assessment Scale (Sunderland et al., 1988) combines direct observations of the patient in different settings and a semistructured interview to obtain information for ratings of depression. Interrater reliability was high for ratings made on 21 adult dementia patients. Although still preliminary, results with these two instruments suggest that it is indeed feasible to overcome the hindrance of cognitive impairment in obtaining sufficient information for making reliable ratings of depressive symptoms, and that a valid instrument for assessing depression in elderly dementia patients may soon be available.

Comorbid Condition of Anxiety and Depression in Elders

Depressive symptomatology in the elderly often co-occurs with anxiety, which can add to the difficulty of the diagnostic process. A category of mixed depression and anxiety is being included provisionally in DSM–IV for patients who do not meet criteria for an already established anxiety or depressive disorder (Liebowitz, 1993). This would include individuals with so-called "subsyndromal" depression and/or anxiety (Liebowitz, 1993). Liebowitz (1993) notes that in the upcoming International Classification of Diseases (ICD–10) such a category is included; thus making the two coding systems compatible in this regard.

Many studies in the literature support a high coexistence of depression and anxiety, with clinical epidemiological studies revealing a prevalence of 4%–20% in the general population (Barrett, Barrett, Oxman, & Gerber, 1988; Hoeper et al., 1979; Schulberg et al., 1985; Von Korff et al., 1987). In reporting data from the Epidemiologic Catchment Area (ECA) sample, Blazer et al. (1988) state that a substantial portion of individuals meeting diagnostic criteria for a major depressive episode may also have symptoms of generalized anxiety. In an earlier article reporting ECA data, Blazer et al. (1987) state that DSM–III-R diagnostic categories did not fully capture the picture of depression presented by geriatric patients; the authors suggest the addition of a mixed depression/anxiety subtype and a symptomatic depression subtype to strengthen diagnostic power with elderly populations.

Both Katon and Roy-Byrne (1991) and Hiller, Zaudig, and Bose (1989) note the greater difficulty in recognizing mild anxiety or dysthymia than in finding either major depression or more severe anxiety disorders such as panic disorder. The tendency of elders to express concerns indirectly, often in the form of somatic complaints, may cause the clinician to overlook milder forms of anxiety or depression. On the other hand, Liebowitz (1993) raises the concern that a mixed depression/anxiety category in DSM–IV would vastly increase the prevalence of psychiatric disorders.

The stability of such a diagnostic construct has not been well delineated in the literature. Indeed, no confirmatory factor analyses testing the separateness of anxiety and depression in the elderly appear in the literature. Thus, as might be expected, no specific instrument for use with this population has yet been developed, nor are there adequate normative data available for this group using more traditional instruments for measuring anxiety and depression. However, recent work emphasizing the comorbidity of these two conditions should encourage continued development of both a conceptual backdrop and more psychometrically sound measures for use in diagnosis, as well as the evaluation of treatment programs for elderly patients.

Depression and Substance Abuse. As in younger and middle-aged persons, depressive disorders may also co-exist with substance abuse problems in older adults, most notably either alcohol dependence or unintentional misuse of prescription and/or over-the-counter medications. Data on the prevalence of substance abuse among the elderly is confusing in itself (ranging from a low estimate of under 1% to a median of 6% across several studies of community-residing elderly; with closer to 20% prevalence being reported for those in institutional and nursing home settings; Bliwise, McCall, & Swan, 1987). Data on the prevalence of the dual diagnosis of depression plus some type of substance abuse is virtually nonexistent, yet patients with both conditions are presenting themselves to medical clinics and mental health services in increasing numbers (Speer, O'Sullivan, & Schonfeld, 1991). Their virtual invisibility until very recently may be due in part to the fact that none of the assessment tools reviewed in this chapter was designed to be sensitive to this issue in the elderly. Although it is true that the DIS, SADS, and SCID interviews contain questions addressing both depressive and substance abuse disorders, none of the three inquires about the kinds of symptoms of substance abuse that have been identified as more common among the elderly, such as unexplained falls, acute cognitive confusion, sexual dysfunction, malnutrition, and incontinence (Solomon, Manepalli, Ireland, & Mahon, 1993). Thus making a correct dual diagnosis in an elder patient can be very difficult; their treatment is complicated by the fact that psychiatric and substance abuse services are typically fragmented in our present system of health care, so that their concurrent treatment, while highly desirable, is often an impossibility (Speer et al., 1991).

Assessment of Depression in Minority Elders

For the most part, the instruments reviewed in this chapter have neither been translated nor validated for use with minority elders, particularly those for whom English is not their native language. Yet with increasing longevity, minority elders are growing proportionally in the United States population and this trend is projected to continue in the future (United States Bureau of the Census, 1988); therefore, it is necessary to consider appropriate methods of assessment for these individuals. In the fields of cross-cultural psychology and psychiatry, there is a substantial body of literature indicating that significant problems occur (either in under-or overreporting of distress and diagnoses) when existing measures are simply applied to groups other than those on whom they were originally developed. For example, use of verbally based intelligence tests with minority children typically results in lowered IQ estimates compared to those obtained with culture-fair tests that are more performance based (Westermeyer, 1987). Similarly, use of most of the measures reviewed here could be inappropriate, unless it can be determined that they have not only been adequately translated (a complex process in itself), but also that the concepts and meanings are relevant to the particular cultural group. For example, the expression of affect is structured in significant ways by cultural conditioning, giving the impassive facial demeanor of many Native Americans and Asian Americans, sometimes misinterpreted as indicating lack of feelings, and the ebullience of many people from Mediterranean countries (Hughes, 1993). Each of the major racial and ethnic groups in this country (and their many distinctive subgroups) has unique culturally determined beliefs about depression; these need to be understood, and the symptoms reported by ethnic elders need to be interpreted within that cultural context (Landrine & Klonoff, 1992; Yeo & Hikoyeda, 1993). Given that the field of "ethnogerontology" is so new, and so little work has been done along the lines suggested here, it will be necessary to use what is available until more ethnically sensitive measures have been developed. Recently, psychometrically based work on item analysis for depression measures has yielded intriguing results. Teresi and Golden (in press), in an analysis of item bias in the CARE, found that the symptoms of headaches, crying, expressed lack of interest, and enjoyment were less severe indicators of depression in Hispanics than in whites. Continued efforts to investigate the psychometric properties of depression measures should result in more accurate assessment of depression in minority groups.

It is noteworthy that of the self-report scales described in this chapter, the GDS has been translated into Chinese, Dutch, French, German, Hebrew, Italian, Japanese, Portuguese, Rumanian, Spanish (including versions used in Spain, Argentine, and Mexico), and Yiddish (Sheikh, Yesavage, Brooks, Friedman, & Gratzinger, 1991); thus it may be the most appropriate one to use at present. Zung and Zung (1986) also report that their Zung SDS currently has been translated into 30 languages and has been used worldwide. In terms of interpretation of information gathered from an interview process, the reader is referred to several recent publications of relevance (Brink, 1992; Gaw, 1993; Jackson, 1988).

SUMMARY

Assessment of depression in the elderly is complicated by the fact that diagnostic classification systems do not completely reflect current problems and issues of late-life depression. For example, prevalence estimates for major depressive disorder are in the order of less than 1% using DSM–III-R criteria, yet serious depressive affect is reported to be as high as 15% in some community samples and ranges to a 50% high in some special elderly populations, such as the medically ill, nursing home residents, or family caregivers. There is also the difficulty that other age-related problems can cause symptoms that may be mistaken for indicators of depression; careful attention is required in the assessment process to make the appropriate differentiation.

Because depression is the most common psychiatric disorder in the elderly, it is frequently useful to screen for this disorder in clinical and research settings. The BDI and GDS have been used effectively as screening devices with the elderly. Both have adequate sensitivity and specificity for detecting level of depression. Recent work evaluating the factor structure of the CES–D in elderly community samples suggests that it also may have value as a clinical screening measure, although it has been used less frequently in this manner. However, none of these instruments provide sufficient information to make a diagnosis, nor do they assess other clinical characteristics of depression, such as duration, subtype, level of reactivity or diurnal variation. The SADS is recommended for diagnostic purposes. The SCID is also a newer structured interview that relates to the DSM–III-R criteria, and it has the added advantage that it provides information about Axis II diagnoses. However, the SCID has been used less frequently with the elderly. Both of these measures are costly in terms of administration and interviewer training time. Further, they do not adequately describe dimensions for the various aspects of late-life depression.

There is still a need for more sensitive and specific measures of late-life depression, both for screening and diagnostic purposes. With the increasing elderly population, this problem should be addressed by professionals with the appropriate clinical and psychometric skills. Their task will be facilitated by continued efforts to provide greater clarification of the criteria for late-life depression and its various types.

REFERENCES

American Psychiatric Association. (1987). *Diagnostic and statistical manual of mental disorders* (3rd ed.). Washington, DC: Author.

Alexopoulos, G. S., Abrams, R. C., Young, R. C., & Shamoian, C. A. (1988). Cornell scale for depression in dementia. *Biological Psychiatry, 23*, 271–284.

Barrett, J. E., Barrett, J. A., Oxman, T. E., & Gerber, P. D. (1988). The prevalence of psychiatric disorders in a primary care practice. *Archives of General Psychiatry, 45*, 1100–1106.

Beck, A. T., & Beck, R. W. (1972). Screening depressed patients in family practice: A rapid technique. *Postgraduate Medicine, 52*, 81–85.

Beck, A. T., Steer, R. A., & Garbin, M. G. (1988). Psychometric properties of the Beck Depression Inventory: Twenty-five years of evaluation. *Clinical Psychology Review, 8*, 77–100.

Beck, A. T., Ward, C. H., Mendelson, M., Mock, J., & Erbaugh, J. (1961). An inventory for measuring depression. *Archives of General Psychiatry, 4*, 561–571.

Berkman, L. F., Berkman, C. S., Kasl, S., Freedman, D. H., Leo, L., Ostfeld, A. M., Cornoni-Huntley, J., & Brody, J. A. (1986). Depressive symptoms in relation to physical health and functioning in the elderly. *American Journal of Epidemiology, 124*, 372–388.

Blazer, D. G., Hughes, D. C., & George, L. K. (1987). The epidemiology of depression in an elderly community population. *Gerontologist, 27*, 281–287.

Blazer, D. G., Swartz, M., Woodbury, M., Manton, K. G., Hughes, D., & George, L. K. (1988). Depressive symptoms and depressive diagnoses in an elderly community population: Use of a new procedure for analysis of psychiatric classification. *Archives of General Psychiatry, 45*, 1078–1084.

Bliwise, N., McCall, M. E., & Swan, S. J. (1987). The epidemiology of mental illness in late life. In E. E. Lurie & J. H. Swan (Eds.), *Serving the mentally ill elderly* (pp. 62–109). Lexington, MA: Lexington Books.

Bradburn, N. M. (1969). *The structure of psychological well-being*. Chicago: Aldine.

Brink, T. L. (1980). Brief psychiatric screening of institutionalized aged: a review. *Long Term Care & Health Services Administration Quarterly, 4*, 253–260.

Brink, T. L. (Ed.). (1992). *Hispanic aged mental health*. Binghamton, NY: Haworth Press.

Brink, T. L., Yesavage, J. A., Lunn, O., Hersema, P. H., Adey, M., & Rose, T. L. (1982). Screening tests for geriatric depression. *Clinical Gerontologist, 1*, 37–43.

Burke, W. J., Houston, M. J., Boust, S. J., & Roccaforte, W. H. (1989). Use of the Geriatric Depression Scale in dementia of the Alzheimer type. *Journal of the American Geriatrics Society, 37*, 856–860.

Butcher, N. J., Dahlstrom, W. G., Graham, J. R., Tellegen, A., & Kaemmer, B. (1989). *Minnesota Multiphasic Personality Inventory (MMPI–2). Manual for administration and scoring*. Minneapolis: University of Minnesota Press.

Copeland, J. R. M., Kelleher, M. J., Kellett, J. M., Gourlay, A. J., Gurland, B. J., Fleiss, J. L., & Sharpe, L. (1976). A semi-structured clinical interview for the assessment of diagnosis and mental state in the elderly. The Geriatric Mental State Schedule: I. Development and reliability. *Psychological Medicine, 6*, 439–449.

Copeland, J. R. M., Dewey, M. E., & Griffiths-Jones, H. M. (1986). A computerized psychiatric diagnostic system and case nomenclature for elderly subjects: GMS and AGECAT. *Psychological Medicine, 16*, 89–99.

Copeland, J. R. M., Dewey, M. E., Henderson, A. S., Kay, D. W. K., Neal, C. D., Harrison, M. A. M., McWilliam, C., Forshaw, D., & Shiwach, R. (1988). The Geriatric Mental State (GMS) used in the community: Replication studies of the computerized diagnosis AGECAT. *Psychological Medicine, 18*, 219–223.

DeForge, B. R., & Sobal, J. (1988). Self-report depression scales in the elderly: The relationship between the CES–D and Zung. *International Journal of Psychiatry in Medicine, 18*, 325–338.

Derogatis, L. R., & Spencer, P. M. (1982). *Administration and procedure—Brief Symptom Inventory (BSI) manual*. Baltimore: Clinical Psychometrics Research.

Dessonville, C., Gallagher, D., Thompson, L. W., Finnell, K., & Lewinsohn, P. (1982). Relation of age and health status to depressive symptoms in normal and depressed older adults. *Essence, 5*, 99–117.

Devins, G. M., Orme, C. M., Costello, C. G., Binik, Y. M., Frizzell, B., Stam, H. J., & Pullin, W. P. (1988). Measuring depressive symptoms in illness populations: Psychometric properties of the Center for Epidemiologic Studies Depression (CES–D) Scale. *Psychology and Health, 2*, 139–156.

Duke University Center for the Study of Aging and Human Development. (1978). *Multidi-*

mensional functional assessment: The OARS methodology. Durham, NC: Duke University Medical Center.

Endicott, J., & Spitzer, R. L. (1978). A diagnostic interview for affective disorders and schizophrenia. *Archives of General Psychiatry, 35*, 837–844.

Feher, E. P., Larrabee, G. J., & Crook, T. H. (1992). Factors attenuating the validity of the geriatric depression scale in a dementia population. *Journal of the American Geriatrics Society, 40*, 906–909.

Futterman, A., Gallagher-Thompson, D., Thompson, L. W., & Moak, G. (in press). Depression in later life. In E. Beckham & R. Leber (Eds.), *Handbook of depression: Treatment, assessment, and research.* New York: Guilford Press.

Gallagher, D. (1986). The Beck Depression Inventory and older adults: Review of its development and utility. *Clinical Gerontologist, 5*, 149–163.

Gallagher, D. (1987). Assessing affect in the elderly. *Clinics in Geriatric Medicine, 3*, 65–85.

Gallagher, D., Nies, G., & Thompson, L. W. (1982). Reliability of the Beck Depression inventory with older adults. *Journal of Consulting and Clinical Psychology, 50*, 152.

Gallagher, D., Breckenridge, J., Steinmetz, J., & Thompson, L. W. (1983). The Beck Depression Inventory and research diagnostic criteria: Congruence in an older population. *Journal of Consulting and Clinical Psychology, 51*, 945–946.

Gallagher, D., Rose, J., Rivera, P., Lovett, S., & Thompson, L. W. (1989). Prevalence of depression in family caregivers. *The Gerontologist, 29*, 449–456.

Gatz, M., Pederson, N. L., & Harris, J. (1987). Measurement characteristics of the mental health scale from the OARS. *Journal of Gerontology, 42*, 332–335.

Gatz, M., & Hurwicz, M. (1990). Are old people more depressed? Cross-sectional data on Center for Epidemiological Studies–Depression Scale factors. *Psychology and Aging, 5*, 284–290.

Gaw, A. C. (Ed.). (1993). *Culture, ethnicity, and mental illness.* Washington, DC: American Psychiatric Press.

George, L. K., & Fillenbaum, G. G. (1985). OARS methodology: A decade of experience in geriatric assessment. *Journal of the American Geriatrics Society, 33*, 607–615.

Golden, R. R., Teresi, J. A., & Gurland, B. J. (1983). Detection of dementia and depression cases with the Comprehensive Assessment and Referral Evaluation Interview Schedule. *International Journal of Aging and Human Development, 16*, 241–254.

Golden, R. R., Teresi, J. A., & Gurland, B. J. (1984). Development of indicator scales for the Comprehensive Assessment and Referral Evaluation Interview Schedule. *Journal of Gerontology, 39*, 138–146.

Graham, J. R. (1990). *MMPI–2: Assessing personality and psychopathology.* New York: Oxford University Press.

Grove, J. R., & Prapavessis, H. (1992). Preliminary evidence for the reliability and validity of an abbreviated Profile of Mood States. *International Journal of Sports Psychology, 23*, 93–109.

Guadagnoli, E., & Mor, V. (1989). Measuring cancer patients' affect: Revision and psychometric properties of the Profile of Mood States (POMS). *Psychological Assessment, 1*, 150–154.

Gurland. B. J., Fleiss, J. L., Goldberg, K., Sharpe, L., Copeland, J. R. M., Kelleher, M. J., & Kellett, J. M. (1976). A semi-structured clinical interview for the assessment of diagnosis and mental state in the elderly. The Geriatric Mental State Schedule: II. A factor analysis. *Psychological Medicine, 6*, 451–459.

Gurland, B., Kuriansky, J., Sharpe, L., Simon, R., Stiller, P., & Birkett, P. (1977–78). The Comprehensive Assessment and Referral Evaluation (CARE)—Rationale, development and reliability. *International Journal of Aging and Human Development, 8*, 9–42.

Gurland, B. J., Golden, R., Teresi, J., & Challop, J. (1984). The SHORT–CARE: An efficient instrument for the assessment of depression, dementia and disability. *Journal of Gerontology, 39*, 166–169.

Hale, W. D., Cochran, C. D., & Hedgepeth, B. E. (1984). Norms for the elderly on the Brief Symptom Inventory. *Journal of Consulting and Clinical Psychology, 52*, 321–322.

Hamilton, M. (1960). A rating scale for depression. *Journal of Neurology, Neurosurgery and Psychiatry, 23*, 56–62.

Hamilton, M. (1967). Development of a rating scale for primary depressive illness. *British Journal of Social and Clinical Psychology, 6*, 278–296.

Harper, R. G., Kotik-Harper, D., & Kirby, H. (1990). Psychometric assessment of depression in an elderly general medical population: over- or underassessment? *Journal of Nervous and Mental Disease, 178*, 113–119.

Hathaway, S. R., & McKinley, J. C. (1951). The Minnesota Multiphasic Personality Inventory manual. New York: Psychological Corporation.

Hertzog, C., Van Alstine, J., Usala, P. D., & Hultsch, D. F. (1990). Measurement properties of the Center for Epidemiological Studies Depression Scale (CES–D) in older populations. *Psychological Assessment, 2*, 64–72.

Hiller, W., Zaudig, M., & Bose, M. (1989). The overlap between depression and anxiety on different levels of psychopathology. *Journal of Affective Disorders, 16*, 223–231.

Himmelfarb, S., & Murrell, S. A. (1983). Reliability and validity of five mental health scales in older persons. *Journal of Gerontology, 38*, 333–339.

Hoeper, E., Nycz, G., Cleary, P., Regier, D., & Goldberg, I. (1979). Estimated prevalence of RDC mental disorder in primary medical care. *International Journal of Mental Health, 8*, 6–15.

Hughes, C. C. (1993). Cultural in clinical psychiatry. In A. C. Gaw (Ed.), *Culture, ethnicity, and mental illness*. Washington, DC: American Psychiatric Press.

Hyer, L., & Blount, J. (1984). Concurrent and discriminant validities of the Geriatric Depression Scale with older psychiatric inpatients. *Psychological Reports, 54*, 611–616.

Jackson, J. S. (Ed.) (1988). *The black American elderly: Research on physical and psychosocial health*. New York: Springer.

Jamison, C., & Scogin, F. (1992). Development of an interview-based geriatric depression rating scale. *International Journal of Aging and Human Development, 35*, 193–204.

Kafonek, S., Ettinger, W. H., Roca, R., Kittner, S., Taylor, N., & German, P. S. (1989). Instruments for screening for depression and dementia in a long-term care facility. *Journal of the American Geriatrics Society, 37*, 29–34.

Katon, W., & Roy-Byrne, P. (1991). Mixed anxiety and depression. *Journal of Abnormal Psychology, 100*, 337–345.

Kaye, J. M., Lawton, M. P., Gitlin, L. N., Kleban, M. H., Windsor, L. A., & Kaye, D. (1988). Older people's performance on the Profile of Mood States (POMS). *Clinical Gerontologist, 7*, 35–56.

Kiernan, B. U., Wilson, D., Suter, N., Naqvi, A., Moltzen, J., Silver, G. (1986). Comparison of the Geriatric Depression Scale and Beck Depression Inventory in a nursing home setting. *Clinical Gerontologist, 6*, 54–56.

Koenig, H. G., & Blazer, D. G. (1992). Epidemiology of geriatric affective disorders. *Clinics in Geriatric Medicine, 8*, 235–251.

Landrine, H., & Klonoff, E. (1992). Culture and health-related schemas: A review and proposal for interdisciplinary integration. *Health Psychology, 11*, 267–276.

Lichtenberg, P. A., Marcopulos, B. A., Steiner, D. A., & Tabscott, J. A. (1992). Comparison of the Hamilton Depression Rating Scale and the Geriatric Depression Scale: Detection of depression in dementia patients. *Psychological Reports, 70*, 515–521.

Liebowitz, M. R. (1993). Mixed anxiety and depression: Should it be included in DSM–IV? *Journal of Clinical Psychiatry, 54*(Suppl.), 4–7.

Lindesay, J. (1990). The Buy's/Age Concern Survey: Physical health and psychiatric disorder in an urban elderly community. *International Journal of Geriatric Psychiatry, 5*, 171–178.

Lubin, B. (1967). *Depression Adjective Check Lists manual.* San Diego: EdITS.

Lubin, B. (1981). *Depression Adjective Check Lists manual* (2nd ed). San Diego: EdITS.

Lubin, B., Zuckerman, M., Hanson, P. G., Armstrong, T., Pinck, C. M., & Seever, M. (1986). Reliability and validity of the Multiple Affect Adjective Check List–Revised. *Journal of Psychopathology and Behavioral Assessment, 8*, 103–117.

Lichtenberg, P. A., Marcopulos, B. A., Steiner, D. A., & Tabscott, J. A. (1992). Comparison of the Hamilton Depression Rating Scale and the Geriatric Depression Scale: Detection of depression in dementia patients. *Psychological Reports, 70*, 515–521.

McNair, D., Lorr, M., & Droppleman, L. F. (1971). *Profile of Mood States: manual.* San Diego: Educational and Industrial Testing Service.

Malgady, R. G., Rogler, L. H., & Tryon, W. W. (1992). Issues of validity in the Diagnostic Interview Schedule. *Journal of Psychiatric Research, 26*, 59–67.

Montgomery, S. A., & Asberg, M. (1979). A new depression scale designed to be sensitive to change. *British Journal of Psychiatry, 134*, 382–389.

Murrell, S. A., Himmelfarb, S., & Wright, K. (1983). Prevalence of depression and its correlates in older adults. *American Journal of Epidemiology, 117*, 173–183.

Myers, J. K., Weissman, M. M., & Tischler, G. L. (1984). Six-month prevalence of psychiatric disorders in three communities, 1980–1982. *Archives of General Psychiatry, 41*, 959–967.

Norris, J. T., Gallagher, D., Wilson, A., & Winograd, C. H. (1987). Assessment of depression in geriatric medical outpatients: The validity of two screening measures. *Journal of the American Geriatrics Society, 35*, 989–995.

O'Hara, M. W., Kohout, F. J., & Wallace, R. B. (1985). Depression among the rural elderly: A study of prevalence and correlates. *Journal of Nervous and Mental Disease, 173*, 582–589.

O'Neill, D., Rice, I., Blake, P., Walsh, J. B., & Coakley, D. (1992). The Geriatric Depression Scale: Rater-administrated or self-administered? *International Journal of Geriatric Psychiatry, 7*, 511–515.

Parmelee, P. A., Katz, I. R., & Lawton, P. (1989). Depression among institutionalized aged: Assessment and prevalence estimation. *Journal of Gerontology, 44*, 22–29.

Parmelee, P. A., Katz, I. R., & Lawton, P. (1992a). Incidence of depression in long-term care settings. *Journal of Gerontology, 47*, 189–196.

Parmelee, P. A., Katz, I. R., & Lawton, P. (1992b). The relation of pain to depression among institutionalized aged. *Journal of Gerontology, 46*, 15–21.

Parmelee, P. A., Lawton, P., & Katz, I. R. (1989). Psychometric properties of the Geriatric Depression Scale among the institutionalized aged. *Psychological Assessment, 1*, 331–338.

Pearson, C., & Gatz, M. (1982). Health and mental health in older adults: First steps in the study of a pedestrian complaint. *Rehabilitation Psychology, 27*, 37–50.

Pfeiffer, E. (1979). A short psychiatric evaluation scale: A new 15-item monotonic scale indicative of functional psychiatric disorder. In F. Hoffmeister & C. Muller (Eds.), *Brain function in old age*. Berlin: Springer Verlag.

Phifer, J. F., & Murrell, S. A. (1986). Etiologic factors in the onset of depressive symptoms in older adults. *Journal of Abnormal Psychology, 95*, 282–291.

Radloff, L. S. (1977). The CES–D scale: A self-report depression scale for research in the general population. *Applied Psychological Measurement, 1*, 385–401.

Radloff, L. S., & Teri, L. (1986). Use of the Center for Epidemiologic Studies–Depression Scale with older adults. *Clinical Gerontologist, 5*, 119–135.

Raft, D., Spencer, R. F., Toomey, T., & Brogan, D. E. (1977). Depression in medical outpatients: The use of the Zung scale. *Diseases of the Nervous System, 38*, 999–1004.

Robins, L. N., Helzer, J. E., Croughan, J., & Ratcliff, K. S. (1981). National Institute of Mental Health Diagnostic Interview Schedule: Its history, characteristics and validity. *Archives of General Psychiatry, 38*, 381–389.

Romano, J. M., & Turner, J. A. (1985). Chronic pain and depression: Does the evidence support a relationship? *Psychological Bulletin, 97*, 18–34.

Roy, R., Thomas, M., & Matas, M. (1984). Chronic pain and depression: A review. *Comprehensive Psychiatry, 25*, 96–105.

Schacham, S. (1983). A shortened version of the Profile of Mood States. *Journal of Personality Assessment, 47*, 305–306.

Schulberg, H. C., Saul, M., McClelland, M., Ganguli, M., Chrusty, W., Frank, R. (1985). Assessing depression in primary medical and psychiatric practices. *Archives of General Psychiatry, 42*, 1164–1170.

Sheikh, J. I., & Yesavage, J. A. (1986). Geriatric Depression Scale (GDS): Recent evidence and development of a shorter version. *Clinical Gerontologist, 5*, 165–173.

Sheikh, J. I., Yesavage, J. A., Brooks, J. O., Friedman, L., & Gratzinger, P. (1991). Proposed factor structure of the Geriatric Depression Scale. *International Psychogeriatrics, 3*, 23–28.

Small, G. W., & Fawzy, F. I. (1988). Psychiatric consultation for the medically ill elderly in the general hospital. *Psychosomatics, 29*, 94–103.

Small, G. W. (1989). Behavioral disorders in Alzheimer's disease: Depression is common. *Bulletin of Clinical Neuroscience, 54*, 2–7.

Solomon, K., Manepalli, J., Ireland, G., & Mahon, G. M. (1993). Alcoholism and prescription drug abuse in the elderly: St. Louis University grand rounds. *Journal of the American Geriatrics Society, 41*, 57–69.

Speer, D. C., O'Sullivan, M., & Schonfeld, L. (1991). Dual diagnosis among older adults: A new array of policy and planning problems. *Journal of Mental Health Administration, 18*, 43–50.

Spitzer, R. L., & Endicott, J. (1977). *SADS–change interview.* New York: New York State Psychiatric Institute.

Spitzer, R. L., Williams, J. B., Gibbon, M., & First, M. B. (1992). The Structured Clinical Interview for DSM–III-R (SCID). I: History, rationale, and description. *Archives of General Psychiatry, 49*, 624–629.

Strassberg, D. S., Clutton, S., Korboot, P. (1991). A descriptive and validity study of the Minnesota Multiphasic Personality Inventory–2 (MMPI–2) in an elderly Australian sample. *Journal of Psychopathology and Behavior Assessment, 13*, 301–311.

Stukenberg, K. W., Dura, J. R., & Kiecolt-Glaser, J. K. (1990). Depression screening scale validation in an elderly, community-dwelling population. *Psychological Assessment, 2*, 134–138.

Sunderland, T., Alterman, I. S., Yount, D., Hill, J. L., Tariot, P. N., Newhouse, P. A., Mueller, E. A., Mellow, A. M., & Cohen, R. M. (1988). A new scale for the assessment of depressed mood in demented patients. *American Journal of Psychiatry, 145*, 955–959.

Teresi, J., & Golden, R. (in press). Latent structure methods for estimating item bias, item validity and prevalence using cognitive and other geriatric screening measures. *Journal of Alzheimer's Disease and Associated Disorders.*

Teresi, J., Golden, R., & Gurland, B. (1984). Concurrent and predictive validity of indicator scales developed for the Comprehensive Assessment and Referral Evaluation (CARE) Interview Schedule. *Journal of Gerontology, 39*, 158–165.

Teresi, J., Golden, R., Gurland, B., Wilder, D. E., & Bennett, R. G. (1984). Construct validity of indicator scales developed for the Comprehensive Assessment and Referral Evaluation (CARE) Interview Schedule. *Journal of Gerontology, 39*, 147–157.

Teri, L., & Wagner, A. (1992). Alzheimer's disease and depression. *Journal of Consulting and Clinical Psychology, 60*, 379–391.

Thompson, L. W., Futterman, A., & Gallagher, D. (1988). Assessment of late-life depression. *Psychopharmacological Bulletin, 24*, 577–586.

Toner, J., Gurland, B., & Teresi, J. (1988). Comparison of self-administered and rater-administered methods of assessing levels of severity of depression in elderly patients. *Journal of Gerontology, 43*, 136–140.

United States Bureau of the Census. (1988). *Statistical abstract of the United States* (108th ed). Washington, DC: U.S. Government Printing Office.

Von Korff, M., Shaprio, S., Burke, J. D., Teitlebaum, M., Skinner, E. A., German, P., Turner, R. W., Klein, L., & Burns, B. (1987). Anxiety and depression in a primary care clinic: Comparison of Diagnostic Interview Schedule, General Health Questionnaire, and practitioner assessments. *Archives of General Psychiatry, 44*, 152–156.

Westermeyer, J. (1987). Cultural factors in clinical assessment. *Journal of Consulting and Clinical Psychology, 55*, 471–478.

Weiss, I. K., Nagel, C. L., & Aronson, M. K. (1986). Applicability of depression scales to the old old person. *Journal of the American Geriatrics Society, 34*, 215–218.

Williams, J. B. W. (1988). A structured interview guide for the Hamilton Depression Rating Scale. *Archives of General Psychiatry, 45*, 742–747.

Williams, J. B., Gibbon, M., First, M. B., Spitzer, R. L., Davies, M., Borus, J., Howes, M. J., Kane, J., Pope, H. G., Rounsaville, B., & Wittchen, W. (1992). The Structured Clinical Interview for DSM–III-R (SCID). II: Multisite test-retest reliability. *Archives of General Psychiatry, 49*, 630–636.

Williamson, G. M., & Schulz, R. (1992a). Pain, activity restriction and symptoms of depression among community-residing elderly adults. *Journal of Gerontology, 47*, 367–372.

Williamson, G. M., & Schulz, R. (1992b). Physical illness and symptoms of depression among the elderly. *Psychology and Aging, 7*, 342–351.

Yeo, G., & Hikoyeda, N. (1993). *Differential assessment and treatment of mental health problems: African American, Latino, Filipino, and Chinese American elders* (Working paper series, no. 13). Stanford, CA: Stanford Geriatric Education Center.

Yesavage, J. A., Brink, T. L., & Rose, T. L. (1983). Development and validation of a geriatric depression scale: A preliminary report. *Journal of Psychiatric Residents, 17*, 37–49.

Zuckerman, M., & Lubin, B. (1965). *Manual for the Multiple Affect Adjective Checklist*. San Diego: EdITS.

Zuckerman, M., & Lubin, B. (1985). *Manual for the Multiple Affect Adjective Checklist–revised*. San Diego: EdITS.

Zuckerman, M., Lubin, B., Rinck, C. M., Soliday, S. M., Albott, W. L., & Carlson, K. (1986). Discriminant validity of the Multiple Affect Adjective Checklist–Revised. *Journal of Psychopathology and Behavioral Assessment, 8*, 119–128.

Zung, W. K. (1965). A self-rating depression scale. *Archives of General Psychiatry, 12*, 63–70.

Zung, W. K. (1975). *The measurement of depression*. Columbus, OH: Merrill.

Zung, W. K., & Zung, E. M. (1986). Use of the Zung Self-Rating Depression Scale in the elderly. *Clinical Gerontologist, 5*, 137–148.

CHAPTER 12

Caregiver Functioning

GARY T. DEIMLING
DEPARTMENT OF SOCIOLOGY
CASE WESTERN RESERVE UNIVERSITY, CLEVELAND

OVERVIEW

An extensive literature has evolved over the past 10–15 years on the effects on caregivers of providing care for impaired older adults (see Barer & Johnson, 1990; Braithwaite, 1992; Wright, Clipp, & George, 1993, for comprehensive reviews). This literature has grown from a few studies on the nature of informal care to a point where caregiving has become a major theme in social gerontology. There are many reasons for the growth of this area. First, it has become recognized that families and friends provide impaired older adults with the bulk of their care (Stone, Cafferata, & Sangl, 1987). Second, it has been shown that informal caregivers are often the major resource that prevents institutional placement of many older adults (Colerick & George, 1986).

Noelker (1990) refers to caregivers as "a valuable but vulnerable resource" (p. 189). She suggests that because family caregivers are the "preeminent and often the only source of community-based long term care" it is important to "prevent or attenuate caregiving's seemingly adverse effects". It is now recognized by formal service providers that it is as necessary to care for the caregivers as it is to care for the older adult patient. For this reason, caregiver assessment is an essential aspect of geriatric assessment (Brown, Potter, & Foster, 1990). Further, with the growth of services specifically targeting caregivers, practitioners need instrumentation to assess caregivers' needs. As respite programs compete for funds with other services for older adults it is essential that comprehensive information is available to evaluate the impact of these services. (See Callahan, 1989, and Lawton, Brody, & Saperstein, 1989, for a discussion of related policy issues.)

This chapter is designed to provide a broad overview of caregiver assessment measures and techniques. These tools serve two purposes. First, they can be used to assess the informal caregiver's capacity to provide or continue to provide care to an impaired older adult. Second, they can be used in evaluation studies of the effectiveness of programs designed to support caregivers.

CAREGIVER ASSESSMENT

To a large degree, caregiver assessment is a subset of the assessment process used with older adult patients. In many regards, it parallels that process and needs to be as comprehensive and multidimensional. This is because caregivers are typically older adults with a broad range of physical and psychosocial needs. Stone et al. (1987) showed that over 35% of caregivers were spouse caregivers with an average age of over 70 years. Further, most adult-child caregivers are either in late middle age or aged.

Given the advanced age of most caregivers and the fact that they often have chronic conditions of their own, the designation of caregiver is at times an artificial distinction. Over time it is not uncommon for caregivers and care recipients to exchange roles. To the degree that the caregiver's own frailty is an issue, many of the techniques and instruments used to assess older adults' physical and mental health are appropriate for caregiver assessment. Because these measures are reviewed elsewhere in this volume they will not be discussed in detail in this chapter (see chapter 2, on physical health; chapter 3, on activities of daily living; and chapter 16, on multidimensional assessment).

The primary intent of this chapter is to review the major assessment techniques that are specifically designed for use with informal caregivers. These measures tend to fall into two broad categories: caregiving effects and caregiver coping and resources. These domains are the focus of this chapter for two reasons. First, they characterize the major themes in the bulk of caregiving research that have been conducted over the past 15 years. Second, they represent important areas for social service interventions designed specifically for caregivers. Hence, the bulk of this chapter will be allocated to a detailed review of the most widely used measures in these areas. In reviewing these measures, the original research that created the measures will be described, the basic conceptual domains identified, and information on the measurement properties provided, where available. Finally, a subjective evaluation of the instrument will be offered based on the instrument's technical merit and suitability for use in caregiver assessment.

While this chapter focuses on the functional assessment of caregivers, it is important to note that very recently there has been promising work in the area of physiological assessment of caregiver stress (Vitaliano, Dougherty, & Siegler, in press). As progress is made in developing standardized testing in that area, and as resources become available for this type of assessment for caregivers, it will become an important part of overall caregiving assessment.

Caregiving Context

The first information necessary as part of a comprehensive, multidimensional assessment of caregiver functioning is the context in which caregiving takes place.

Considerable research has demonstrated the importance of the relationship of the caregiver to the care recipient, that is whether the caregiver is a spouse, an adult child, or other family or friend (Cantor, 1983; Deimling, Bass, Townsend, & Noelker, 1989; Walker & Allen, 1991; Young & Kahana, 1989), and the living arrangement (Deimling et al., 1989), that is, whether or not the caregiver lives with the care recipient. In addition to information on family structure and the care setting other personal information about the caregiver, such as employment status, is also important. For adult-child caregivers, their employment status reflects potentially competing responsibilities and role conflicts that might occur.

Obtaining information on the care setting and personal characteristics of the caregiver doesn't require extensive or caregiver-specific instrumentation. This information can be accurately and reliably documented using items in any multidimensional assessment such as the Older Americans Resources and Services (OARS) (Duke University Center for Study of Aging and Human Development, 1978) or the Comprehensive Assessment and Referral Evaluation (CARE) (Gurland & Wilder, 1984; Golden, Teresi, & Gurland, 1984). Chapter 16 in this volume also provides an extensive discussion of alternative instrumentation in this area.

Beyond the basic structural features of the care setting, the history of the caregiving situation is equally important. This includes for how long care has been provided, the expected duration of the caregiving situation (temporary or permanent), whether either the caregiver or care recipient changed residences to establish the care setting, and the onset of caregiving. Many of the major caregiving studies have incorporated such items, and these should also be part of any comprehensive assessment of caregivers.

Another aspect of the caregiving context that is of potential importance from a clinical perspective is the occurrence of other stressful life events for the caregiver. Other recent stressful life events may exacerbate the strain associated with caregiving. For example, adult-child caregivers who have recently been divorced may be dealing with the aftermath of that major stressor at the same time they are needed to provide care to a seriously impaired parent. There have been no life events scales specifically tailored to caregivers' life circumstances. However, the Geriatric Scale of Recent Life Events developed by Kiyak, Liang, and Kahana (1976) is an adaptation of the Holmes and Rahe life events scale (1967) that is appropriate for older adults. This and other measures of life events such as those reviewed in chapter 15 of this volume may be adapted for use with caregivers.

Caregiving Effects

The second major category of measures that are typically part of a comprehensive, multidimensional assessment and are the primary focus of this chapter, is caregiving effects. The effects of caregiving can be organized into three categories: The global physical health, mental health effects and well-being caregivers experience, the negative effects that caregivers attribute to caregiving (burden or strain), and the positive effects that caregivers attribute to caregiving (caregiving satisfaction). Each of these three different, but complementary types of effects and the specific indicators that operationalize them will be reviewed in the following subsections.

Caregiver Physical Health, Mental Health, and Well-Being

Measures of caregiver health and well-being are essential features of caregiver assessment. George and Gwyther (1985) have argued convincingly that global measures of physical health and psychosocial well-being, that is those that are not caregiving specific, have several advantages. First, global measures often have established norms for the general population with age-specific norms available in some cases. Second, using global measures makes it possible to compare the health and functioning of caregivers with noncaregivers of similar age, gender, and racial characteristics. Third, the use of global measures resolves another problem that has been raised concerning most caregiving effects measures, which might be termed *attribution ambiguity.*

This ambiguity results from asking caregivers to attribute the cause of an effect they perceive, such as a change in health or well-being, directly to caregiving. Attribution is often operationalized by prefacing measures with the phrase "Because of caregiving . . .". Measures such as these invite the caregiver to attribute an outcome that may have many possible causes to caregiving. The use of global measures avoids this problem because caregivers are asked only to characterize their health and well-being, not to attribute it to care-related events. However, in order to determine causality using global measures, change over time must be established using longitudinal panel designs.

In the area of physical health several widely used global measures that are appropriate for caregiver assessment are self-reported health, health conditions and symptoms such as those found in the OARS (Duke University, 1975) and the National Health and Nutrition Examination Survey (NHANES–II) National Center for Health Statistics, 1981). Chapter 2 of this volume provides a thorough review of items such as these.

An important related area of caregiver health is the ability to perform daily activities. Caregivers' ability to perform these basic tasks for themselves is one indicator of ability to assist impaired relatives. Therefore, traditional indicators of activities of daily living (ADL) such as the Physical Self Maintenance (PSM) and Instrumental Activities of Daily Living (IADL) (Lawton & Brody, 1969) should be considered for inclusion in a comprehensive, multidimensional caregiver assessment.

The argument for assessing caregivers' mental health and well-being parallels that made with regard to physical health and functioning. An extensive number of instruments developed for the general population or for older adults are potentially useful for caregiver assessment. Schulz, Visintainer, and Williamson (1990) provide an extensive review of these measures including measures of depression such as the Beck Depression Inventory (BDI; Beck & Beck, 1972); the Center for Epidemiological Studies–Depression Scale, CES–D (Radloff, 1977), and Self-Rated Depression Scale (SDS; Zung, 1965). Chapter 11 in this volume reviews these and other related instruments.

One of the most comprehensive and widely used measures of mental health symptomatology appropriate for older adults is the Hopkins Symptom Checklist (Derogatis, Lipman, Rickels, Uhlenhuth, & Covi, 1974) and variations such as the Symptom Checklist–90 (SCL) (Derogatis, Lipman, & Covi, 1973). This multidimensional instrument assesses five areas of mental health and psychiatric symptoms including depression, anxiety, and hostility. A number of variations and adaptations of this basic instrument have been used in the caregiving literature (Young & Kahana, 1989).

Three other areas of caregiver well-being that have typically been considered are life satisfaction, morale, and affect. One measure of life satisfaction often used with caregivers is the Life Satisfaction Index (LSI) (Havighurst, Neugarten, & Tobin, 1961) in its several variations—the LSI–A, LSI–B, and LSI–Z (Wood, Wylie, & Sheafor, 1969). The Philadelphia Geriatric Center (PGC) Morale Scale (Lawton, 1975) has become one of the most widely used instruments to assess older adults' emotional well-being and is appropriate for use with caregivers. Two widely used measures of affect, the Bradburn Affect Balance Scale (Bradburn, 1969) and the Positive and Negative Affect Scale (PANAS; Watson, 1988) are appropriate for caregivers. (See Kercher, 1992, and chapter 10 of this volume for a discussion of these measures.)

Measuring Burden and Strain: Conceptual Issues

Much of the considerable research on caregivers has focused on the burden or strain that they have experienced related to the care they provide. This literature has included an ongoing debate concerning the conceptualization, labeling and measurement of these care-specific effects. Although it is not the purpose of this chapter to continue or extend that debate (see Barer & Johnson, 1990; Braithwaite, 1992; George & Gwyther, 1986; Miller, McFall, & Montgomery, 1991; Montgomery, Gonyea, & Hooyman, 1985; Pearlin, Mullan, Semple, & Skaff, 1990; Poulshock, & Deimling, 1984; Pratt, Schmall, Wright, & Cleland, 1985; Schulz et al., 1990), there are several aspects of that debate that need to be discussed before proceeding with a review of specific instruments.

The study of care-related strain and burden continues to be bogged down in terminological problems. The first of these is the issue of subjective versus objective burden/strain. Because caregiver assessment typically takes the form of caregivers' reports, it is inherently subjective. Even when caregivers are asked about seemingly factual changes in their lives related to caregiving, what is recorded is their subjective perceptions of those events or effects. Labeling "objective" the more concrete effects caregivers experience and report, although not particularly useful, is not necessarily problematic as long as the researcher/evaluator is clear that these represent the caregivers' perceptions. And, in fact, caregiver's perceptions have their own inherent validity and represent important clinical information on which interventions may be based.

To some degree this labeling debate concerning burden/strain is related to the attribution ambiguity discussed earlier. The use of attributed effects measures has often been relied on by researchers and evaluators because of the limitations imposed by cross-sectional designs. With the cross-sectional research that has typically been used to study caregiving, researchers have not had pre- or postcaregiving measures of the care-related effects available to them; nor have they had measures at two or more points in time during the caregiving process. In the absence of longitudinal measurement, causality has often been used to explain observed linkages. The risk is that this invites the caregiver to attribute strain in areas such as family relationships, or role conflicts to caregiving that may, in fact, have other or multiple causes.

Another conceptual/measurement issue in understanding caregiver strain is the degree to which characteristics of care receivers, such as their physical and mental impairment, are viewed as burden. In several of the measures reviewed below care recipient characteristics are part of the determination of the degree of burden experienced. Care recipient impairment clearly characterizes the nature of the stressor but should not be confused with the burden experienced by caregivers. Indeed, a specific level of impairment in one care receiver may translate into either lower or higher levels of perceived burden or strain for different caregivers depending on a variety of other factors including the caregiver's personality, coping and social resources.

Several of the measures reviewed below present a similar conceptual/measurement ambiguity that confounds the understanding of care-related burden or strain. In some measures the caregiver is asked to report the occurrence of an event, and then is asked to rate the problematic nature of that event. The dilemma that this type of measure poses is that when separate measures are used for the occurrence of these events and caregivers' reactions to the event, these two measures are intrinsically confounded and have high intercorrelation. In addition to ambiguity in the interpretation of the findings, it also presents problems of multicollinearity in multivariate analyses.

One strategy that in part resolves this problem is to ask the questions separately but to score the nonoccurrence as 0 and the caregiver's response to the event with a numeric rating of 1 or higher, corresponding to the degree of bother. This combined score unfortunately also has shortcomings. A low total score across a number of items may reflect either the relative nonoccurrence of these events or their occurrence but at a low level of bother. Whichever approach is used, the researcher/evaluator needs to take these issues into account in interpreting the results obtained using this type of measure.

Probably the most important issue that needs to be considered in reviewing the measures presented below is the presence or absence of an overriding conceptual model. Most of the measures reviewed here were developed as single constructs, or as measures that have several dimensions within a larger construct. Although it has been increasingly recognized that caregiver strain and burden are multidimensional constructs, only a few of the measures reviewed incorporate a larger conceptual framework.

The use of a broader conceptual model may also help to resolve the labeling and attribution issues noted above. Models such as the one proposed by Pearlin et al. (1990) are very useful. In this model primary stressors such as the characteristics of the care receiver are treated separately from attributed secondary sources of strain such as caregiving effects. Global health and well-being are seen as the ultimate outcomes. Several of the caregiving effects measures reviewed below use this type of sophisticated conceptual approach and the primary benefit is clear, unconfounded measurement.

The development of measures within a larger paradigm has important practice advantages besides the obvious theoretical and methodological sophistication involved. The ability of those conducting assessments to separate out broader mental health issues from those unique to the caregiving context could be an essential part of developing a clinical intervention that can either focus on resolving the broader mental health issues of the caregiver or, alternatively, providing support for care-related activities.

Caregiving-Specific Measures of Burden and Strain

Labelling and conceptual issues notwithstanding, research has shown that caring for a seriously ill or impaired older adult does have effects on specific aspects of caregivers' lives. As a result, assessing caregiver strain is a central feature of caregiver assessment. This section will review in detail the measures and techniques that have been employed, including evaluation of their conceptual sophistication and practical utility from the perspective of both the researcher and practitioner.

Historically the first, and the most widely used, approach to measuring caregiving effects has examined the burdens and strain attributed by caregivers to care provision. Research conducted by the Zarits and their colleagues (Zarit, Reever, & Bach-Peterson, 1980; Zarit, Todd, & Zarit, 1986; Zarit & Zarit, 1982) in the early 1980s focused on caregivers' reports of specific types of burdens they experienced. Much of the work that followed during the next 10 years provided substantive and methodological variations on this theme. Specifically, a number of researchers and clinicians added items to tap additional dimensions of care-related burden, organized care-related burden into conceptually distinct dimensions, or tested the multidimensionality of this concept. However, most of these measures have one feature in common: they represent the caregivers' perceptions and the attribution of specific burdens and strains to caregiving. As noted above, this approach requires caregivers to sort through the numerous responsibilities and stressors that impact on them and to identify the specific burdens and strains that are the result of caregiving.

Measures using this approach, aside from being the most widely used measures of caregiving effects, have been shown to correlate with global measures of physical and mental health and with specific care-related stressors such as the care recipient's physical and mental impairments and behaviors. This review will begin with the original measures devised by Zarit and colleagues and continue with 14 additional measures, presented in alphabetical order by the last name of the first author.

Burden Interview (Zarit et al.). In its original form (Zarit, Reever, & Bach-Peterson, 1980) the Burden Interview contained 29 items which cover problematic areas most frequently mentioned by caregivers in their research. The items include areas such as caregiver's emotional health, psychological well-being, finances, social life, and the relationship between the caregiver and care recipient. Caregivers are asked to indicate how much discomfort these caused them. The Burden Interview was designed to be used as a single total score without subdimensions or factors. The total score was shown to correlate weakly with caregiver stressors, such as care recipient's impairment.

The strength of this measure lies in the broad range of care-related strain issues that it taps in its large number of items. In spite of its length, it has been extensively used in its entirety with no reported difficulty. Although the original work by the authors does not report on the psychometric properties of the instrument, subsequent use by a number of researchers has demonstrated its internal consistency (Young & Kahana, 1989) and content validity. Perhaps its greatest strength from a research standpoint lies in the fact that there are dozens of caregiver studies and program evaluations published using either the original index or comparable reformulations. As a result there are numerous studies with varying subpopulations of caregivers available for comparison.

Quality of Caregiver–Care Receiver Relationship and Degree of Strain Experienced by Caregivers (Cantor). Following the work of Zarit and his colleagues, the field of gerontology began a more intense and comprehensive assessment of the attributed effects that caregiving has on family and friends providing that care. One of the earliest studies to recognize the complexity and multidimensional nature of care-related strain was the work of Cantor (1983) using data drawn from a larger study entitled "The Impact of the Entry of the Formal Organization on the Informal Support System of Older Americans." In reporting on that research, Cantor organized the items into two broad categories, the quality of the caregiver–care-receiver relationship and the strain experienced by the caregiver.

In Cantor's research seven separate items were used to measure the quality of caregiver–care receiver relationships. Caregivers were asked whether they agree or disagree with statements that describe different aspects of the relationship such as getting along well, understanding each other, treating each other well, having similar views on life and being close. Substantial differences were found in the reported quality of the relationship depending on the type of relationship (spouse, adult child, other relative, or friend/neighbor).

Caregiver strain was measured using an extensive series of items that were categorized as worry (care receivers' health, state of mind, financial condition, help sufficiency), strain arising from the caregiving role (emotional, physical, and financial) and impact on caregivers' lives (everyday chores, time for other family, social activities, hobbies, ability to keep a job, vacations, free time, and other family relationships). Composite scores were constructed for the latter two categories. However, neither the method used to create these scores nor information on validity/reliability were reported. Multivariate analyses demonstrated that both of these measures were significantly related to type of caregiver (spouse caregivers showing greatest strain and impact followed by adult children and other relatives and nonrelatives) and to other important aspects of caregiving such as amount of assistance and caregiver gender.

Because these items were not empirically validated and their potential internal consistency is unknown, they cannot be recommended for use in their current form as part of a multidimensional caregiver assessment. However, because of the conceptual themes they represent and the breadth of specific aspects of caregiving effects they cover, this work by Cantor should be reviewed as part of the process of constructing a comprehensive caregiver assessment.

Caregiver Hassles Scale (Kinney and Stephens). Kinney and Stephens (1989a; 1989b) developed a multidimensional scale designed to assess caregivers' perceptions of daily hassles associated with caring for an impaired older adult. The authors indicate that this scale differs from other burden and strain scales because it focuses on the minor events comprising the day-to-day experiences of caregivers. Caregivers are asked to indicate whether any of 42 hassles (defined as "things that annoy or bother you, make you angry or upset") have occurred during the past week (nonoccurrence scored as 0). For those hassles that occurred, they are then asked to indicate how much of a hassle it was on a 4-point continuum ranging from *it wasn't* to *a great deal.*

The scale can be used either as a total score by summing across all items or as five subscales. The five subscales represent different areas including: Basic ADL (9 items), Instrumental ADL (7 items), Cognition (9 items), Behavior (12 items), and the Caregiver's Support Network (5 items). The α reported for the total scale was .91 with subscale α reliability ranging from .74 to .89. The full scale correlates moderately with other measures of psychiatric symptoms such as anxiety, hostility, and depression.

The authors suggest that the scale offers a means of identifying the general level of stress among caregivers as well as pointing to the source of that stress. They further suggest that it is this type of information that can be used by health care professionals in planning interventions and services for caregivers. The measure's strengths lie in its link to specific caregiver stressors, its multidimensional structure established using factor analysis, and relatively high internal consistency for the total scale and subscales. Although lengthy, clinicians and practitioners could selectively use subscales where time of administration presents a problem.

Cost of Care Index (CCI; Kosberg and Cairl). Kosberg and Cairl (1986) introduced a 20-item, multidimensional scale to assess the impact of caregiving. Four items are used to tap each of five dimensions that were identified by factor analysis: Personal and Social Restrictions, Physical and Emotional Problems, Economic Costs, Value Investment in Caregiving, and the Perception of the Older Individual as a "Provocateur." Caregivers are asked whether they strongly disagree, agree, or strongly agree with each statement in the index.

The authors reported high internal consistency with an α for the total index of .91. The total index and its five dimensions vary in their correlation from weak to moderate with caregiver stressors such as patient functioning and other global dimensions of caregiver mental health. This instrument is recommended by the authors as part of an overall assessment of older adults and their families and has been used for screening and counseling family caregivers. It was designed specifically as a tool for case managers to use as they work with families in making nursing home placement decisions. The authors suggest that one of its primary advantages is that it measures specific dimensions of burden that are perceived by the caregiver to be adversity directly attributable to care responsibilities. Once the sources of adversity are identified, the professional working with the caregiver can address the problems through counselling, education or other programmatic interventions (Kosberg, Cairl, & Keller, 1990).

The strengths of this instrument lie in the broad content covered by the items, the empirically derived multidimensionality, and high internal consistency. It is relatively brief, and because it has defined subscales and was designed as a tool for practitioners, is easy to administer.

Subjective Caregiver Burden and Caregiving Impact (Lawton et al.). Lawton, Kleban, Moss, Rovine, and Glicksman (1989) developed five measures of caregiving appraisal based on extensive exploratory and confirmatory factor analysis. Two of these indicators, drawn from Zarit's Burden Interview (Zarit et al., 1980), may be categorized as strain or burden measures. The first of these, entitled Subjective Caregiver Burden, is comprised of 10 items that operationalize the caregiver's appraisal that areas such as his or her health and emotional well-being have been affected. The second indicator, entitled Caregiving Impact, includes four items that tap caregivers' perceptions that their social life and family relationships have been affected by caregiving.

The authors indicated that the Subjective Burden measure and Caregiving Impact measure are moderately correlated with each other ($r = .31$ and .40 in two different samples), and have moderate internal consistency as indicated by α coefficients of .85 and .87 for the former and .65 and .70 for the latter.

These two measures have the advantage of being part of a larger conceptual model that views burden in the broader context of caregiving appraisal. The fact that the measures are derived from sophisticated factor analyses with demonstrated construct validity is a major strength. The fact that the individual items that make up these indices have been previously part of other validated instruments provides comparability with prior research and enhances content validity. The relative brevity of these two indicators, combined with acceptable reliability, also recommends these for use as part of caregiver assessment.

Personal and Interpersonal Burden (Miller et al.). Miller, McFall, and Montgomery (1991) constructed two measures of caregiver burden from an array of items included in the Informal Caregiver Survey, a companion to the National Long Term Care Survey. The first indicator they constructed, Personal Burden, represents the caregiver's appraisal of limitations in personal actions and activities due to providing care. This six-item scale includes the caregiver's perception of declining health, the financial cost of care, emotional strains, and limitations in social activities. The Interpersonal Burden scale contains four items that measures caregivers' reactions to specific problematic behaviors such as yelling and embarrassing behavior by the care recipient. The two scales were shown to be highly correlated ($r = .75$) with personal burden having an α reliability of .76 and interpersonal burden having an α of .68. The authors indicate that confirmatory factor analysis supports the use of two separate factors in spite of this high intercorrelation.

The strength of these indicators lies in the breadth of content contained in the relatively brief scale and the fact that they are derived from a major national data base. Another strength is the multidimensional nature of the scale that allows personal and interpersonal burden to be measured separately. Another strength of this instrument is the considerable follow-up research conducted by these investigators using these instruments to study caregiver stress after nursing home admission (McFall & Miller, 1992) and in relation to service use (Miller & McFall, 1991).

Objective and Subjective Burden (Montgomery et al.). Montgomery, Gonyea, and Hooyman (1985) developed one of the first measures used to operationalize caregiver burden that distinguishes between objective and subjective burden. This dichotomous conceptualization was put forth earlier by Thompson and Doll (1982) and has been widely adopted in the caregiving literature. The Objective Burden indicator is a nine-item measure in which respondents report on a 5-point continuum the extent to which caregiving impacts areas of their lives such as time for themselves, privacy, finances, health, and relationship with family members. Subjective Burden is a multi-item inventory in which respondents use a 5-point continuum (ranging from rarely to most of the time) to indicate how often they have experienced each of 13 specific feelings such as depression, lack of appreciation, nervousness, and so forth.

The two dimensions of burden are conceptually defined rather than being based on empirical factor structures. The authors reported α reliability of .85 for objective burden and .86 for subjective burden and moderate intercorrelation between the two measures (.34). They further reported that the two types of burden are differentially correlated with specific caregiving tasks such as nursing, bathing, and transportation. Because the two types of burden correlate differently with specific caregiving tasks, the authors suggest that they are useful in assisting the caseworker in prescribing specific caregiver interventions.

The strength of these indicators lie in their relative brevity and simplicity of administration. They have been widely used, were designed with the needs of practitioners in mind, and have demonstrated reliability. Although not developed using empirically derived factor structures, they are based on conceptualizations that are prominent in the caregiving literature.

Family Strain Scale/Global Burden (Morycz). Morycz (1985) developed two indicators of care-related strain as part of a larger conceptual model of caregiver strain. The first of these indicators is a single-item global burden measure that asks the caregiver if "having to watch the patient is a strain," and is scored on a 4-point continuum from *not at all* to *a great deal.* The second indicator is a 14-item scale which asks if the caregiver experiences specific burdens such as disturbed household routine and changes in relationships and health using the same 4-point scale.

The author suggests that the first six items relate to caregivers' feeling states such as "feeling blue" or "angry," that the second five items reflect perceived changes in living patterns, and that the final two items reflect perceived changes in their own health. However, these distinctions are conceptually based and not empirically grounded in factor analyses. Internal consistency is demonstrated by a relatively strong reliability coefficient of .77 obtained for the total scale. The scale correlates strongly with the Zung Depression Scale and correlates moderately with the single-item summary burden indicator they created.

With regard to its clinical utility, the author states that data analysis indicated that the family strain indicator was a strong predictor of the desire to institutionalize for daughter caregivers but less strong for spouse and son caregivers. The strengths of these indicators are the breadth of caregiving effects that they tap and their multidimensional character. The second and third dimensions that measure changed living patterns and health change could be used separately, with feeling states used as substitute for a global measure of depression or omitted in favor of a standardized depression measure. Because the author does not report the reliability of the separate indicators, and because the factor structures have not been empirically derived, such an approach should be used with caution.

Caregiver Burden Index (CBI; Novak and Guest). Novak and Guest (1989b) developed a 24-item multidimensional measure of caregiver burden entitled the Caregiver Burden Index (CBI), which the authors describe as sensitive to caregivers' feelings and accurate in its picture of caregivers' responses to the demands of caregiving. Caregivers are asked to indicate how accurately each statement describes their feelings on a 5-point continuum ranging from *not at all descriptive* to *very descriptive.* Based on factor analysis, the index was shown to contain five factors: Time-Dependence Burden (5 items), Developmental Burden (5 items), Physical Burden (4 items), Social Burden (5 items) and Emotional Burden (5 items), which are weakly to moderately intercorrelated. They report α reliability coefficients of between .73 and .86 for these factors.

The strength of this index is that it provides empirically derived subscales which cover a wide range of problems reported by caregivers. The subscales all have demonstrated high internal consistency and factor loadings, and moderate intercorrelations between subscales. Further enhancing its utility for practitioners, the authors provide a strategy for using the CBI with caregivers by creating a Caregiver Burden Profile (CBP) in which each caregiver's scores on the separate subscales can be graphically portrayed using standardized scores calculated from the raw scores. This five-factor profile can then be used in clinical settings to compare clients and to make clinical decisions regarding interventions.

Consequences of Caregiving (Pearlin et al.). Pearlin, Mullan, Semple, and Skaff (1990) provide a theoretically based and conceptually sophisticated model for assessing the consequences of caregiving. They provide a model in which the primary stressors that arise out of caregiving give rise to secondary effects entitled "role strains" and "intrapsychic strains." These, in turn, are viewed as having an impact on global mental health outcomes. The authors created seven indicators that reflect burden or strain. They are: Overload (four items, $\alpha = .80$), Relational Deprivation (six items, $\alpha = .77$), Family Conflict (three subscales with α coefficients ranging from .80 to .86, Job Conflict (five items, $\alpha = .75$), Economic Strain (three separate items), Role Captivity (three items, $\alpha = .83$), and Loss of Self (two items, $r = .76$).

This set of indicators represents one of the most conceptually sophisticated and empirically grounded measurement models of the effects of caregiving found in the literature. The overall model not only encompasses the negative effects of caregiving noted above but also includes measures of the positive effects of caregiving as well (see section 4 in this chapter). Although the total set of indices is quite lengthy and hence, not practical for most clinical settings, these highly reliable and brief subscales could be used independently to address specific caregiver issues.

Caregiver Burden/Caregiving Impact (Poulshock and Deimling/Deimling and Bass). Over the course of several studies, staff at the Benjamin Rose Institute have developed a number of measures of caregiver strain. The first group of four measures corresponds to the burden that the caregiver perceives is the direct result of the care recipient's ADL impairment, cognitive incapacity, disruptive behavior, and social functioning (Poulshock & Deimling, 1984). Scores on each of these items ranged from 0 (no burden) to 3 (greatest burden).

The second set of indicators were derived from factor analyses of 34 items that measure the impact caregivers perceive that caregiving has had on their lives.

From these items two indicators were derived. The first of these, Negative Impact on Elder/Caregiver/Family Relationships, contains 11 items, subsequently reduced to eight items with an α .88 (Deimling & Bass, 1989). The second indicator, labeled Activity Restriction, measures the degree to which caregiving has reduced the caregiver's participation in social and recreational activities. Originally containing eight items, it also was revised to contain five items with an α reliability of .80 (Deimling & Bass, 1986).

A third indicator was developed by the Benjamin Rose research team (Deimling et al., 1989) to tap the caregivers' perceptions that their physical and/or emotional health had declined as a result of caregiving. Six items that covered areas such as the frequency of illness, irritability, aches and pains, and general health decline had an α reliability of .95.

These indicators were among the earliest developed that recognize the multidimensional nature of care-related strain/burden and that separated the caregivers' perceptions of caregiving and related strain from other changes in their lives. Their strength lies in their established construct validity using factor analysis and in the content validity demonstrated by their moderate to strong correlation with care-related stressors and global measures of caregiver well-being. From a clinical perspective they are relatively easy to administer due to their brevity and simplicity.

Burden 1 and Burden 2 (Pruchno and Resch). Pruchno and Resch (1989) developed two indicators of caregiver burden. The first, entitled Burden 1, is a single item that asks the caregiver how burdened they feel, overall, on a 5-point continuum ranging from *not at all burdened* to *very greatly burdened.* The second indicator, entitled Burden 2, is a 17-item index in which caregivers were asked how often (*never, sometimes, often*) during the past month they experienced a range of feelings including isolation, irritability, nervousness. The authors reported an α of .89 on the Burden 2 index. However, no subdimensions or factors were identified by the authors.

The authors report moderate to strong intercorrelation of the two burden measures and weak to moderate correlation of the burden scores with caregiver stressors, such as care recipient impairment. The indicators are both moderately correlated with other global indicators of mental health such as depression.

The strength of these two indicators is that when taken together they cover a broad range of caregiving strain symptoms, with the single item tapping the subjective burden dimension, and the second measure documenting the occurrence of caregiving effects. The latter measure has strong internal consistency.

Caregiver Strain Index (Robinson). Robinson (1983) developed a 13-item list of statements that reflect the difficulties that caregivers face after the hospitalization of an older relative. The caregiver is asked to indicate whether these difficulties apply (yes = 1) or do not apply to them (no = 0), including sleep disturbance, changes in personal plans, financial strain, and feelings of being emotionally overwhelmed or physically strained. The index in its original form was designed to be used as a single total score and subdimensions or specific factors were not provided.

The author reports an α reliability of .86; the index was shown to correlate weakly with global measures such as affect, self-rated health, and depression. It was shown to be moderately correlated with other psychiatric symptoms such as anxiety. The author suggests that the internal consistency of the index items and correlation with important criterion variables such as care recipient impairment makes this instrument useful as a screening instrument for caseworkers, preventive clinical practice, or in designing educational materials for caregivers.

As such, the instrument's strength lies in that it was designed with clinical and practice interventions in mind and has acceptable reliability and content validity. However, because it is unidimensional and incorporates diverse items, it may not be as useful in distinguishing specific areas of caregiver need as other multidimensional indicators.

Screen for Caregiver Burden (Vitaliano et al.). Vitaliano, Russo, Young, Becker, and Maiuro (1991) developed an indicator entitled the Screen for Caregiver Burden (SCB). This measure includes 25 items tapping several domains, including care recipient behaviors, disruptions in family and social life, and caregiver affective responses. It is designed to assess both the prevalence (objective burden) of caregivers' experiences and their appraisal of the emotional distress associated with these experiences (subjective burden). Objective Burden (OB) is determined by the number of experiences that the caregiver indicated has occurred from among the 25 items. A Subjective Burden (SB) score was created by summing across all items using the following response categories: *no occurrence,* or *occurrence but no distress* (1); *mild distress* (2); *moderate distress* (3); *severe distress* (4).

The authors report α reliabilities of .84 and .85 for OB and .88 and .89 for SB at two different points in time with a single sample. Test/re-test reliabilities of .70 and .64, respectively, for SB and OB were obtained. Moderate SB and moderate to strong OB correlations with indicators of caregiver functioning were shown. Both OB and SB correlated moderately with global indicators of caregiver mental health such as depression, anxiety, anger, and morale. The primary strength of these two indicators is their conceptual and demonstrated empirical link to major care-related stressors and relatively strong psychometric properties.

Caregiving Costs (Walker et al.). As part of a larger measurement model of caregiving/care-receiving outcomes, Walker, Martin, and Jones (1992) developed a measure of Caregiving Costs. Caregiving daughters were asked how often they experienced each of 28 specific feelings or events that reflect the potential costs associated with caregiving—feelings of guilt or resentment, less time for family, friends or work, and loss of sleep. Responses were coded from 1 to 5, with higher score indicating greater perceived cost. Based on factor analysis, three subscales were identified: Insufficient Time, Frustration, and Anxiety. The first subscale contained eight items and was shown to have an α reliability of .86. The second subscale contained six items with an α of .82. The third subscale contained five items with an α of .61.

The index's strength lies in the breadth of issues that are tapped in the extensive number of items, and the fact that these costs are examined within a larger conceptual framework that includes caregiving benefits. Even though the index is lengthy, the fact that it has subdimensions that exhibit high internal consistency (with the exception of the anxiety subscale) makes it possible to selectively use these components when duration of administration is important. However, it should be noted that the scale was originally developed for research with daughter caregivers. Its properties when used with other groups, such as spouse or male adult-child caregivers, remain to be demonstrated.

Caregiver Satisfaction

Although the literature on caregiving has, in general, focused on the negative impact of caregiving, there has been some research and development of measures that examine the positive aspects of caregiving. These measures recognize that the caregiving situation, even in very difficult cases, provides the opportunity for benefits for those providing care. Although the positives may or may not balance out the negatives, it is important for a comprehensive assessment to identify these positive effects so that practitioners can build on the strengths in the caregiving setting.

Unfortunately, most caregiving research has used the absence of negative effects as a surrogate measure for positive effects. Just as with measures of positive and negative affect, which have been shown to be distinct and orthogonal dimensions (Bradburn, 1969), positive and negative caregiving effects may exist simultaneously and be orthogonal. Three measures of caregiving satisfaction are reviewed here.

Uplifts (Kinney and Stephens). Kinney and Stephens (1989b) developed a companion instrument to their Caregiving Hassles scales which they labeled Caregiving Uplifts. This index in its most recent form includes 42 items that represent events that are potential uplifts, that is those that make the caregiver feel "good, joyful, glad or satisfied." Like its companion Hassles Index, this measure scores both the occurrence of the event and the degree that the caregiver perceives it as an uplift on a 4-point continuum ranging from *not at all* to *a great deal*. Also, like the Hassles scale, the Uplifts are anchored in the tasks associated with caregiving and the impairment of the care recipient. The total index contains subdimensions that reflect the caregivers uplifts related to Activities of Daily Living, Instrumental Activities of Daily Living, Cognitive Performance, Behaviors, and Social Network.

Test–retest reliability for the total index was reported to be .89 (Kinney and Stephens, 1987, 1989) with α reliability ranging from .71 to .91 for specific dimensions. Further, they reported that the Uplifts Scale was virtually uncorrelated with their Hassles Scale.

The strength of this index lies in the fact that it is conceptually linked to care-related stressors, and is a companion to the Caregiver Strain Index. Taken together with its companion index, it provides a very complete picture of the caregiver's response to care-related events. The total index has relatively strong psychometric properties, and because the subdimensions have similar strengths, they may be used independently if the length of complexity of the total index is not practical from a clinical standpoint.

Caregiving Satisfaction (Lawton et al.). Lawton, Kleban, Moss, Rovine, and Glicksman (1989) developed a Caregiver Satisfaction Index as part of a multidimensional caregiving appraisal model, which includes measures of caregiver strain discussed above. This five-item measure was derived from factor analysis of the 47 items in their total measurement model. The items in the satisfaction index reflect some of the positive aspects of caregiving, such as the companionship of the care recipient or the appreciation shown by the care recipient, and demonstrated an α reliability of .68. The index was weakly but significantly correlated with positive affect for adult-child caregivers and more strongly correlated with the help given by caregivers. The index was moderately and negatively correlated with several caregiver strain and burden measures as well as global measures of well-being such as positive affect and depression.

Uplifts (Pruchno and Resch). Pruchno and Resch (1990) developed an Uplifts Index as a companion to their two burden indices. This six-item index measures the frequency of positive, uplifting care recipient behaviors, for example, providing companionship, being enjoyable to be with, and expressing appreciation. An α reliability of .82 for this indicator was shown to be significantly and negatively correlated with the desire to institutionalize the care recipient.

The strength of this indicator is that it is part of a broader conceptualization of caregiving effects that includes positive effects and reflects strengths in the caregiving situation that practitioners can build on as they work with the family. It also has strong psychometric properties, and its negative correlation with the desire to institutionalize is of clinical importance.

Caregiver Coping Resources

While the primary purpose of this chapter has been to review measures of caregiving effects, it should be recognized that from clinical and practice perspectives a comprehensive assessment requires documentation of caregiver resources. A caregiver's resources are important because to a large degree they determine the capacity to continue caregiving. Unfortunately, caregiver resources and the positive effects of caregiving have received much less attention than caregiver strain. Caregivers bring to the care setting a variety of resources, and some caregivers have notable resource deficits. From a clinical perspective, building on existing resources and shoring up the resource deficits are important practice goals. In this way, caregiver assessment continues to parallel assessment of the care recipient.

Coping Resources

There are several measures in the stress and coping literature that have been widely used or adapted for use with caregivers. The F–COPES developed by Olson and McCubbin (1982) was originally designed for use with families in general. However, the F–COPES has been adopted by gerontological researchers in the area of family caregiving (Pratt et al., 1985). The F–COPES consists of 30 items that tap eight coping strategies that individuals and families use in response to problems. Three are internal: reframing, problem solving confidence, and passivity; and five are external, focusing on social support, which includes spiritual support and support from extended family, friends, neighbors, and social services. It has high internal consistency ($\alpha = .86$) and test re-test reliability (.81).

Barber (1988), in a study of the correlation between coping and caregiver burden, found that two dimensions of the F–COPES, confidence in problem solving and spiritual support, were moderately and negatively associated with caregiver burden. Pratt et al. (1985) found that two external coping strategies, spiritual support and extended family support, were negatively and significantly associated with caregiver burden, and that all three internal coping strategies were significantly negatively associated with burden.

In addition to the research that is based on the F–COPES, other researchers in the field of aging have developed instrumentation to assess the coping resources of older adults and their families. Three of these are reviewed below.

ECRC Coping Index (Kahana et al.). The Elder Care Research Center (ECRC) Coping Index (Kahana, Kahana, & Young, 1987), unlike the F–COPES, was developed specifically to identify the coping resources of older adults, though not necessarily of caregivers. The most recent 22-item version of the scale asks respondents the likelihood of employing diverse strategies when facing a prototypical stressful event, for example, hospitalization. Respondents indicate on a 4-point continuum how likely they are to choose each strategy.

The index was designed to be used as three subscales representing different coping styles: Instrumental (10 items), Escape (7 items), and Affective (5 items). Intercorrelations of individuals' coping scores at two points in time demonstrate that the coping styles endorsed by respondents were relatively stable over time, with affective coping showing the greatest consistency and escape strategies being the least consistent over time.

The strength of this index lies in the content, which is appropriate for older adults who have faced a health-related stressor. Its multidimensional character and brevity make it useful for practitioners who need to document the type of personal coping resources the caregivers have available to deal with care-related stressors.

Coping Management (Pearlin et al.). Pearlin, Mullan, Semple, and Skaff (1990) provide 21 coping items organized into three subareas that operationalize coping within the caregiving context. These indicators are an integral part of the model of the relationship between caregiver stress and coping that they have developed (see also Pearlin, Turner, & Semple, 1989). In the first group of four items, entitled Management of the Situation, the caregiver indicates on a 5-point continuum how often specific things are done to manage the care setting. Alpha reliability is not reported, and the authors suggest use of the individual items.

The second group consists of three sets of three items and is entitled Management of Meaning. These items ask the caregiver to indicate how often they think in specific ways. These are grouped as reduction of the caregiver's expectations, positive comparisons, and placing the illness in a larger context. Reported α coefficients for these three sets of items range from .48 to .63. The third group of items, entitled Management of Distress, are designed to be used collectively or as separate items and ask the caregiver to indicate the frequency of each of eight behaviors such as getting exercise, eating, or smoking.

The strength of the coping indicators provided by Pearlin and his colleagues is that they were designed specifically for the caregiving context and are part of a larger conceptual model of coping and care-related stress. The fact that they have a strong conceptual grounding that was empirically tested makes them unique. Because the items are grouped into useful conceptual categories it is possible for the clinician to use subsets of items to meet particular needs of individual caregivers. The fact that several of the coping subscales have unknown or weak psychometric properties, however, limits their utility.

Coping (Pruchno and Resch). Pruchno and Resch (1989) developed a 15-item scale designed to operationalize the coping strategies of caregivers based on the prior work of Kiyak, Montgomery, Borson, and Teri (1985) and of Kahana et al. (1987). This index contains four dimensions identified by the authors through factor analysis. The first dimension, Wishfulness, contains three items that assess the degree to which the caregiver wished that they could change things. This index has an α of .73. The second dimension, Acceptance, also contains three items ($\alpha = .69$). The third dimension, comprised of four items, represents the caregiver's use of intrapsychic coping. This subscale has an α of .71. The fourth dimension measures the caregiver's use of instrumental coping strategies. It is a five-item index with a reported α of .77.

The strength of these measures lies in the fact that they were designed specifically for caregivers, are multidimensional, have reasonably good internal consistency and, because of their brevity, can be easily administered.

Social Support as a Caregiver Resource

One important source of coping resources is the social support available to and used by the caregiver. Indeed a comprehensive caregiver assessment needs to include a thorough review of the quantity and quality of support available and used by the caregiver. Several of the coping measures discussed above include one or more items about the role of social support. However, a more exhaustive assessment of social support, such as that provided by Clipp and George (1990) is clearly desirable and should be a major part of a comprehensive caregiver assessment. Measures that reflect social support of caregivers largely parallel those designed for use with older adults in general. These are reviewed elsewhere in this volume and will not be reviewed here.

SUMMARY AND CONCLUSION

This chapter has proceeded under the assumption that a comprehensive assessment of caregiver functioning includes questions that document the context and setting in which caregiving takes place. Along with information on the history of the caregiving situation, these facts provide an important frame of reference on which practitioners can base clinical decisions. However, the core of most caregiver assessments will focus on the effects of caregiving and the resources of the caregiver that allow him or her to continue to meet the demands of the role.

With regard to caregiving effects, the first step in designing an assessment protocol will be to select a limited number of items that operationalize the caregiver's physical health, mental health, and well-being from among the numerous standardized global measures in these areas. The initial assessment scores on these measures, which are not caregiving specific, can serve as baseline measures for later comparison with reassessment scores on these same items. The choice of measures should reflect the substantive areas that will best inform clinical intervention and later serve to document program impact.

The second step in designing an assessment protocol is to select from among the numerous caregiving specific measures of burden or strain. Of the 15 measures reviewed here the most conceptually sophisticated, substantively exhaustive, and empirically grounded are those developed by Lawton, Kleban, et al. (1989), Novak and Guest (1989b), Pearlin et al. (1990), Vitaliano et al. (1991), and Walker et al. (1992). The number of items included in these measures, if used in their entirety, may be problematic in some clinical or practical situations. Since these measures are multidimensional, with most subscales having acceptable reliability, assessors may choose to be selective and administer only portions of these measures.

Those who wish to tap both the positive and negative effects of caregiving may want to use measures developed by Kinney and Stephens (1989a), Lawton, Kleban, et al. (1989), or Pruchno and Resch (1989). Although each of these has specific strengths and weaknesses, as noted above, the fact that in each of these cases both the strengths and weaknesses of caregivers can be examined with a common methodology makes them worth consideration.

Many of the remaining measures have as their strength brevity, simplicity of administration, and/or development within a clinical context. As a result of these strengths, they have received wide usage. They do vary widely in the strength of their psychometric properties, as noted above. However, measures such as those developed by Zarit et al. (1980), Kosberg and Cairl (1986), Montgomery et al. (1985), Morycz (1985), Poulshock and Deimling (1984)/Deimling and Bass (1986), and Robinson (1983) because of their prior usage, have the advantage of extensive findings in a variety of contexts, subgroups, and samples. Others, such as Cantor (1983) and Miller and McFall (1991), have been part of major national studies and therefore also have extensive comparability. Selection from among this group will depend on the desired substantive content, the importance of specific measurement properties, and ease of administration.

With regard to coping resources, the range from which to choose is more limited. The original F–COPES has been widely used and has well-established measurement properties and extensive published findings for comparative purposes. However, the measures developed by Kahana et al. (1987) and Pruchno and Resch (1989) tap similar dimensions and have been developed specifically for older adults. Finally, the measures developed by Pearlin et al. (1990) were specifically developed to examine coping within a larger caregiving measurement model that includes the positive and negative effects of caregiving. Choices of measures in this area can be made between a context for coping that is specific to caregiving or one that is more general, as in the Pearlin et al. (1990) model of stress and coping.

Certainly, in most practice settings it is not possible to use detailed multi-item indicators from all the areas that have been suggested in this chapter. However, the indicators reviewed provide a relatively comprehensive resource file from which clinicians and researchers can selectively draw in order to create a profile of the needs and resources of the caregiver so that supportive services can be implemented and evaluated.

REFERENCES

Barber, C. E. (1988). Correlates of subjective burden among adult sons and daughters caring for aged parents. *Journal of Aging Studies, 2*, 133–144.

Barer, B. M., & Johnson, C. L. (1990). A critique of the caregiving literature. *The Gerontologist, 30*, 26–29.

Bradburn, N. M. (1969). *Structure of psychological well being*. Chicago: Aldine.

Brown, J. J., Potter, J. F., & Foster, G. B. (1990). Caregiver burden should be evaluated during geriatric assessment. *Journal of the American Geriatrics Society, 85*, 455–456.

Beck, A. T., & Beck, R. W. (1972). Screening depressed patients in family practice: A rapid technique. *Postgraduate Medicine,* 1–85.

Braithwaite, V. (1992). Caregiving burden: Making the concept scientifically useful and policy relevant. *Research on Aging, 14*, 3–27.

Callahan, J. J. (1989). Play It Again Sam—There is no impact. *The Gerontologist, 29*, 5–6.

Cantor, M. (1983). Strain among caregivers: A study of the experience in the United States. *The Gerontologist, 24*, 597–504.

Clipp, E. C., & George, L. K. (1990). Caregiver needs and patterns of social support. *Journals of Gerontology: Social Sciences, 45*, S102–S111.

Colerick [Clipp], E. J., & George, L. K. (1986). Predictors of institutionalization among caregivers of patients with Alzheimer's disease. *Journal of the American Geriatrics Society, 34*, 493–498.

Deimling, G. T., Bass, D. M., Townsend, A. L., & Noelker, L. S. (1989). Care-related stress: A comparison of spouse and adult-child caregivers in shared and separate households. *Journal of Aging and Health, 1*, 67–82.

Deimling, G. T., & Bass, D. M. (1986). Symptoms of mental impairment among elderly adults and their effects on family caregivers. *Journal of Gerontology, 41*, 778–784.

Derogatis, L. R., Lipman, R. S., Rickels, K., Ulenhuth, E. H., & Covi, L. (1974). The Hopkins symptoms checklist (HSCL): Self-report symptom inventory. *Behavioral Science, 19*, 1–15.

Derogatis, L. R., Lipman, R. S., & Covi, L. (1973). SCL–90: An outpatient psychotic rating scale. Preliminary report. *Psychopharmacology Bulletin, 1*, 13–28.

Duke University Center for Study of Aging and Human Development. (1978). Older Americans Resources and Services (OARS): Multidimensional Assessment Survey. Durham, NC: Duke University.

George, L. K., & Gwyther, L. P. (1986). Caregiver well-being: A multidimensional examination of family caregivers of demented adults. *The Gerontologist, 26*, 253–259.

Golden, R. R., Teresi, J. A., & Gurland, B. J. (1984). Development of indicator scales for the Comprehensive Assessment and Referral Evaluation (CARE) Interview Schedule. *Journal of Gerontology, 39*, 138–146.

Gurland, B. J., & Wilder, D. E. (1984). The CARE instrument revisited: Development of an efficient systematic clinical assessment. *Journal of Gerontology, 39*, 129–137.

Havighurst, R. J., Neugarten, B. L., & Tobin, S. S. (1961). The measurement of life satisfaction. *Journal of Gerontology, 16*, 134–143.

Holmes, T. H., & Rahe, R. H. (1967). The social readjustment rating scale. *Journal of Psychosomatic Research, 11*, 213–218.

Kahana, E. F., Kahana, B., & Young, R. (1987). Strategies of coping and post-institutional outcomes. *Research on Aging, 9*, 182–199.

Kercher, K. (1992). Assessing subjective well-being in the old old. The PANAS as a measure of orthogonal dimensions of positive and negative affect. *Research on Aging, 14*, 131–168.

Kinney, J. M., & Stephens, M. A. P. (1989a). Caregiving Hassles Scale: Assessing the daily hassles of caring for a family member with dementia. *The Gerontologist, 29*, 328–332.

Kinney, J. M., & Stephens, M. A. P. (1989b). Hassles and uplifts of giving care to a family member with dementia. *Psychology and Aging, 4*, 402–408.

Kiyak, H. A., Liang, J., & Kahana, E. (1976, September). *A methodological inquiry into the Schedule of Recent Life Events*. Paper presented at the annual meeting of the American Psychological Association, Washington, DC.

Kiyak, H. A., Montgomery, R., Borson, S., & Teri, L. (1985, November). *Coping patterns among patients with Alzheimer's disease and non-demented elderly.* Paper presented at the annual meeting of the Gerontological Society of America, New Orleans, LA.

Kosberg, J. I., & Cairl, R. E. (1986). The Cost of Care Index: A case management tool for screening informal caregivers. *The Gerontologist, 26*, 273–278.

Kosberg, J. I., Cairl, R. E., & Keller, D. M. (1990). Components of burden: Interventive implications. *The Gerontologist, 30*, 236–240.

Lawton, M. P. (1975). The Philadelphia Geriatric Center Morale Scale: A revision. *Journal of Gerontology, 30*, 85–89.

Lawton, M. P., & Brody, E. M. (1969). Assessment of older people: Self maintenance and instrumental activities of daily living. *The Gerontologist, 9*, 179–186.

Lawton, M. P., Brody, E. M., & Saperstein, A. R. (1989). A controlled study of respite service for caregivers of Alzheimer's patients. *The Gerontologist, 29*, 8–16.

Lawton, M. P., Kelban, M. H., Moss, M., Rovine, M., & Glicksman, A. (1989). Measuring caregiving appraisal. *Journals of Gerontology: Psychological Sciences, 44*, P61–P71.

McFall, S., & Miller, B. H. (1992). Caregiver burden and nursing home admission of frail elderly persons. *Journals of Gerontology: Social Sciences, 47*, S73–S79.

Miller, B., McFall, S. (1991). The effect of caregiver's burden on change in frail older person's use of formal helpers. *Journal of Health and Social Behavior, 32*, 165–179.

Miller, B., McFall, S., & Montgomery, A. (1991). The impact of elder health, caregiver involvement, and global stress on two dimensions of caregiver burden. *Journals of Gerontology: Social Sciences, 46*, S9–S19.

Montgomery, R., Gonyea, J., & Hooyman, N. (1985). Caregiving and the experience of subjective and objective burden. *Family Relations, 34*, 19–26.

Morycz, R. K. (1985). Caregiving strain and the desire to institutionalize family members with Alzheimer's disease: Possible predictors and model development. *Research on Aging, 7*, 329–361.

National Center for Health Statistics. (1981). *National health and nutrition examination survey II.* Hyattsville, MD: Public Health Service.

Noelker, L. S. (1990). Family caregivers: A valuable but vulnerable resource. In Z. Harel, P. Ehrlich, P., & R. Hubbard (Eds.), *The vulnerable aged: People, services, and policies* (pp. 189–206). New York: Springer.

Novak, M., & Guest, C. (1989a). Caregiver response to Alzheimer's disease. *International Journal of Aging and Human Development, 28*, 67–79.

Novak, M., & Guest, C. (1989b). Application of a multidimensional caregiver burden inventory. *The Gerontologist, 29*, 798–803.

Olson, D., & McCubbin, H. (1982). Circumplex model of marital and family systems: Application to family stress and crisis intervention. In H. McCubbin & D. Olson (Eds.), *Family stress, coping and social support.* Springfield: Thomas.

Pearlin, L. I., Mullan, J. T., Semple, S. J., & Skaff, M. M. (1990). Caregiving and stress process: An overview of concepts and their measures. *The Gerontologist, 30*, 583–591.

Pearlin, L. I., Turner, H., & Semple, S. (1989). Coping and the mediation of caregiver stress. In E. Light & B. Lebowitz (Eds.), *Alzheimer's disease treatment and family stress: Directions for research* (pp. 198–217). Rockville, MD: U.S. Department of Health and Human Services.

Poulshock, S. W., & Deimling, G. T. (1984). Families caring for elders in residence: Issues in the measurement of burden. *Journal of Gerontology, 39*, 230–239.

Pratt, C., Schmall, V., Wright, S., & Cleland, M. (1985). Burden and coping strategies of caregivers of Alzheimer's patients. *Family Relations, 34*, 27–34.

Pruchno, R., & Resch, N. L. (1989). Mental health of caregiving spouses: Coping as mediator, moderator, or main effect? *Psychology and Aging, 4*, 454–463.

Radloff, L. S. (1977). The CES–D scale: A self-report depression scale for research in the general population. *Applied Psychological Measurement, 1*, 385–401.

Robinson, B. C. (1983). Validation of a caregiver strain index. *Journal of Gerontology, 38*, 344–348.

Schulz, R., Visintainer, P., & Williamson, G. M. (1990). Psychiatric and physical morbidity effects of caregiving. *Journals of Gerontology: Psychological Sciences, 45*, P181–P191.

Stone, R., Cafferata, G. L., & Sangl, J. (1987). Caregivers of frail elderly: A national profile. *The Gerontologist, 27*, 616–626.

Thompson, E. H., & Doll, W. (1982). The burden of families coping with the mentally ill: An invisible crisis. *Family Relations, 3*, 379–388.

Vitaliano, P., Dougherty, C., & Siegler, I. (in press). Biopsychological factors and impaired quality of life as risks for the outcome of CVD in caregivers of people with Alzheimer's disease. In R. Abeles, H. Gift, & M. Ory (Eds.), *Aging and quality of life: Charting new territories in behavioral science research.* New York: Springer.

Vitaliano, P. P., Russo, J., Young, H. M., Becker, J., & Maiuro, R. D. (1991). The screen for caregiver burden. *The Gerontologist, 31*, 76–81.

Vitaliano, P. P., Young, H. M., & Russo, J. (1991). Burden: A review of measures used among caregivers of individuals with dementia. *The Gerontologist, 31*, 67–75.

Walker, A. J., & Allen, K. R. (1991). Relationship between caregiver daughters and their elderly mothers. *The Gerontologist, 31*, 389–396.

Walker, A. J., Martin, S. S. K., & Jones, L. L. (1992). The benefits and costs of caregiving and care receiving for daughters and mothers. *Journals of Gerontology: Social Sciences, 47*, S130–S139.

Watson, D. (1988). Development and validation of brief measures of positive and negative affect: The PANAS scale. *Journal of Personality and Social Psychology, 54*, 1063–1070.

Wood, V., Wylie, M. L., & Sheafor, B. (1969). An analysis of a short, self-report measure of life satisfaction: Correlations with raters judgments. *The Gerontologist, 6*, 31 (Abstract).

Wright, L., Clipp, E., & George, L. (1993). Health consequences of caregiver stress. *Medicine, Exercise, Nutrition and Health, 2*, 181–195.

Young, R. F., & Kahana, E. (1989). Specifying caregiver outcomes: Gender and relationship aspects of caregiving strain. *The Gerontologist, 29*, 660–666.

Zarit, S. H., Reever, K. E., & Bach-Peterson, J. (1980). Relatives of the impaired elderly: Correlates of feelings of burden. *The Gerontologist, 20*, 649–655.

Zarit, S. H., Todd, P. A., & Zarit, J. M. (1986). Subjective burden of husbands and wives as caregivers: A longitudinal study. *The Gerontologist, 26*, 260–266.

Zarit, S. H., & Zarit, J. M. (1982). Families under stress: Interventions for caregivers of senile dementia patients. *Psychotherapy: Theory, Research, and Practice, 19*, 461–471.

Zung, W. (1965). A self-rating depression scale. *Archives of General Psychiatry, 12*, 63–70.

CHAPTER 13

Assessment of Pain in the Elderly

PATRICIA A. PARMELEE
POLISHER RESEARCH INSTITUTE
PHILADELPHIA GERIATRIC CENTER

Folk wisdom tells us that aging is accompanied by aches and pains: that joints grow stiffer, muscles tire more easily, and the cumulative, minor ailments of normal aging cause at least transient discomfort. Yet surprisingly little is known about older persons' experience of pain and particularly about the assessment of pain in this group. There is a large general literature from which to draw and at least some demonstration of the generalizability of pain assessment methods to the elderly, but surprisingly little research has directly examined pain and its measurement among older people. Furthermore, a number of special considerations recommend against simply assuming that methods and measures that have proven successful with younger persons will be equally as useful with the elderly.

Thus, unlike many in this volume, this chapter can offer no comprehensive review of assessment methods known to be suitable for use with older adults. Instead, it begins with a brief overview of the prevalence and experience of pain among older persons. Non-age-specific methods for assessing pain will then be examined, with special emphasis on their applicability to older populations.

THE EPIDEMIOLOGY OF PAIN IN THE ELDERLY

A number of common health conditions, both chronic and acute, may be associated with pain in old age. Osteoarthritis, osteoporosis, postherpetic neuralgia, diabetic neuropathies, cardiovascular problems, and a variety of other chronic disorders are both more common among older than younger persons and characterized by persistent or intermittent pain. These and other disorders, in turn, contribute to the general frailty that accounts for increased risk of falls and susceptibility to fractures, another relatively common source of pain among the elderly.

Yet despite this panoply of inherently painful, age-related disorders, the notion that old age is accompanied by increased pain is at best an oversimplification. Sternbach (1986) found, in a stratified random sample of adults in the United States, that persons over age 65 were less likely than younger adults to complain of headache, backache, muscle pains, stomach pain, and dental pain but more apt to report joint pain (see also Brattberg, Thorslund, & Wikman, 1989; Von Korff Dworkin, Le Resche, & Kruger, 1988). In contrast, Crook, Rideout, and Browne (1984) surveyed patients of a group family practice clinic and found that the prevalence of persistent, but not temporary, pain increased significantly with age. Harkins and Price (1992), analyzing data from the National Health and Nutrition Examination Survey 1982–1984 Follow-Up, similarly found that the percentage of persons reporting musculoskeletal pain as well as their ratings of the severity of that pain increased across ascending age cohorts. Of course, the question is clouded by measurement issues such as older persons' differential sensitivity to or tolerance of pain; these will be discussed shortly. For now, it is unclear from current knowledge whether older persons in fact are subject to greater or more frequent pain than younger individuals.

The extent of the problem is more clearly depicted by surveys of pain specifically among older people. Thomas and Roy (1988) found that 73% of a sample of members of a community center for the aged reported chronic pain. Studies in nursing homes revealed that between 71% and 83% of elderly residents are troubled by pain (Roy & Thomas, 1986; Ferrell, Ferrell, & Osterweil, 1990). Our own data for nursing home and congregate apartment residents indicates that 82% report at least one persistent pain complaint. Thus, pain appears to be a major problem for older persons, particularly the frail elderly.

DEFINITION AND MEANING OF PAIN

Thus far, I have not attempted to define *pain*; surprisingly few authors do so. Because pain is a human universal—we all experience it at one time or another—it is often assumed that no "textbook definition" is necessary. Nonetheless, some consideration of what pain is and how it is experienced is crucial to discussion of its measurement.

The Dual Nature of Pain

Perhaps the single most frequently cited definition of pain is that offered by the International Association for the Study of Pain (Merskey, 1986): "An unpleasant sensory and emotional experience associated with actual or potential tissue damage or described in terms of such damage" (p.1). This definition nicely portrays the hybridization of the concept of pain that has taken place over the years, moving from primary (if not sole) emphasis on physiological processes toward recognition of the subjective nature and multiple causes of pain. Today, not only basic perceptual processes but also complex affective, motivational, and psychosocial factors are accepted as contributors to the experience of pain. Yet the central core of this contemporary definition—*actual or potential tissue damage*—remains strongly physiological.

During the past few decades, great strides have been made in explicating the neurological bases of pain experience, in terms of both central and peripheral mechanisms (see Cailliet, 1993). But there has been much less progress in developing physiologically based means of measuring pain. Although such indices as cortical evoked potentials, cardiovascular stress response, and electromyograms have been used with varying success in laboratory settings (see Flor, Miltner & Birbaumer, 1992, for a review), they have not been adapted for use in routine clinical assessment of pain. The logistic problems of obtaining and interpreting such measures are compounded by the specificity of certain physiological measures to discrete types of pain. In addition, in many pain syndromes, there is no direct correspondence between anatomical state and subjective experience of pain. Persons report pain in the absence of any detectable physical cause, and tissue damage can occur without pain (see Fernandez & Turk, 1992; Trief, Elliott, Stein, & Frederickson,1987, for review and discussion). Even where there is a clear physical cause for pain, objective disease severity and/or degree of tissue damage are at best only moderately correlated with persons' reported experience of pain (Greenwald, Bonica, & Bergner, 1987; Keefe et al., 1987).

In short, the relationship between physiological basis for and subjective experience of pain remains, at this stage of knowledge, ill defined. Even in clinical settings, assessors have limited access to physiological evidence that would support pain complaints, and that evidence appears to correspond only roughly to the individual's experienced discomfort. The following discussion, therefore, emphasizes the subjective qualities and experience of pain, and introduces some important distinctions among types and aspects of pain.

Dimensions of Pain Experience

A first aspect of pain is its *intensity*, or the degree of subjective discomfort experienced. Although intensity is probably the most frequently measured, it is by no means the only dimension on which pain may be characterized. This section briefly examines four aspects of pain that, in addition to intensity, are central to its measurement: its sensory, affective, motivational, and behavioral components.

The notion that pain stimuli differ qualitatively as well as quantitatively, first explicated by Dallenbach (1939), has led to a great deal of interest in the distinct varieties of *sensory* experience associated with pain. For example, if one thrusts her finger into a candle, she may describe the sensation as "burning." The same finger, upon being hit by a hammer, may "throb," and should the hapless digit next encounter a hypodermic needle, the result might be labeled "pricking" or "piercing." Thus, as Melzack (1983) cogently framed the issue,

> The word "pain" refers to an endless variety of qualities . . . , not to a specific, single sensation that varies only in intensity.... Describing pain solely in terms of intensity is like specifying the visual world only in terms of light flux without regard to pattern, color, texture, and the many other dimensions of visual experience.(p. 2)

This focus on the qualitative sensation of pain has been accompanied by acknowledgment of its emotional or *affective* dimension. Pain is inherently aversive, and the unique bodily sensations that make a given stimulus painful generate negative affect as well. Although there is some controversy over the distinguishability of sensory and affective dimensions of pain, a recent review (Fernandez & Turk, 1992) argues convincingly that the two are separate, albeit not necessarily independent, elements. Its unpleasant sensory and affective qualities lend a third, *motivational* dimension to pain, in that organisms seek both to avoid and to stop pain as quickly as possible. Perhaps the foremost explication of this position is the gate-control theory of Melzack and Wall (1965; also, Melzack & Casey, 1968), which postulates distinct but interactive sensory-discriminative and motivational-affective systems that, together with central control processes within the nervous system, determine the experience and meaning of pain.

Fordyce (1976), in his seminal explication of the *behavioral* dimension of pain, argues that expressions of pain are operant behaviors that respond like any other to reinforcement. Although they are initially displayed spontaneously in reaction to sensory and affective experience, behavioral expressions of pain may come over time to depend more on their consequences—specifically, others' response to them—than on the stimulus conditions that originally produced them. Although this model underpins much of the extant research on pain behavior, this chapter defines the behavioral component of pain more broadly, as the array of overt and cognitive responses persons make to pain of any sort: verbal and nonverbal expressions of pain, behavioral attempts to ease or prevent pain, cognitions about its meaning, and strategies for coping with pain.

In sum, pain is a complex and multifaceted experience, of which actual physical sensation is only a small part. Before turning to issues of assessment, it is important to qualify this broad definition with a few distinctions of types and sources of pain: experimental versus clinical pain and, within the latter category, acute versus chronic and organic versus functional pain.

Clinical Versus Experimental Pain. Much of our knowledge of the basic qualities of pain experience comes from laboratory studies in which carefully calibrated techniques are used to induce pain. Methods of inducing *experimental pain* are quite varied, including electrical shock to various parts of the body, focusing a beam of radiant heat on the skin, exposure of the hand or arm to extreme cold, and use of a tourniquet to exert pressure on the arm or other extremity. Research on experimental pain has been central in establishing basic psychophysical dimensions of pain; the most heavily studied dimensions are threshold, or the intensity at which a stimulus is first experienced as painful, and tolerance, the point at which the individual finds stimulation unbearable. Such research has also yielded very useful information regarding, for example, the effects of temporary mood states and situational cues, demographic and personality characteristics, and the analgesic properties of a surprising variety of drugs (see review by Wolff, 1983).

Many of these studies are immediately relevant and may relatively easily be extended to clinical settings. Nonetheless, experimentally induced pain is not a clear analog of *clinical pain*, that is, pain that is experienced in daily life. Although there has been considerable effort to validate laboratory methods against clinical pain experience and develop experimental techniques that effectively mimic "real life" pain (see Wolff, 1983, for review and discussion), basic differences between the two complicate generalization. Specifically, the acute, time-limited nature of experimental pain, along with subjects' knowledge of its source, escapability, and ultimately benign character, offers only a rough analog to the pain one encounters in everyday life. In particular, although I could find no empirical evidence on this matter, it is likely that subjects' ability to explain and control pain in the laboratory diminishes the affective response that is so strong a component of clinical pain. Thus, care must be taken in extrapolating from the artificiality of laboratory research to the very real consequences of clinical pain for daily life.

Acute Versus Chronic Pain

I have just implied that one central contributor to people's tolerance of experimental pain is their knowledge that it will soon be over. The duration of clinical pain is similarly crucial both historically, in terms of how long a person has experienced pain, and prognostically, in terms of expectations for relief. Thus, the distinction of *acute pain*, usually defined as pain of 6 or fewer months' duration, from more persistent *chronic pain* is a central one.

Because of its intractability and consequent implications for physical and psychological functioning, chronic pain has received considerably more attention than acute pain. Although there is some information on factors that influence such acute phenomena as postoperative and labor pain, current understanding of pain and its effects is strongly based on such disorders as chronic low back pain, temporomandibular joint syndrome, and selected diseases such as rheumatoid arthritis. The exact causes of many of the most heavily studied types of chronic pain are often unclear, and the term *chronic pain* is often used as a synonym for "pain of unknown origin." This raises a further necessary distinction: that of *organic pain*, which has an identifiable physiological basis, from *functional* or *psychogenic pain*, for which no physical cause can be found. Note that functional pain is not to be confused with what some call the "psychic" pain of depression or other emotional distress. Rather, it is a physical phenomenon, albeit without identifiable cause.

Functional pain is generally considered to be a manifestation more of personality disturbance than of physical disorder and has been the subject of numerous studies describing the typical "pain-prone" personality (Blumer & Heilbronn, 1982; see Trief et al., 1987, for review and critique of the concept). I could find no research addressing the prevalence of functional pain syndromes or their distinction from organic pain in the elderly. However, there are several streams of thought that, by calling into doubt the validity of at least some older persons' pain reports, effectively bring into play the issue of functional pain complaints. The following section therefore outlines some general considerations in assessing pain among older persons.

ASSESSING PAIN IN THE ELDERLY: GENERAL ISSUES

A number of pain measures have been shown to be reliable and valid among younger persons, but few have been systematically tested with the elderly. Although many will likely prove equally as effective with older persons, certain characteristics of the aging process and today's cohort of older persons recommend caution. It will therefore be helpful, before turning to specific measures, to examine some general problems and issues pertinent to pain and its assessment in late life: thresholds for experiencing and reporting pain, response and reporting biases, psychological influences on the experience and reporting of pain, and cognitive status.

Sensory and Reporting Thresholds

A first, very central question is whether the elderly experience pain differently than do young adults. There is some biological basis to support the notion that older persons may show diminished sensitivity to painful stimuli. However, it appears that, unlike age-linked losses in vision, hearing, smell, and taste, any age changes in pain sensitivity may be caused by changes not in receptors themselves but in the processing of nerve impulses (see reviews by Kenshalo, 1977; Devor, 1991). Such processes would help account for the fact that, despite the increasing rates of potentially painful disorders with increasing age, pain complaints generally decline across persons in their 60s, 70s, and 80s (Lavsky-Shulan et al., 1985; Thomas & Roy, 1988). As yet, however, there has been little direct link of these basic nervous system changes to the experience of pain in late life.

The question is further complicated by the absence of longitudinal work on this issue. Cohort effects, whether cultural or biological, becloud interpretation of available evidence on age differences in sensory thresholds and pain tolerance, and even within this relatively small literature, one must proceed with caution: At least one study compared young adults with an "old" group whose average age was 46!

Harkins, Kwentus, and Price's 1984 review of the literature yielded 10 studies of age differences in sensitivity to pain that included truly elderly persons. Results were contradictory even in studies using the same criterion variable, leading Harkins and colleagues to conclude that there are no meaningful differences in pain sensitivity across age groups (see also Harkins & Price, 1992). A closer look at this literature suggests that there may in fact be age differences, but they may be more complex than a simple linear trend. For example, Evans and colleagues (1992) found age differences in pain sensitivity among diabetics but not in healthy older and younger persons. This suggests a need to assess pain within the context of overall physical health. Harkins and colleagues (Harkins & Chapman, 1976, 1977; Harkins, Price, & Martelli, 1986) have shown a consistent interaction of age with stimulus intensity such that, as compared with younger adults, older persons were less likely to say a low intensity stimulus was painful but more likely to label higher intensity stimuli as painful. Outside the laboratory, pilot research by Harkins and Price (1992) suggests that, although the sensory experience of pain may not be markedly different among aged versus younger chronic pain sufferers, older individuals experience less marked negative affective responses to pain. Thus, obtained age differences may be due not so much to changes in sensory processes per se as to cognitive labeling of a given sensation as painful. Harkins and colleagues' (1984) literature review further led them to attribute observed age differences to a type of reporting bias similar to Botwinick's (1978) generalized cautiousness in responding.

In short, even the basic experience of a stimulus as painful may depend as much on general health and psychological and cognitive factors as on stimulus characteristics. Therefore, we next consider several factors that may influence older persons' experience and expression of pain.

Response Sets and Biases

A first set of pertinent factors are basic questions of methodology and the sophistication of older persons regarding test formats in general. I have already alluded to the problem of cautious responding. More generally, many of the standard methods for assessing pain are rather complex, requiring some degree of abstract thinking and/or fine discrimination among response alternatives. Such tasks may be difficult for the elderly because of sensory and cognitive changes as well as lack of experience with psychometric tests. It is beyond the scope of this chapter to enumerate such factors; interested readers may consult Thompson (1980) for a general overview and Herr and Mobily (1991) for discussion with specific reference to standardized pain measures.

In addition to these very basic kinds of problems, older persons' interpretations of the effects of aging may color self-reports of pain. Some individuals may accept chronic aches and pains as intrinsic to aging and, consequently, not worth reporting; others may feel it is unacceptable to show pain (see, e.g., Greenlee, 1991; Leventhal & Prohaska, 1986). Some, fearing the implications of pain for continued good health or dreading intensive treatment for pain-related disorders, may purposely de-emphasize pain (Clinton & Eland, 1990). Conversely, pain may in some circumstances be used as a "cover" for functional deficits arising from cognitive impairment or other causes (Fordyce, 1978; McIntosh, 1990). Fordyce's (1976) analysis and subsequent research on social influences on pain behavior (e.g., Lousberg, Schmidt, & Groenman, 1992) further suggest that pain complaints may be used to gain others' sympathy or maintain one's "sick role" in interpersonal relationships.

In sum, both instrumentation and a wide variety of response sets and biases may color older persons' self-reports of pain. Some of these, such as cautiousness and interpretations of and projections about pain, are directly linked with age. Others, such as use of pain complaints to justify inactivity or to maintain role relationships, occur among persons of all ages; however, the direction and strength of such effects is quite likely linked to life-cycle differences in social roles and activity patterns. Clearly, more research is needed to investigate the exact manifestations of such effects and variables that influence them, among older persons.

Depression, Affect, and the "Mask of Pain"

A strong potential confound in assessing pain is affective state, particularly depression. Although major depression is no more common than in younger age groups, rates of minor depression are markedly higher in the elderly (Blazer, Hughes, & George, 1987), and depression is strongly associated with acute or chronic illness and disability (Kukull et al., 1986; Parmelee, Katz, & Lawton, 1992). Thus, depression is frequently concomitant with the kinds of health and functional limitations that may be associated with pain in late life.

A large literature (reviewed by Romano & Turner, 1985) documents the positive relationship between pain and depression among persons of all ages; several recent studies (e.g., Parmelee,Katz,& Lawton,1991; Williamson & Schulz, 1992) confirm the phenomenon among older persons. However, the causal paths in this association are unclear. It is quite logical that persons who experience severe, chronic pain and consequent functional limitations may become depressed. More disturbing in its implications for assessment of pain is the possibility that depression may play a causal role. It has been argued that, particularly in late life, complaints of pain and other generalized somatic symptoms may substitute for expressions of depressed affect in the syndrome called *masked depression* (Goldfarb, 1974; Williamson, 1978). That is, to avoid being stigmatized as having emotional problems, older persons may mask depression by presenting instead a complaint of pain or other physical symptoms.

Available evidence, though scant, calls into question this conventional wisdom. Our own research in a geriatric residential institution (Parmelee, Katz, & Lawton, 1991; see also Williamson & Schulz, 1992) yielded significant associations of pain with depression even when physical health and functional disability were controlled statistically. However, this appeared to be due not to pain complaints' masking depression, but to depression's exacerbating real physical pain. Specifically, the association of pain complaints with depression was significant only where there was an identifiable physical cause for a specific complaint (e.g., heart problems among persons complaining of chest pain).

Thus, there is at present no reason to assume that pain complaints of depressed older persons are any less valid that those of affectively "normal" individuals. At the same time, it is clear that depression and other affective disturbances—most notably, anxiety (e.g., Casten & Parmelee, under review)—may affect older persons' perception and reporting of pain. Hence, the same caveat offered earlier with respect to physical health and functioning applies to psychological status as well: Pain assessment must be made within the overall health context, taking into account the range of affective and motivational factors that may influence older persons' experience and description of pain.

Cognitive Status

A last, but by no means insignificant, concern is cognitive status. Although only a small minority of older persons suffer from Alzheimer's disease and other dementing illnesses, cognitive impairment becomes more prevalent with increasing age and rates are much higher among institutionalized older persons (Parmelee, Katz, & Lawton, 1989). Furthermore, chronic pain itself may lower concentration and attention span, exacerbating basic problems of pain assessment. Communication disorders may further impair demented individuals' capacity to report pain. Thus, it is not surprising that, in long-term care facilities, chronic pain is less likely to be identified among cognitively impaired residents than among more alert individuals (Sengstaken & King, 1993).

One likely source of underdiagnosis of pain among cognitively impaired aged is our tendency to assume that even relatively mild cognitive deficits compromise the reliability or validity of symptom self-reports. Yet, a recent examination of pain self-reports in geriatric residential facilities argues against such an assumption (Parmelee, Smith, & Katz, 1993). Cognitively impaired persons were somewhat less likely than their intact counterparts to endorse a variety of pain complaints. However, the validity of impaired respondents' self-reports, operationalized as presence of an identifiable physical cause for a particular complaint, equalled that of cognitively intact persons. Of course, problems of response sets and test sophistication may be especially pertinent to those with declining cognitive abilities. It is unlikely that persons with significant impairment would be able to negotiate some of the more complex assessment methods typically used with younger persons. Nonetheless, our research strongly suggests that when questions are phrased simply and straightforwardly, even moderately demented individuals can give valid, reliable information about their pain experience. Thus, as long as older persons can responsibly respond to queries, their self-reports of pain should not be discounted.

STANDARD METHODS FOR PAIN ASSESSMENT AND THEIR APPLICATION TO THE ELDERLY

Having identified some general barriers to assessing older persons' pain, we now turn to existing measures and methods. Because of the dearth of research on these techniques specifically with the elderly, much of the following discussion will draw speculatively from concerns just outlined. Assessment approaches will be examined in two general areas: basic pain experience and the effects of pain on daily life.

Pain Experience

The complex of qualities that make up basic pain experience—intensity, sensory qualities, affect and motivation—is by far the most intensively studied aspect of pain in any age group. The several standard means of assessing pain experience can be grouped for convenience into three basic categories: self-report, observational methods, and third-party ratings.

Self-Report Measures: *Verbal Scales*. The single most widely-used self-report measure of pain is the McGill Pain Questionnaire (MPQ; Melzack, 1975). Developed in conjunction with Melzack and Wall's (1965) gate-control theory, the MPQ was designed to assess that model's postulated three dimensions of pain experience. Specifically, the Pain Rating Index (PRI) uses 78 adjectives grouped into 16 categories assessing sensory-discriminative qualities (e.g., temporal, thermal, punctate pressure), the motivational-affective dimension (e.g., tension and punishment), and an overall evaluative dimension addressing the "bearability" of the pain. Respondents check as many of the 78 terms as apply to their own pain. Other scales tap present pain intensity (PPI) on a 6-point labeled scale, the location of pain, and its temporal quality. Melzack (1975) recommended a scoring technique that yielded measures of (a) pain intensity, as indicated by the single-item PPI; (b) a summated pain rating index (PRI-S), representing the total scale values of all endorsed descriptors within or across the 16 subclasses, using values obtained by Melzack and Torgerson (1971); (c) a ranked pain rating index (PRI-R), using rank orders within classes rather than scale values, and (d) the total number of pain descriptors endorsed (number of words chosen).

Despite its widespread acceptance, intensive study (see, e.g., Fernandez & Turk, 1992), and prolific use with clinical pain populations, the validity of the MPQ with older populations has received little attention. Corran, Helme, and Gibson (1991) did include the MPQ among an array of instruments used in a small sample of geriatric pain clinic patients. Test-retest reliability was good for the PRI total scale but only moderate to low for the pain intensity measure. The latter scale did, however, show substantial correlations with other measures of pain intensity, was sensitive to effects of pain treatment, and was independent of summary scores for the PRI, confirming the divergent validity of pain intensity and sensory qualities in this elderly population. Although this is, to my knowledge, the only validation of the MPQ with the aged, a few additional studies have used predominantly older persons, with apparent success (Burckhardt, 1984; Ferrell & Schneider, 1988; Lichtenberg, Skehan, & Swensen, 1984). Unfortunately, none of these studies examined response rates or biases, completeness of data, or age effects. Because the MPQ is fairly long and requires some degree of verbal sophistication, it may pose problems for some older persons. At this point,

TABLE 13.1 The Philadelphia Geriatric Center Pain Intensity Scale

With the exception of item 4, for which the number of days is recorded, all items use the following scale:

1 = Not at all
2 = A little
3 = Moderately
4 = Quite a bit
5 = Extremely

1. In general, how much have you been bothered by pain over the past few weeks?
2. How much are you bothered by pain right now?
3. How much are you bothered by the pain when it is at its worst?
4. How many days a week does the pain get really bad?
5. How much are you bothered by the pain when it is at its least?
6. How much has the pain interfered with your day-to-day activities?

however, the extent of such problems is unclear, and further validation of the MPQ with the aged is much needed.

The many variants of the MPQ Present Pain Intensity and related scales also have not been validated with elderly populations. However, my colleagues and I (Parmelee, Katz, & Lawton, 1991; Parmelee, Smith & Katz, 1993) have had considerable success among elderly institution residents using a two-component pain measure of our own construction.[1] The pain intensity component, based very loosely on questions contained in the MPQ, uses six brief questions to assess the prevalence, persistence, and intensity of experienced pain. It appears as Table 13.1. A second checklist taps 11 specific *pain complaints* common among older persons (e.g., joint pain, chest pain). The pain intensity measure shows good test-retest reliability (r=.84), but further research is needed to affirm the validity of this instrument, particularly with more able older persons.

Self-Report Measures: *Graphic Scales*. Equally as popular as the MPQ is the visual analog scale (VAS), in which the rater is presented with a line representing the full range of possible pain intensity, usually from *"pain as bad as it could be"* to *"no pain,"* and asked to mark the point along that line that best indicates his or her own pain level. Visual analog scales may be horizontal or vertical and may or may not include intermediate descriptors along the continuum. Variants include boxed and simple numerical rating scales. Most commonly used to tap pain intensity, VASs show good reliability and validity vis-à-vis other self-report measures and have been successfully used to assess affective and other dimensions of pain in nonelderly populations (see Huskisson, 1983). Nonetheless, VASs are not without problems, including high noncompletion rates relative to verbal scales. Of particular interest is Kremer, Atkinson and Ignelzi's (1981) finding that VAS noncompleters were significantly older (mean age 75 years) than completers (54 years). Thus, the level of abstraction required by VAS, along with the sensory deficits of normal aging and older persons' general lack of experience with graphic scales, may cause problems with all but the most able and test-savvy older persons. Some of these difficulties might be circumvented through adaptation of the basic VAS to make it inherently more meaningful, for example, construction of a pain "thermometer," but this has yet to be explored systematically.

Observational Measures. A second class of measures that has enjoyed considerable attention in recent years is observational techniques. Several systems have been developed for rating pain behaviors (and inferring pain intensity from them) either in vivo or from videotaped segments of behavior. The majority were developed for use in clinical settings, including during physical examinations, and call for ratings to be made over a few minutes' time under each of several conditions, for example, sitting, standing, reclining, walking. The most heavily studied is Keefe and Block's (1982) five-category system (guarding, bracing, rubbing, grimacing, and sighing), which has been adapted and validated with a variety of clinical populations (e.g., Ahles et al., 1990; Anderson et al., 1992). This approach offers strong interrater reliability, concurrent and discriminant validity, and sensitivity to effects of treatment.

A related approach focuses more narrowly on facial expressions of pain (e.g., LeResche & Dworkin, 1988; Prkachin & Mercer, 1989). Research with these systems has shown that facial expressions differ as a function of sources of pain, the social context in which pain occurs, and personality characteristics, and that observers can reliably differentiate genuine from "faked" facial expressions of pain (Craig, Hyde, & Patrick, 1991; Parker, Calahan, & Smarr, 1993).

The advantages of observational approaches are obvious in that they avoid such pitfalls of self-report measures as response sets and biases, comprehension problems, and ecological validity of responses. Although such pain assessment methods have not been specifically tested with older adults, general work on late life facial expression and its decoding (e.g., Levenson, Carstensen, Friesen, & Ekman, 1991; Malatesta, Fiore, & Messina, 1987) suggests that observational techniques should generalize without problem. Indeed, all the samples among whom this method was developed and validated included at least some elderly subjects. This approach may be especially useful for assessing pain among individuals whose cognitive or communicative impairments preclude effective self-report. Preliminary evidence on nonverbal affective communication of demented older persons (Albert, Cohen, & Koff, 1991; Allender & Kasniak, 1989) is encouraging and recommends further exploration with specific reference to pain assessment.

Of course, because behavioral observation is both technically demanding and time consuming, it is likely to be difficult to generalize from laboratory to clinical settings. Technological problems are compounded by context effects. Building on Fordyce's (1976) behavioral model of chronic pain, several observational studies (e.g., Block, Kremer, & Gaylor, 1980; Romano et al., 1991) indicate that behavioral expression of pain may be based as strongly in social as in sensory or affective processes. Thus, careful consideration must be given the social context in which pain behavior is observed.

Third-Party Ratings. A final group of measures bypass the pain sufferer completely, relying instead on the report of others who know the person well. Although I could find no standard instruments for third-party rating of pain, a variety of ad hoc measures have been used to obtain either medical staff's ratings of patients' pain, usually in acute hospital settings, or family caregivers' ratings of their relatives' pain.

The evidence on medical professionals' pain assessments is somewhat discouraging. Care providers rarely espouse a consistent approach to pain assessment, show only moderate interrater reliability, and often make inaccurate assessments vis-à-vis patient self-reports (Camp, 1988; Grossman, Sheidler, Swedeen, Mucenski, & Piatadosi, 1991; Teske, Daut, & Cleeland, 1983). Although errors occur in both directions, the general tendency is toward underestimating patients' self-reported pain.

It has become increasingly popular to use family members as proxy informants not only on factual, externally verifiable information (see discussion by Magaziner, Simonsick, Rashner, & Hebel, 1986), but on pain and other subjective states as well (e.g., Morris et al., 1986; Moss, Lawton, & Glicksman, 1991). The few formal efforts to assess the validity of such ratings offer a somewhat more heartening picture than that for medical professionals. Morris and colleagues (1986), in a study of predominantly elderly cancer patients, reported a concordance of 67.7% between patients' own pain ratings and estimates made by family caregivers. In contrast to medical professionals, caregivers' errors were generally in the direction of overestimates of the presence and degree of pain. Although they did not examine pain per se, Magaziner and associates (1986) similarly found that family members tended to overestimate the extent of their elder relatives' self-reported functional deficits, and that this tendency increased as a function of increased contact with the older person. O'Brien and Francis (1988), also in a cancer population, found good agreement on presence of pain, but far less concordance on the degree and qualities of pain as measured by the McGill Pain Questionnaire. In all these and other, similar, studies, there was a tendency for agreement to decline as the behavior in question became less immediately observable and as response formats became more complex.

In sum, family members do appear to offer fairly valid proxy data on pain, presumably because of their close acquaintance with and frequent opportunity to observe the patient. Yet regardless of the rater's identity, observational ratings of pain are clearly contaminated by such variables as the nature of the patient's illness, demographic and personality characteristics of both patient and rater, the nature of their relationship, the setting in which observations and ratings are made, and the structure of the rating scale. Standardized third-party measures of pain and its effects would clearly be an attractive alternative for use with older persons, particularly those in whom severe cognitive or physical impairments preclude self-report. To date, however, there has been little concerted effort to develop and validate such measures.

Functional and Psychological Effects of Pain

Another major area of interest is the behavioral consequences of pain, that is, the effects of pain on functional abilities and daily life. Of particular interest are measures that tap disability consequent to pain and strategies for coping with pain.

An increasingly popular alternative to the MPQ for generalized pain assessment is the West Haven-Yale Multidimensional Pain Inventory (WHYMPI; Kerns, Turk, & Rudy, 1985). Although the WHYMPI does assess pain intensity and subjective qualities, its primary focus is on the effects of pain on everyday life. Thus, the pain experience section addresses not only pain severity and emotional responses to pain, but also interference with functioning, activities, and satisfaction derived from them; sense of control over pain; and the supportiveness of significant others. Others' responses to pain are further delineated in three realms (punishing, solicitous, and distracting), and a range of daily activities are catalogued. Although this instrument has been used with a variety of chronic pain populations, there has, as with other methods, been little exploration of its performance among older persons. At face value, however, the length of the instrument (52 items) and its 7-point, Likert-type response format may cause some problems, especially with cognitively less intact individuals. A much less lengthy alternative that addresses many of the same issues is the Pain Disability Index (see Tait, Chibnall, & Krause, 1990), which taps the degree to which pain interferes with family and home responsibilities, recreation, social activity, occupation, sexual behavior, self-care, and life-support activity. However, this measure, too, needs further exploration with elderly samples.

There are a few disease-specific assessment tools that nicely address pain and its impact on daily life. Perhaps the most immediately relevant to the elderly is the Arthritis Impact Measurement Scales (AIMS2 [second version]; Meenan, Mason, Anderson, Guccione, & Kazis, 1992), which assesses arthritis pain and consequent disability. The five-item pain scale addresses general pain frequency and severity as well as symptoms specific to arthritis. Additional subscales assess functional effects of arthritis in terms of various basic and instrumental activities of daily living, social functioning, and affective state. The AIMS has been used successfully with elderly osteoarthritis sufferers (Keefe et al., 1987), and a recent revision especially for geriatric assessment (GERI-AIMS; Hughes, Edelman, Change, Singer, & Schuette, 1991) offers the added advantage of distinguishing arthritis-specific pain from that caused by comorbid health problems.

A final group of measures are designed specifically to assess coping with pain and its effects. By far the most widely used is Rosenstiel and Keefe's (1983) Coping Strategies Questionnaire (CSQ), which has been used in numerous non-age-specific studies as well as a few investigations of osteoarthritis among older persons (e.g., Keefe et al., 1987). The CSQ does not assess pain per se, but focuses instead on the frequency with which individuals rely on each of eight different tactics for coping with pain: diverting attention, reinterpreting pain sensations, coping self-statements, ignoring pain sensation, praying and hoping, catastrophizing, increasing activity level, and pain behaviors. Unfortunately, despite several factor analytic studies (e.g., Keefe et al., 1987; Stewart & Knight, 1991; Tuttle, Shutty, & DeGood, 1991), there is little evidence about response problems and completion rates. However, the CSQ's length (50 items) and unlabeled 7-point response format have caused problems in my own pilot work with middle-aged and elderly medical outpatients. A similar but less heavily studied measure is the revised Survey of Pain Attitudes (SOPA; Jensen & Karoly, 1989), which uses 24 five-point scales to assess reliance on medication, hope for a medical cure, need for solicitude, sense of pain control, perceived disability, and emotional response to pain. A third alternative is the Vanderbilt Pain Management Inventory (VPMI; Brown & Nicassio, 1987), 18 five-point items that were originally developed to differentiate active and passive coping strategies among rheumatoid arthritis sufferers. Although they tap many of the same dimensions as the CSQ, the SOPA and the VPMI have enjoyed much less attention and have not, to my knowledge, been used with predominantly elderly populations. Other measures of coping with chronic illness, although not oriented specifically toward pain, may be useful in assessing how elderly persons cope with pain and its effects. One good example is Felton and Revenson's (1984) adaptation of the Ways of Coping Checklist.

SUMMARY AND CONCLUSIONS

Perhaps the single most clearcut conclusion to be drawn from this somewhat cursory overview is that, at this point, we know far too little about the experience of pain among the elderly to make strong recommendations about how to assess it. It is likely that the myriad existing instruments will prove quite easily generalizable to relatively healthy, cognitively intact older persons. However, for the frail aged (who, unfortunately, are the most likely to experience severe and persistent pain), many of the assessment approaches currently available may prove too long and too complex for easy use. Of course, one's choice of research measures depends on not only the particular population with whom one is working but also the question posed. For basic research on, for example, age changes in the psychophysics of pain experience, such relatively complex measures as the McGill Pain Questionnaire or multiple visual analog scales may be necessary to capture the complexities of the phenomenon. For epidemiologic work or studies of the psychosocial concomitants of pain, simpler and more straightforward indices such as our own pain inventory or subscales of longer instruments such as the WHYMPI and the AIMS may more parsimoniously capture the intensity and effects of experienced pain.

The length and complexity of many popular standardized measures makes them unwieldy for use in clinical settings, where the need is perhaps greatest for a simple, consistent, and comprehensive measurement approach. Here, a few simple and straightforward questions, coupled with careful attention to nonverbal indicators and facial expressions, may prove the most expedient means of identifying persistent pain. For clinical purposes, perhaps the clearest indication from the existing literature is that older persons' pain complaints—or, for that matter, the absence of complaints—must be evaluated within the overall context in which they occur. Although no pain complaint should be dismissed, each should be evaluated with a careful eye toward cognitive biases, affective responses, and interpersonal circumstances that may color presenting complaints of discomfort.

It would be easier to make recommendations about pain assessment if there were some "gold standard" against which the construct validity of existing instruments could be judged. Unfortunately for assessors, the subjective nature of pain experience renders it intrinsically elusive and subject to the kinds of personal, social, and situational biases enumerated earlier. Thus, for example, it seems logical that functional disability should be a relatively objective indicator of pain intensity; yet existing evidence strongly indicates that the pain-disability link, like more straightforward self-reported pain, is closely associated with personality, coping strategies, and interpersonal factors (Hagglund, Haley, Reveille, & Alarcon,1989; Summers, Haley, Reveille, & Alarcon,1988). In the search for a template against which to judge assessment approaches, ongoing development of physiological indicators of pain response is worth watching closely. In particular, syndrome-specific techniques such as electromyographic measurement of muscle tension, seem quite promising. With respect to any single, generalized biophysical marker of pain response, however, the specter of psychosocial biases again rears its head in terms of individiual differences in generalized physiological reactivity. Although this approach is certainly worth pursuing, it appears doubtful at this point that any such generalized standard measure will soon be forthcoming.

In closing, then, I repeat the call for more research on pain in older persons: its unique nature, factors that influence its experience and expression and, of course, means of validly and reliably assessing it.

NOTE

1. Primary credit for development of this scale goes to Ira Katz and Powell Lawton, who have most graciously permitted me to collaborate on its validation and substantive application.

ACKNOWLEDGMENTS

Preparation of this chapter was supported by National Institute of Mental Health grants 40380 (I. R. Katz, principal investigator) and 49846 (P. Parmelee, principal investigator).

REFERENCES

Ahles, T. A., Coombs, D. W., Jensen, L., Stukel, T., Maurer, L. H., & Keefe, F. J. (1990). Development of a behavioral observation technique for the assessment of pain behaviors in cancer patients. *Behavior Therapy, 21*, 449–460.

Albert, M. S., Cohen, C., & Koff, E. (1991). Perception of affect in patients with dementia of the Alzheimer type. *Archives of Neurology, 48*, 791–795.

Allender, J., & Kaszniak, A. W. (1989). Processing of emotional cues in patients with dementia of the Alzheimer type. *International Journal of Neuroscience, 46*, 147–155.

Anderson, K. O., Bradley, L. A., Turner, R. A., Agudelo, C. A., Pisko, E. J., Salley, A. N. Jr., & Fletcher, K. E. (1992). Observation of pain behavior in rheumatoid arthritis patients during physical examination: Relationship to disease activity and psychological variables. *Arthritis Care and Research, 5*, 49–56.

Blazer, D., Hughes, D. C., & George, L. K. (1987). The epidemiology of depression in an elderly community population. *The Gerontologist, 27*, 281–287.

Block, A. R., Kremer, E. F., & Gaylor, M. (1980). Behavioral treatment of chronic pain: The spouse as a discriminative cue for pain behavior. *Pain, 9*, 243–252.

Blumer, D., & Heilbronn, M. (1982). Chronic pain as a variant of depressive illness: The pain–prone disorder. *Journal of Nervous and Mental Disease, 170*, 381–406.

Botwinick, J. (1978). *Aging and behavior.* New York: Springer.

Brattberg, G., Thorslund, M., & Wikman, A. (1989). The prevalence of pain in a general population. The results of a postal survey in a county of Sweden. *Pain, 37*, 215–222.

Brown, G. K., & Nicassio, P. M. (1987). Development of a questionnaire for the assessment of active and passive coping strategies in chronic pain patients. *Pain, 31*, 53–64.

Burckhardt, C. S. (1984). The use of the McGill Pain Questionnaire in assessing arthritis pain. *Pain, 19*, 305–314.

Cailliet, R. (1993). *Pain: Mechanisms and management.* Philadelphia: Davis.

Camp, L. D. (1988). A comparison of nurses' record assessment of pain with perceptions of pain as described by cancer patients. *Cancer Nursing, 11*, 237–243.

Casten, R., & Parmelee, P. A. (1994, August). *Path analysis of anxiety, depression and pain among institutionalized elderly.* Presented at the annual meeting of the American Psychological Association, Los Angeles.

Clinton, P., & Eland, J. (1990). Pain. In M. Maas & K. Buckwalter (Eds)., *Nursing diagnoses and intervention for the elderly* (pp. 348–368). Reading, MA: Addison-Wesley.

Corran, T. M., Helme, R. D., & Gibson, S. J. (1991). An assessment of psychometric instruments used in a geriatric outpatient pain clinic. *Australian Psychologist, 26*, 128–131.

Craig, K. D., Hyde, S. A., & Patrick, C. J. (1991). Genuine, suppressed and faked facial behavior during exacerbation of chronic low back pain. *Pain, 46*, 161–171.

Crook, J., Rideout, E., & Browne, G. (1984). The prevalence of pain complaints in a general population. *Pain, 18*, 299–314.

Dallenbach, K. M. (1939). Somesthesis. In E. G. Boring, H. S. Langfeld, & H. P. Weld (Eds.), *Introduction to psychology* (pp. 608–625). New York: Wiley.

Devor, M. (1991). Chronic pain in the aged: Possible relation between neurogenesis, involution and pathophysiology in adult sensory ganglia. *Journal of Basic & Clinical Physiology and Pharmacology, 2*, 1–15.

Evans, E. R., Rendell, M. S., Bartek, J. P., Bamisedun, O., Connor, S., & Giitter, M. (1992). Current perception thresholds in ageing. *Age and Aging, 21*, 273–279.

Felton, B. J., & Revenson, T. A. (1984). Coping with chronic illness: A study of illness controllability and the influence of coping strategies on psychosocial adjustment. *Journal of Consulting and Clinical Psychology, 52*, 343–353.

Ferrell, B. A., Ferrell, B. R., & Osterweil, D. A. (1990). Pain in the nursing home. *Journal of the American Geriatrics Society, 38*, 409–414.

Ferrell, B. R., & Schneider, C. (1988). Experience and management of cancer pain at home. *Cancer Nursing, 11*, 84–90.

Fernandez, E., & Turk, D. C. (1992). Sensory and affective components of pain: Separation and synthesis. *Psychological Bulletin, 112*, 205–217.

Flor, H., Miltner, W., & Birbaumer, N. (1992). Psychophysiological recording methods. In D. C. Turk & R. Melzack (Eds.), *Handbook of pain assessment* (pp. 169–190). New York: Guilford.

Fordyce, W. E. (1976). *Behavioral methods for chronic pain and illness.* St. Louis: Mosby.

Fordyce, W. E. (1978). Evaluating and managing chronic pain. *Geriatrics, 33*, 59–62.

Goldfarb, A. I. (1974). Masked depression in the elderly. In S. Lesse (Ed.), *Masked depression* (pp. 236–249). New York: Jason Aronson.

Greenlee, K. K. (1991). Pain and analgesia: Considerations for the elderly in critical care. *AACN Clinical Issues in Critical Care Nursing, 2*, 720–728.

Greenwald, H. B., Bonica, J. J., & Bergner, M. (1987). The prevalence of pain in four cancers. *Cancer, 60*, 2563–2569.

Grossman, S. A., Sheidler, V. R., Swedeen, K., Mucenski, J., & Piantadosi, S. (1991). Correlation of patient and caregiver ratings of cancer pain. *Journal of Pain and Symptom Management, 6*(2), 53–57.

Hagglund, K.J., Haley, W. E., Reveille, J. D., & Alarcon, G. S. (1989). Predicting individual differences in pain and functional impairment among patients with rheumatoid arthritis. *Arthritis and Rheumatism, 32*, 851–858.

Harkins, S. W., & Chapman, C. R. (1976). Detection and decision factors in pain perception in young and elderly men. *Pain, 2*, 253–264.

Harkins, S. W., & Chapman, C. R. (1977). The perception of induced dental pain in young and elderly women. *Journal of Gerontology, 32*, 428–435.

Harkins, S. W., & Price, D. D. (1992). Assessment of pain in the elderly. In D. C. Turk & R. Melzack (Eds.), *Handbook of pain assessment* (pp. 315–331). New York: Guilford.

Harkins, S. W., Kwentus, J., & Price, D. D. (1984). Pain and the elderly. In C. Benedetti, C. R. Chapman, & G. Morcca (Eds.), *Advances in pain research and therapy* (Vol. 7, pp. 103–121). New York: Raven.

Harkins, S. W., Price, D. D., & Martelli, M. (1986). Effects of age on pain perception: Thermonociception. *Journal of Gerontology, 41*, 58–63.

Herr, K. A., & Mobily, P. R. (1991). Complexities of pain assessment in the elderly: Clinical considerations. *Journal of Gerontological Nursing, 17*(4), 12–19.

Hughes, S. L., Edelman, P., Change, R. W., Singer, R. H., & Schuette, P. (1991). The GERI-AIMS: Reliability and validity of the Arthritis Impairment Measurement Scales adapted for elderly respondents. *Arthritis and Rheumatism, 34*, 856–865.

Huskisson, E. C. (1983). Visual analog scales. In R. Melzack (Ed.), *Pain measurement and assessment* (pp. 33–37). New York: Raven.

Jensen, M. P., & Karoly, P. (1989, March). *Revision and cross-validation of the Survey of Pain Attitudes (SOPA)*. Presented at the annual meeting of the Society of Behavioral Medicine, San Francisco, CA.

Keefe, F. J., & Block, A. R. (1982). Development of an observational method for assessing pain behavior in chronic low back pain patients. *Behavior Therapy, 13*, 363–375.

Keefe, F. J., Caldwell, D. S., Queen, K. T., Gil, K. M., Martinez, S., Crisson, J. E., Ogden, W., & Nunley, J. (1987). Pain coping strategies in osteoarthritis patients. *Journal of Consulting and Clinical Psychology, 55*, 208–212.

Kenshalo, D. (1977). Age changes in touch, vibration, temperature, kinesthesis, and pain sensitivity. In J. E. Birren & K. W. Schaie (Eds.), *Handbook of the psychology of aging*, 1st ed., pp. 562–601). New York: Van Nostrand Reinhold.

Kerns, R. D., Turk, D. C., & Rudy, T. E. (1985). The West Haven-Yale Multidimensional Pain Inventory (WHYMPI). *Pain, 23*, 345–356.

Kremer, E. F., Atkinson, J. H., & Ignelzi, R. J. (1981). Measurement of pain: Patient preference does not confound pain measurement. *Pain, 10*, 241–248.

Kukull, W. A., Koepsell, T. C., Inui, T. S.,Borson, S., Okimoto, J., Raskind, M. A., & Gale, J. A. (1986). Depression and physical illness among elderly general medical clients. *Journal of Affective Disorders, 10*, 153–162.

Lavsky-Shulan, M., Wallace, R. B., Kohout, F. J., Lemke, J. H., Morris, M. C., & Smith, I. M. (1985). Prevalence and functional correlates of low back pain in the elderly: The Iowa 65+ Rural Health Study. *Journal of the American Geriatrics Society, 33*, 23–28.

LeResche, L., & Dworkin, S. F. (1988). Facial expressions of pain and emotions in chronic TMD patients. *Pain, 35*, 71–78.

Levenson, R. W., Carstensen, L. L., Friesen, W. V., & Ekman, P. (1991). Emotion, physiology, and expression in old age. *Psychology and Aging, 6*, 28–35.

Leventhal, E. A., & Prohaska, T. R. (1986). Age, symptom interpretation and health behavior. *Journal of the American Geriatrics Society, 34*, 185–191.

Lichtenberg, P. A., Skehan, M. W., & Swensen, C. H. (1984). The role of personality, recent life stress and arthritic severity in predicting pain. *Journal of Psychosomatic Research, 28*, 231–236.

Lousberg, R., Schmidt, A. J. M., & Groenman, N. A. (1992). The relationship between spouse solicitousness and pain behavior: Searching for more experimental evidence. *Pain, 51*, 75–79.

Magaziner, J., Simonsick, E. M., Kashner, T. M., & Hebel, J. R. (1986). Patient-proxy response comparability on measures of patient health and functional status. *Journal of Clinical Epidemiology, 41*, 1065–1074.

Malatesta, C. Z., Fiore, M. J., & Messina, J. J. (1987). Affect, personality, and facial expressive characteristics of older people. *Psychology and Aging, 2*, 64–69.

McIntosh, I. B. (1990). Psychological aspects influence the threshold of pain. *Geriatric Medicine, 20*, 37–41.

Meenan, R. F., Mason, J. H., Anderson, J. J., Guccione, A. A., & Kazis, L. E. (1992). AIMS2: The content and properties of a revised and expanded Arthritis Impact Measurement Scales health status questionnaire. *Arthritis and Rheumatism, 35*, 1–10.

Melzack, R. (1975). The McGill Pain Questionnaire: Major properties and scoring methods. *Pain, 1*, 277–299.

Melzack, R. (1983). Concepts of pain measurement. In R. Melzack (Ed.), *Pain measurement and assessment* (pp. 1–5). New York: Raven.

Melzack, R., & Casey, K. L. (1968). Sensory, motivational, and central control determinants of pain: A new conceptual model. In D. Kenshalo (Ed.), *The skin senses* (pp. 423–439). Springfield, IL: Thomas.

Melzack, R., & Torgerson, W. S. (1971). On the language of pain. *Anesthesiology, 34*, 50–59.

Melzack, R., & Wall, P. D. (1965). Pain mechanisms: A new theory. *Science, 150*, 971–979.

Merskey, H. (1986). Classification of chronic pain: Description of chronic pain syndromes and definition of pain terms. *Pain* (Supp. 3), 1.

Morris, J. N., Mor, V., Goldberg, R. J., Sherwood, S., Greer, D. S., & Hiris, J. (1986). The effect of treatment setting and patient characteristics on pain in terminal cancer patients: A report from the National Hospice Study. *Journal of Chronic Disease, 39*, 27–35.

Moss, M. S., Lawton, M. P., & Glicksman, A. (1991). The role of pain in the last year of life of elderly persons. *Journals of Gerontology: Psychological Sciences, 46*, P51–P57.

O'Brien, J., & Francis, A. (1988). The use of next-of-kin to estimate pain in cancer patients. *Pain, 35*, 171–178.

Parker, J. C., Callahan, C. D., Smarr, K. L., et al. (1993). Relationship of pain behavior to disease activity and health status in rheumatoid arthritis. *Arthritis Care and Research, 6*, 71–77.

Parmelee, P. A., Katz, I. R., & Lawton, M. P. (1989). Depression among institutionalized aged: Assessment and prevalence estimation. *Journals of Gerontology: Medical Sciences, 41*, M22–M29.

Parmelee, P.A., Katz, I.R., & Lawton, M.P. (1991). The relation of pain to depression among institutionalized aged. *Journals of Gerontology: Psychological Sciences, 46*, P15–P21.

Parmelee, P. A., Katz, I. R., & Lawton, M. P. (1992). Incidence of depression in long-term care settings. *Journals of Gerontology: Medical Sciences, 46*, M189–M196.

Parmelee, P. A., Smith, B. D., & Katz, I. R. (1993). Pain complaints and cognitive status among elderly institution residents. *Journal of the American Geriatrics Society, 41*, 517–522.

Prkachin, K. M., & Mercer, S. R. (1989). Pain expression in patients with shoulder pathology: Validity, properties and relationship to sickness impact. *Pain, 39*, 257–265.

Romano, J. M., & Turner, J. A. (1985). Chronic pain and depression: Does the evidence support a relationship? *Psychological Bulletin, 97*, 18–34.

Romano, J. M., Turner, J. A., Friedman, L. S., Bulcroft, R. A., Jensen, M. P., & Hops, H. (1991). Observational assessment of chronic pain: Patient-spouse behavioral interactions. *Behavior Therapy, 22*, 549–567.

Rosenstiel, A. K., & Keefe, F. J. (1983). The use of coping strategies in chronic low back pain patients: Relationship to patient characteristics and current adjustment. *Pain, 17*, 33–44.

Roy, R., & Thomas, M. R. (1986). A survey of chronic pain in an elderly population. *Canadian Family Physician, 32*, 513–516.

Sengstaken, E. A., & King, S. A. (1993). The problem of pain and its detection among geriatric nursing home residents. *Journal of the American Geriatrics Society, 41*, 541–544.

Sternbach, R. S. (1986). Survey of pain in the United States: The Nuprin Pain Report. *Clinical Journal of Pain, 2*, 49–53.

Stewart, M. W., & Knight, R. G. (1991). Coping strategies and affect in rheumatoid and psoriatic arthritis. *Arthritis Care and Research, 4*, 116–122.

Summers, M. N., Haley, W. E., Reveille, J. D., & Alarcon, G. S. (1988). Radiographic assessment and psychologic variables as predictors of pain and functional impairment in osteoarthritis of the knee or hip. *Arthritis and Rheumatism, 31*, 204–209.

Tait, R. C., Chibnall, J. T., & Krause, S. (1990). The Pain Disability Index: Psychometric properties. *Pain, 40*, 171–182.

Teske, K., Daut, R. L., & Cleeland, C. S. (1983). Relationships between nurses' observations and patients' self-reports of pain. *Pain, 16*, 289–296.

Thomas, M. R., & Roy, R. (1988, July/August). Age and pain: A comparative study of the "younger and older" elderly. *Pain Management*, 174–179.

Thompson, L. W. (1980). Testing and mnemonic strategies. In L. W. Poon, J. L. Fozard, L. S. Cermak, D. Arenberg, & L. W. Thompson (Eds.), *New directions in memory and aging* (pp. 367–377). Hillsdale, NJ: Erlbaum.

Trief, P. M., Elliott, D. J., Stein, N., & Frederickson, B. E. (1987). Functional vs. organic pain: A meaningful distinction? *Journals of Clinical Psychology, 43*, 219–226.

Tuttle, D. H., Shutty, M. S. Jr., & DeGood, D. E. (1991). Empirical dimensions of coping in chronic pain patients: A factorial analysis. *Rehabilitation Psychology, 36*, 179–188.

Von Korff, M., Dworkin, S. F., Le Resche, L., & Kruger, A. (1988). An epidemiologic comparison of pain complains. *Pain, 32*, 173–183.

Williamson, G. M., & Schulz, R. (1992). Pain and depression among community-residing elderly. *Journals of Gerontology: Psychological Sciences, 46*, P367–P372.

Williamson, J. (1978). Depression in the elderly. *Age and Aging, 7*(Supp.), 35–40.

Wolff, B. B. (1983). Laboratory methods of pain measurement. In R. Melzack (Ed.), *Pain measurement and assessment* (pp. 7–13). New York: Raven.

CHAPTER 14

Assessing the Environment

FRANCES M. CARP
THE WRIGHT INSTITUTE, BERKELEY

This chapter deals with the environments in which older persons spend most of their time. The large majority are homes in communities. About 5% are institutions, and a similar number are planned facilities, highrise or campus style, low cost or expensive. Assessment developed inversely to prevalence. Most assessment has been of special housing and institutions.

As is clear from the table of contents of this volume, the environment influences, is influenced by, and interacts with other domains of assessment. An elder's remaining in the community is affected by health, activities of daily living (ADL), life events, cognition, mobility, pain, caregiving, and personality, as well as by the environment. Living alone or in an institution leaves one vulnerable to depression and to functional decrements. The environment affects health, ADL, mobility, cognitive functions, social behavior and affect.

Environmental assessment is important because the environment is more accessible to change than are factors such as health, personality, or cognition. Assessment involves three issues: identifying salient variables, measuring them, and collecting and analyzing data on the measures to achieve a purpose (e.g., to specify design defects or to test theory). Some measures are single items; others, multi-item scales. They use various types of information: views of residents, ratings by observers, and technical measures. Whether measures are single items or sophisticated scales and either subjective or objective, they should cleanly assess the environment, not confounding it with other influences on outcomes under study.

Environmental assessment includes investigation of effects of the environment on residential satisfaction and overall well-being. These outcomes have many determinants, and such studies must be carefully designed. Housing satisfaction is influenced by health, social behavior, personality and affect. Life satisfaction is related to health, social behavior, affect, personality, and life events, as well as to living environment. The issue is: Does the environment make a significant additional contribution, directly, and/or in what sort of interaction with which other variables?

Study design must insure that effects attributed to the environment do not spuriously reflect other variables. Otherwise, knowledge is misled and interventions are ineffective or even deleterious. With valid, reliable measures of all variables, such inquiries may be managed by statistical procedures, such as regression analysis into which environmental variables are entered after other known or likely influences on the outcome are in the equation. However, with any new issue, observational studies must define the parameters, lest further work be misdirected. In the long run, some assessors' goals are better met by informal approaches without scale development or other statistical treatment.

The organization of the chapter is roughly temporal: This assessment field began in special housing, continued in institutions, and turned belatedly to the community environments where most older persons live. Coverage is not comprehensive. The goal is to portray the history of the field and give examples of various types and stages of assessment within each of three areas: special housing, institutional settings, and the community. This chapter presents the historical context, substantive findings as they relate to the development of measures, evaluation of the emergent measures, and theoretical models underlying both the measures and the studies which generated the measures.

ASSESSMENTS IN SPECIAL HOUSING

The First Public Housing for the Elderly

There was little interest in assessing environments of older people until the late 1950s. Consensus among social scientists was that by the end of adolescence the personality was pretty well fixed. As persons aged, their capacity for adaptation decreased; they became rigid, and environmental change was thought to be harmful. These conclusions of academe were challenged by social policy after the Great Depression. Public housing was initiated in the late 1930s, and due to poverty, the extending life span, and alterations in the extended family, many of its tenants were elderly. Sensitive managers (e.g., Thompson, 1992) noted design features that were problematic for older tenants, and in the late 1950s the federal Public Housing Administration approved projects designed for the elderly.

A pre-post study (Carp, 1966) of the first such facility assumed that older people can adapt to a better environment, and that effects on individuals depend on the congruence between the new milieu and the person. Influences of other variables that might affect outcomes were controlled by using a comparison group of similar persons who remained in the original housing. Those who moved in adapted readily and improved in life satisfaction and in physical and mental health compared to similar nonmovers. Tenants' satisfaction with garbage disposal, maintenance and repairs, laundry, housekeeping, sleeping, eating, and shopping increased from applicant status levels; nonmovers' satisfaction remained about the same. There were no measures of specific changes in environment that might underlie these effects. Applicants lived in substandard housing, but there was no quantification of its deficiencies. Physical measures were limited to the new building and to study of minor issues (e.g., distance between apartment doors affected social behavior, distance to the elevator affected participation in activities on the ground floor). On a brief visit prior to moving in, applicants spontaneously noted design features that were to prove undesirable. The investigator recommended that designers have prospective residents assess "mock-ups" prior to construction of facilities.

In regard to the personal environment, all residents of this facility moved from individual (and often isolating) living situations to congregate housing. Applicants' extraversion scores predicted their interpersonal behavior as residents. Applicants high in extraversion became sociable tenants, and extremely introverted applicants became more seclusive and withdrawn than at applicant status (Carp & Carp, 1980). Results were similar for activities and desire for activities: applicants with high scores in extraversion became busy, involved residents; those with low scores became even less active than the least active comparison persons (Carp, 1978).

This was a study of one facility, the first of its kind, which had a highly qualified and motivated staff, and was the focus of local and national attention. In less unique situations, such positive effects on residents might not occur. To check generalizability, Lawton and Cohen (1974) studied five projects selected for diversity. they found favorable effects in housing satisfaction, involvement in activities, satisfaction with the status quo, and perceived change for the better. This and other studies confirmed the capacity of older persons to adapt, but they shared the limitation of environmental assessments based on subjective judgments. Tenant evaluations are open to a variety of biases, staff have their own, and even outside observers view the world through personal preconceptions. To understand the person-environment relationship and to improve environmental design, it is desirable to have objective measures of environmental attributes.

A National Sample of Federally Assisted Housing

Lawton and Nahemow (1979) added objective measures of the environment to tenant, administrator, and observer judgments in a test of the utility of traditional behavioral science methods in assessing the impact of design features. Their national sample of 3,654 elderly tenants of 154 sites in 22 states was representative of all tenants, housing sites, and geographic locations of federally assisted housing.

Sponsorship (public housing vs. FHA Section 202, nonprofit-sponsored low rent housing) and size of the community as well as length of residence, age, marital status, gender, race, and health of tenants were partialed out. Objectively measured characteristics that accounted for significant additional variance in one or more of three tenant well-being criteria were kitchen size, cabinet space, kitchen counter space, closet space, carpeted halls (high rise), private balcony (high rise) or yard (low rise), electric stove, heat control in unit, shower or tub plus shower, and good lobby/hall lighting (high rise).

To obtain these design-relevant results, collection of objective data was costly and statistical analysis "an extremely untidy process" (Lawton & Nahemow, 1979, p. 8). The investigators recommended alternatives—observation of tenants' use of special design features and open-ended discussions with tenants—without quantification or statistical analysis.

Human Factors Approaches

"Adaptable housing" is Steinfeld's (1987) model: Anthropometric tolerances of older persons should determine housing design. Using flexible, full-scale mockups, which allowed a variety of arrangements and configurations, to examine a range of design solutions, persons with various limitations simulated tasks of everyday living. Goal-oriented task performance often exceeded traditional anthropometric measurements, and Steinfeld recommends use of the former. Results are specific design suggestions at various cost levels.

Czaja, Weber, and Nair (1993) used task analysis to break down activities of daily living into subtasks and each subtask into actions and compared task demands with personal capabilities. Using videotapes, 25 tasks (e.g., meal preparation, grocery shopping, laundry) were decomposed into actions, postures, grips, products, and locations. Objective environmental measures yielded estimates of performance demands. An example of the findings: In kitchens, high shelves average 73 inches and middle shelves, 65 inches, with shelves 12 inches deep. The average overreach of older women is 68 inches. There is need for expanded human factors task analysis of this type to promote a better engineering response to environmental design for older persons.

Retirement Communities

Retirement communities for the more affluent became an industry after World War II, particularly in Florida, California, and Nevada (Baldwin, 1984). Current studies tend to be designed as marketing research for developers of specific retirement communities.

ASSESSMENTS IN INSTITUTIONS

Following closely and overlapping with the burst of studies in special housing came environmental assessments in institutions.

Some Congruence Models

For Kahana, Liang, and Felton (1980) the optimal environment is that in which congruence between a person's needs and the environment's supplies is maximal. Measures of congruence were discrepancies between patient preference and staff ratings on five aspects of nursing homes considered relevant to patient well-being: segregate, congregate, institutional control, affect display, and impulse control. Resident preferences and staff ratings entered regressions before congruence scores, which had three variants: nondirectional incongruencies (effects of over- and undersupply are the same), and two one-directional incongruencies (oversupply and undersupply). Two nondirectional difference scores accounted for an increment of 8% in morale; oversupply along two dimensions and undersupply along three explained 10%. Contrary to prediction, incongruence on the congregate dimension was positively related to morale. Results were clearest in the most institutional settings, suggesting that the model and/or dimensions may be relevant primarily to them. A problematic issue is whether staff ratings reflect the environment as experienced by the resident.

Kiyak (1978) chose three different dimensions: physical privacy, isolation, and social solitude. She defined congruence as the difference between resident preferences and resident ratings of the nursing home. Congruence so defined made a significant contribution beyond that of preferences and ratings for amount of physical privacy and isolation. Kiyak's definition of congruence avoids the criticism that staff ratings do not reflect the environment as experienced by the patient, but it compounds the statistically problematic nature of the difference score by obtaining both components from the same source.

The findings from Kahana's study were not replicated in Veterans Administration domiciliaries and other care facilities studied by Nehrke et al. (1981). On the basis of empirical clustering of items, they developed 15 dimensions: Responsive Health Care; Excitement and Continuity; Staff Support for Personal Autonomy; Institutional Support for Religiosity; Personal Privacy; Tolerance for Restlessness; Freedom of Choice; Lack of Respect from Staff; Social Stimulation; Homogeneity; Physical Barriers to Mobility and Interaction; Discontinuity; Resident Interaction Level; Change versus Sameness; and Aloofness of Residents. Congruence was, again, the discrepancy between patient preference and patient evaluation. Congruence scores contributed to resident well-being, beyond their contributions to component preference and evaluation scores. These scales share the same source of data criticism with Kahana et al.'s (1980) study. Prediction was best in the most institutional settings, suggesting limitation of applicability.

Therapeutic Environment Screening Scale (TESS)

A large proportion of institutionalized older persons are cognitively impaired (Van Nostrand, Miller, & Furner, 1993; Weisman, Calkins, & Sloane, in press), and there is consensus that the environment plays an important role in their care (Calkins, 1988; Coons, 1987; Hiatt, 1979; U.S. Congress, 1987). The physical environment is identified as a major factor (Hiatt, 1979; Teresi, Lawton, Ory, & Holmes, in press; U.S. Congress, 1992; Weisman et al., in press). The special care unit (SCU) for the cognitively impaired is a growing response in need of empirical assessment

(Ohta & Ohta, 1988). Gold, Sloane, Mathew, Bledsoe, and Konanc (1991) decided, "What is needed now is an evaluation of multiple care settings for Alzheimer's patients, some of which are SCUs and some of which are more traditional nursing home units" (pp. 467–468). The environmental docility hypothesis was the conceptual basis of Lawton and Simon's 1968 study: They assume that individuals with dementing illnesses respond more intensely to the environment than do their cognitively unimpaired peers, and, therefore, will benefit more from environmental improvements relevant to their dementia (e.g., better orienting cues, less confusion and distraction).

A 12-item Therapeutic Environment Screening Scale (TESS) was developed to assess the physical environment (Sloane & Mathew, 1990; Mathew & Sloane, 1991). The rationale for its development includes Lawton's (1982) docility hypothesis plus Hiatt's (1979) distinction of four environments (social, psychological, cultural, and physical), with Hiatt's caveat that "only the physical environment affects the individual 24 hours a day" (Sloane & Mathew, 1990, p. 22). Comparison of 31 SCUs with 32 matched comparison units in integrated facilities found significant differences in 5 of the 12 items; homelike aspects, amount of personal items, access to an enclosed outdoor area, kitchen appliances for resident use, and non-use of television in the public area. The difference on a composite score using all items was significant. The results encouraged further scale development.

The study that used the TESS (Gold et al., 1991; Sloane & Mathew, 1991) showed advantages for the demented in SCUs over traditional units; for example, there was less use of physical restraint in SCUs (Coons, 1991). However, there may be problems with the TESS and with the study design. The TESS item, patient use of television, is questionable as a descriptor of the physical environment. Other TESS items that showed significant differences between features of the physical environments in SCUs versus usual units may be questioned in terms of their special relevance to dementia: SCUs had more homelike atmospheres, patients were allowed to have more personal items, there was greater access to sheltered outdoor areas and more availability of kitchen equipment for patient use. Do these items fit the usual desiderata for physical environments specific to the demented? To Sloane, the purpose of the TESS is "to evaluate the appropriateness of the physical environment for persons with dementia," and "In sum, including elements that may work for the nondemented does not represent a design flaw" (Sloane, personal communication, February 1994).

The study had variance on the environment side (SCUs vs. usual) but none on the person side (all were demented); it does not address the issue of whether nondemented patients might benefit as much or more from features of SCUs, not only in the TESS items and other differences in physical settings that minimize distracting and conflicting stimuli (Calkins, 1988; Hall, Kirschling, & Todd, 1986; U.S. Congress, 1987), but also from more intensive staffing (Weisman, Calkins, & Sloane, in press) by staff with special training (Coleman, Barbaccia, & Crouchton-Minihane, 1990; Coons, 1987; Maas, 1988), more individuation of activities

(Grossman, Weiner, Salamon, & Burros, 1986), more work with families (Ackerman, 1985; Hansen, Patterson, & Wilson, 1988), smaller size and newer construction (Mathew & Sloane, 1991), more selective admission criteria, fewer patients, and more private rooms (Sloane, Mathew, Desai, Weissert, & Scarborough, 1990). The study demonstrated that demented patients in SCUs fared better than demented patients in traditional units; it leaves open the question of whether SCUs are simply better nursing home units. If it becomes policy to admit the demented to SCUs and the nondemented to traditional units, questions of equity and fairness may arise. Already families are weighing the stigma of an Alzheimer's diagnosis against the better care that label is likely to procure.

Moreover, design of research in this area must take into account the many SCU-versus-usual differences that may confound results of studies on any one difference. For example, to assess the role of differences in physical environments, nonphysical aspects of the environment must be controlled to insure against attributing to the physical environment the effects of other variables. Gold et al. (1991) acknowledged the limitations of their design: "It is possible that more money is channelled into SCUs than into control units; therefore differences may be based primarily on financial abilities and considerations" (p. 475). Due to stricter admission criteria in many SCUs, they noted, "It would be important in future research to carefully control the composition of patients" (p. 475).

Teresi, Holmes, and Monaco (1993) noted that one goal of SCUs is to enhance the quality of life for residents who are not demented and studied that effect. In integrated units of four long-term care facilities, they studied the impact on cognitively intact residents of living with or adjacent to demented persons. They concluded that "facilities placing cognitively impaired persons with nonimpaired persons may be putting the nonimpaired persons at risk in terms of poor quality of life as measured by dissatisfaction with life and the environment and possible 'excess' demoralization" (pp. 357–358). However, there is "an important caveat," the impossibility of controlling possible bias due to staff decisions regarding placement. The reality of such a bias is suggested by the fact that cognitively intact residents placed next to demented residents tended to be those with fewer kin contacts and in poorer health, which "may indicate that noncognitively impaired residents assigned cognitively impaired roommates are weaker advocates for themselves by virtue of their own physical frailty and by lack of relatives who could act as intermediaries" (p. 357).

When the National Institute on Aging (NIA) Collaborative Studies on Special Care Units for Alzheimer's Disease was funded, Philip Sloane, Department of Family Medicine, The University of North Carolina, had TESS 2 still under development. Revisions were made by Sloane, Gerald Weisman and Maggie Calkins, special consultants, School of Architecture and Urban Planning, University of Wisconsin, and by NIA Steering Committee members, Jeanne Teresi, Mildred Ramiriz, and others; to produce TESS-2+ for the NIA studies (draft manual written by Calkins & Weisman, 1992). TESS-2+ is the most detailed and comprehensive protocol for assessing environments of people with dementia on which data are currently being collected. It may still be too coarse-grained, and its psychometric properties are as yet unknown. "TESS-2+ is best suited to assessing physical environments as potential co-variates in studies which are looking at something else" (Calkins, personal communication, August 1993). Results of the NIA studies should yield additional information on TESS-2+.

The completed TESS 2 (Sloane, unpublished data) includes not only an Environmental Checklist but also an Administrative Questionnaire (which includes issues such as physical plant, administration and personnel) and a Resident and Staff Observation Checklist (a measure of the process of care that is being used by three of the NIA studies). "The concept behind three instruments is to capture physical, administrative, and programmatic (interpersonal) aspects of the environment" (personal communication, 1994, February). Sloane intends to evaluate the instrument package during the next year.

Multiphasic Environmental Assessment Procedure (MEAP)

The MEAP (Moos & Lemke, 1984, in press) is based on a model of residential facilities as dynamic systems with four domains: resident and staff characteristics, physical features, policies and services, and social climate. The assessment involves five scales. The standardization sample for the 1992 revision was 262 community facilities (135 nursing homes, 60 residential care facilities, 67 congregate apartments) and 81 veterans' facilities (24 domiciliaries and 57 nursing homes) in various regions of the nation. Reliabilities (α, test-retest) and validities (construct, criterion) are generally good.

Together, the five instruments give a comprehensive view of a facility. They enable monitoring of change, comparing of facilities and comparing an existing situation with the ideal of residents, owner, staff, or others. Subscales can be combined for eight indices of quality: Staff Resources, Staffing Level, Physical Comfort, Security, Autonomy, Services, Rapport, and Control (Lemke & Moos, 1986). Instruments can be used separately (e.g., an architect may be interested only in Physical Features).

The MEAP is applicable in a range of supportive facilities from nursing homes to congregate housing with services, and the procedure may be adaptable to the environments of independently living elderly in congregate settings (Scheidt, in press).

ASSESSMENT IN THE COMMUNITY

Housing

Not until the late 1970s did attention turn to the environments occupied by most older persons (Montgomery, Stubbs, & Day, 1980; Struyk, 1977). The Annual

Housing Survey (AHS) (Office of Policy Development and Research, 1980) begun in 1976 by the Department of Housing (HUD) and the Census Bureau, provides national sample data for many studies. Lawton (1981) used a single-item approach to cross-tabulate housing deficiencies (e.g., exposed wiring) with marital status for older persons who were married, living alone, or who lived in households with 2 or more persons. Married couples and people living with younger family had better housing. The housing of older persons living alone was worse; and housing of men living alone, worst.

HUD set standards for housing adequacy based on six types of amenities: plumbing, kitchen, structure, common areas, heating, and electrical (Simonson, 1981). For relevance to intervention, Struyk and Turner (1984) divided items into Structural Adequacy and Maintenance Adequacy. Structural Adequacy accounted for 4.7% to 6.1%, and Maintenance Adequacy for 2.2% to 8.4% of the variance in housing satisfaction, with personal variables controlled. However, scores are dichotomous and therefore insensitive to possible important variations within the *adequate* and *inadequate* categories.

Standard scaling procedures were applied to the Struyk and Soldo (1980) categories to increase sensitivity by developing measures with multiple scale points and to eliminate noncontributing items (Christensen, Carp, Cranz, & Wiley, 1992). Scaling was done on data not used in the main analyses. Original and revised measures were compared as predictors of housing satisfaction, using 4,534 cases in the 1978 Annual Housing Survey Core and Supplement File for which the household head was over 75, and for which there were criterion data in the 1983 AHS Supplement, allowing prediction across 5 years.

Analyses were performed for household heads over 80 ($N = 2{,}165$) and replicated for those 75–79 ($N = 2{,}369$). Controls were personal characteristics plus household composition and housing cost/income (Baer, 1976). Analyses were performed separately for owners and renters, who differ in reporting housing problems (Newman & Struyk, 1983, 1984) and in the amount of variance in housing satisfaction explained by physical housing attributes (O'Bryant & Wolf, 1983).

The revised assessments were significantly superior as predictors of housing satisfaction. The new Structural Adequacy Scale explained from 4.8% to 9.6% of additional variance; and the revised Maintenance Quality Scale, 5.8% to 18.5%. Variance contributions of the new scales are not large. However, they represent cross-validated predictions across 5 years, using easily obtainable data. Advantages of psychometric scaling are apparent in the improved predictive power. Moreover, it is wasteful to continue collecting data on items to which over 99% of people give the same answer.

Assessing Neighborhoods

Studies on the importance of neighborhood disagree. One criticism of this research is its usual focus on the global concept of neighborhood. Defining the dimensions of neighborhood quality might clarify the situation. Using large sample data ($N1$ = 1,520, $N2$ = 1,021) Carp and Carp (1982a) developed scales that are reliable (Cronbach's α) and cross-validated on 11 dimensions of neighborhood quality as perceived by residents (perceived environmental quality indices, or PEQIs): Safety, Accessibility, Air Quality, Privacy, City Maintenance, Neighbors' Maintenance, Neighbors' Characteristics, Noise Disturbing Activities in Home, Noise Disturbing Outdoor Activities, Noise From Traffic and Industry, and Noise From Neighbors.

These scales were developed on a full adult age range, and are age-unbiased in the sense that the underlying factor structure was shown to be the same for six age groups from 18 through 70+. This is an advantage in testing hypotheses regarding older people. For example, the much touted tendency of the old to give "rosy" answers was confirmed—but, importantly, it was a linear trend throughout adulthood, not a difference between old and young. This questions whether the rosy response is particular to old age, and requires new explanations of this response tendency.

Independent of respondents, objective (technical) environmental measures were taken in their neighborhoods to see whether objective features account for significant variance in residents' perceptions of their neighborhood and in their overall well-being (Carp & Carp, 1982b). Measures were taken from U.S. Geological Survey (USGS) maps to which other information was added. USGS maps include elevation relative to sea level and locations of railroads, highways, freeways, and arterial roads. Routes and stations of the rapid-transit system were added, as were land use and population data from the U.S. Census, and the location of the resident of each respondent. Distances from respondents' homes were measured with engineering rulers. To count the number of items within a given distance of a home, plastic overlays were used. Nine factors were derived and cross-validated from the 21 measures of the physical environment and the eight descriptors of the population surround. To test the contribution of these technical environmental assessment indices (TEAIs) to residents' perceptions (PEQIs) and well-being (Carp & Carp, 1982b), nine factors that included Residents' Backgrounds, Environmental Attitudes, and Age and Sex were partialed out. TEAIs made significant additional contributions to variance in all PEQIs and both well-being indices. Interestingly, TEAIs and person factors made complementary rather than duplicative contributions.

La Gory, Ward, and Sherman (1985) explored objective environmental conditions, subjective definitions, and the person's environmental docility (Lawton & Simon, 1968) as determinants of neighborhood satisfaction. Objective data were from the Census. Likert-type items measured perceptions of neighborhood safety, convenience, maintenance, and the kind of people seen as living in one's area. Two aspects of environmental docility were tapped: ability to receive and respond to environmental stimuli (health and mastery) and ability to change environments (view of ability to move to another residence). Respondents were 11,185 persons over 60. All three general factors were significant contributors to satisfaction, with "mental portraits" (perceptions) most potent. The investigators concluded that the "ecological actor" should become a basic theoretical and empirical unit of analysis, and that survey research should be superseded by intensive interviews with selected subgroups of older persons.

The Ideal Neighborhood

Adults aged 25 and older rated the importance of 15 environmental characteristics as if they "were looking for another place to live" (Carp & Carp, 1982c). Using an exploratory-confirmatory approach ($N1 = 1{,}218$, $N2 = 815$), three factors were extracted and cross-validated: Access to Services and Facilities, Relationships to Others, and Esthetics. In regard to Access to Services and Facilities, there are highly significant age trends in regard to school and work. Not surprisingly, access to both is very important to younger adults, but not to older persons. Esthetics shows no age difference. General attractiveness, cleanliness, lack of litter, quietness, nice landscaping, and minimal air pollution are "very important" to the majority at all ages. Assessment across age clarifies understanding by documenting consistencies as well as differences between age groups.

Proximity to services, facilities, and other people seem favorable neighborhood characteristics. The importance of proximity has been emphasized particularly with regard to service utilization (Lawton, 1980). However, there are negative trade-offs. Older women living alone (vulnerable to neighborhood conditions) described the ideal in terms of 37 services and amenities (Carp & Carp, 1982c). The respondent chose whether she would have each within walking distance, farther away, it did not matter, or she did not know. The task was repeated for "within a block of home."

Provision of the response option *don't care* as well as *don't know* was informative. Few respondents didn't know, but many found irrelevant the location of such facilities as a dentist, doctor, lawyer, bank, beauty shop, church or synagogue, H&R Block office, etc., other than their own. Response options of both inclusion and exclusion clarified the negative concomitant aspects of proximity. Despite high fear of crime, 73% would not have a police station within a block because of the concomitant noise, "type of people," and detriment to esthetic quality. Results were similar for a fire station. Proximity to senior centers and nutrition sites had positive valences of needed services, activities and sociability but negative valences with regard to the appearance of such facilities and their attraction of "a lot of (poor) old people." Senior facilities should be within walking distance, but not on one's block. Generalization from the study is limited by including data only on older women living alone.

Assessment of Community Housing and Neighborhood

Jirovec, Jirovec, and Bossé (1985) studied only men. They, too, speculated that contradictory findings regarding the impact of nearness of goods and services on neighborhood satisfaction may reflect a trade-off: access to needed facilities versus undesirable concomitants. They studied both housing and neighborhood conditions as correlates of residential satisfaction, which proved to be largely a function of the latter. Neighborhood beauty, safety, interest level, and quietness were significantly related to residential satisfaction when controls for demographic, family, and personal variables were used. The investigators advise studying both housing and neighborhood environment as determinants of residential satisfaction because of the relationships between characteristics of the two and the trade-off involved.

According to our complementary/congruence model (Carp & Carp, 1984), residential satisfaction and psychological well-being depend upon the extent to which the environment (physical and personal) meets residents' demands and provides the supplies for human needs in the home and in the neighborhood. Following Murray (1938), these can be divided into life-maintenance or viscerogenic (Nutrition, Sleep/Rest, Personal Hygiene, Laundry, Housecleaning) and higher-order or psychogenic (Harm avoidance, Avoidance of unpleasantness, Order, Affiliation, Privacy, Esthetics), with Self-Others Similarity an additional neighborhood factor. Life-maintenance needs are universal; outcomes should be determined by the degree of complementarity between the person's competence and the environment's provision for meeting basic needs through the activities of daily living (Lawton's docility hypothesis). In regard to higher order needs, individual differences are salient: Outcomes depend upon the degree of congruence between the strength of the psychogenic need and the resources of the environment for meeting it. Modifiers that may affect relationships of predictors to outcomes and increase the amount of variance accounted for in outcomes include Locus of Control, Coping Style, Social Supports, Status Resources (e.g., income, education) and Life Events.

Valid and reliable multi-item measures were selected or developed for all components. Separate environmental assessment scales were based on three data sources: respondent evaluations, observer ratings, and technical measures. For the last, an environmental protocol was developed, field tested, and revised until satisfactory in terms of interrecorder reliability within items and Cronbach's α among items in a scale (TEAI). For homes, the protocol includes such data as area measures of rooms, areas and heights of workspaces, volumes of storage spaces at various heights, instrumental readings of light and sound, and inventories of appliances and fixtures. For neighborhoods, the census provided data on land use, population characteristics, and housing conditions; the health department provided data on mortality and morbidity; and the police department provided data on crime rates. Environmental data were coded on maps, and measures were taken with rulers and plastic overlays.

Funds for a pilot study limited sample size and the number of variables. Older women living alone were selected because of their prevalence and environmental vulnerability. Predictors were TEAIs relevant to viscerogenic and psychogenic needs in homes and neighborhoods. Outcomes were Housing Satisfaction, Neighborhood Satisfaction and Well-Being (Carp & Carp, 1983). Other variables were Personal Competence, which represents 12 measures (e.g., cognition, range-of-motion) and Status Resources, which represents 18 items.

Lawton's docility hypothesis is probably the most often cited and influential concept in the area of environmental assessment. Therefore, considerable effort was expended to demonstrate some sort of interaction between personal competence and environmental resource, at either overall score or component level, in affecting any outcome. No such effect was observed. TEAIs and competence measures had good response distributions and alphas. Competence components were standard measures in general use with established psychometric respectability. Environmental docility did not apply to persons capable of living alone in the community.

Remaining funds did not allow testing effects of congruence between strength of psychogenic needs and quality of relevant environmental resources. Predictors were TEAIs relevant to viscerogenic and psychogenic needs in home and neighborhoods. Personal Competence and Status Resources entered equations first. They accounted for 10% of variance in Housing Satisfaction, 5% of variance in Neighborhood Satisfaction, 17% of variance in one index of Well-Being (depression), and 21% in the other (Contentment). TEAIs accounted for an additional 30% of Housing Satisfaction (for a total of 40%), an additional 28% of Neighborhood Satisfaction (for a total of 33%), an additional 26% in one index of Well-Being (for a total of 43%), and an additional 17% in the other (for a total of 38%; Carp & Christensen, 1986a, 1986b).

Recent analyses tested the theoretical assumption regarding psychogenic needs (Carp, forthcoming). For higher order needs, predictors were congruences between respondent need scores and relevant TEAIs. Personal Competence and Status Resources entered equations first. Predictors accounted for 41% of additional variance in Housing Satisfaction (for a total of 51%), 42% in Neighborhood Satisfaction (for a total of 47%), and 34% (for a total of 51%) and 29% (for a total of 50%) in Well-Being.

This is a sound battery of environmental, personal, mediating, and outcome measures, carefully developed and scaled on the basis of existing instruments and using large ad hoc samples. Analyses of pilot data suggest its utility to test the theoretical model for which it was developed and demonstrate the ability of parts of the model to account for meaningful proportions of variance in residential satisfaction and well-being. The power of the environmental assessments in combination with all other variables in the model has not been tested. The hypothesis that level of personal competence determines the role of environmental docility cannot be tested without data on this battery from persons incapable of living alone in the community. The predicted roles of resident and observer and technical assessments of home and neighborhood have not been investigated. Cost is the obstacle to adequate testing of this environmental assessment paradigm. A large sample is needed. Collection of technical environmental data consumes several hours at each home and neighborhood. Several interviews are necessary to obtain background, mediator, competence, needs, and outcome data. The limitation of pilot study data to women living alone limits generalizability of the results that were obtained. (However, limitation to women alone and small sample size were not present in scale development.)

A series of studies (Scheidt, 1984; Scheidt & Windley, 1982, 1983, 1987; Windley & Scheidt, 1982, 1985, 1988) sought to develop a taxonomy of sociological and psychological dimensions of small towns and environmental measures of the dimensions (based on first- and second-order factor analysis of data from standardized instruments and traditional questionnaires) to predict housing and neighborhood satisfaction and psychological well-being, using standard statistical procedures. Now Scheidt is using the concept of "community covenant" (Schroeder, 1980) and an "experiential field approach" for insights into ways to sustain residents of small towns experiencing drastic changes in their physical, social, and cultural environments (Norris-Baker & Scheidt, 1990, 1991; Scheidt & Norris-Baker, 1990). Qualitative assessment is the goal, and case study is the method: open-ended conversations with a dozen older residents, additional structured but informal conversations, observations in selected behavior settings, tours with residents, archival research on the community, and photo-documentation.

Programs for Home Modification and Repair

Programs for home modification and repair to enable persons to remain at home proliferate. Pynoos, Overton, Liebig, & Calvert (in press) studied 300 programs nominated by area agencies on aging, state units on aging, and departments of rehabilitation. They found environmental assessment to be a weak link in in-home services. Assessors tend to look only at aspects of the environment for which their programs are responsible (e.g., weatherization). Many programs look only at the home, with no functional assessment of the resident. Case managers, social workers, and nurses may not be adept at environmental assessment. Coordination among programs is poor. When client payment plays a role, residents are often involved in assessment, but they tend to underreport deficiencies. Occupational therapists, who are best trained to analyze person-environment interactions, are rarely used. There is need for standard assessment procedures, coordination among programs, and attraction of the private sector into participation.

One home assessment of Pynoos and Cohen (1992a) presents a checklist guide for a tour of one's home, specifying hazards for special areas (entry, kitchen, bathroom, bedroom, all living areas) plus general concerns (fire safety, fall prevention, security, cleaning, dressing). The resident marks each item "yes" or "no," then sets priorities among "yeses." The second chapter suggests solutions to each problem by environmental and/or behavioral alteration. Finally, a resource guide gives names and addresses of organizations and publications and suggests types of local stores that may be helpful in solving particular problems. Older homeowners tend not to report needed repairs (Chen & Newman, 1987). Some questions that are intended to evoke environmental evaluations are worded "Can you . . .?" They focus the respondent's attention on his or her own personal competence and tend to evoke defensive responses that minimize the environmental problem (Carp & Carp, 1981). However, for mentally, physically, and financially competent persons, the Pynoos and Cohen home safety guide seems useful.

Another Pynoos and Cohen publication (1992b) takes the reader on an imaginary tour of six houses and apartments with a volunteer at an agency that helps older persons make their homes more livable. Readers help the character identify problems and recommend solutions that might apply to their own homes. Problems and solutions are presented in cartoons; there are games, puzzles, a quiz on myths and realities about the home; a list of sources of products, information, and funding; and tips on how to find reliable repair persons.

In the private sector Enhancements Adapting Senior Environments (EASE) program, a physical therapist performs a functional assessment of the person and an environmental assessment of the home using a checklist (Christenson, private publication). The information is integrated by computer into a room-by-room plan of adaptation. Recommendations are accompanied by names of product and service suppliers and a toll-free phone number for additional information or to place orders is listed.

A conference of experts convened by the American Association of Retired Persons (1993), focused on the question of life span design of residential environments for a population that is aging: How to design new and retrofit old housing to promote independence as strengths and capacities change over the years of longer living. They concluded that features older persons need (e.g., grab bars) are also beneficial for others, and that original design should incorporate provisions for easy modifications.

CONCLUDING REMARKS

After a volatile rise and expansion, environmental assessment hit the doldrums in the past 5 years. During the period of special interest for this volume, publication in scientific journals decreased and the tenor of work altered. Tests of theoretically derived hypotheses diminished. Practical efforts such as guidelines for professional interventions and self-help guides for the elderly to improve their own environments grew.

From its inception, environmental assessment was directed by the search for solutions to human problems. Early investigators tested concepts from theory systems in their disciplines that seemed relevant to gerontological problems (e.g., housing the elderly) and devised measures for such testing, using current statistical methods. Lately, work aims more directly at solutions to problems (e.g., changes in small towns, housing maintenance) using less formal methodologies.

Lawton and Nahemow (1979) purposefully studied the utility of traditional behavioral science methodology to this field. They documented significant effects of objective environmental assessments, but, in view of the effort of data collection and the complexity of analysis, they recommended less arduous and costly alternatives that avoid quantification or statistical analysis. After completing a study with traditional methodology, La Gory et al. (1985) concluded that the ecological actor should become the focus of attention and that the methodology should be interviews. After years of work to develop an environmental taxonomy and valid, reliable measures to make it operational using sophisticated statistical analyses, Scheidt and Norris-Baker (1990) have turned to an experiential field approach to explore ameliorations of the rural crisis of the past decade for elderly residents of small towns.

Some investigators find environmental assessment with informal data and no statistics suited to their goals. Where this proves satisfactory, well and good. However, experience in other fields suggests that in many instances such approaches, necessary in early stages of investigating any new area, should be superseded by theory-directed research using measures and procedures that allow replication of studies, which increased both confidence in the findings and confidence in recommending interventions. Some investigators have left the field because they no longer felt they were "doing science."

Cost may be a major deterrent to statistically rigorous studies. There were once funds for extensive scale and model development (Carp& Carp, 1984) but funds for an adequate test of this paradigm are unavailable.

Nevertheless, the soundest way toward solution of some practical problems may be through research based in theory and using refined measures. There is now available a repertoire of environmental assessment procedures. Many protocols have not been published in full in the literature (e.g., MEAP, TESS-2+, TESS 2, PEQIs, TEAIs), but they are available commercially or from their developers. Use of existing instruments saves work and guards against chance factors in one's data. Some of the following suggestions may assist in selection or development of environmental measures and their use in research.

Environmental variables must be relevant to people, for example, to their competence and/or needs. The study purpose, theory, and previous research provide guidance in the selection of variables. Environments are assessed through various sources: resident evaluations, observer judgments, and technical measures. Each has a different role. Only residents can report on a home as it affects them, but they often give sanguine ratings and understate deficiencies. Observers' ratings avoid some resident response biases, but they cannot reflect the 24-hour-a-day experience of residents, and as outsiders they observe through their own preconceptions regarding qualities of homes and neighborhoods. Neither residents' nor observers' evaluations are technical enough to provide information requisite to alter the environment. For example, assessing and ameliorating neighborhood noise require data in terms of sound levels, and in the location of sources of noise and the possibility of sound baffling elements such as intervening walls or land barriers (Carp & Carp, 1982b).

Differences among resident, observer, and technical assessments can be enlightening. In nursing homes, tenant versus staff rating differences should alert management. In communities, strategies to ameliorate the situation of older persons trapped at home due to fear of crime on the streets may be developed by comparing scores of residents with technical assessments such as one TEAI Harmavoidance item, Safety from Crime in the Neighborhood (Carp & Carp, 1982b).

Question and answer format is important. Environmental assessments may be confounded with respondent competence and/or defensiveness if questions are worded, "How well can *you* . . .?" when the aim is to assess the living unit. Some environmental components have both positive and negative valences, and response options should allow expression of the trade-off.

The sample of environments and persons for data collection must be appropriate to the study purpose, theory base, and number of variables in analyses. One pitfall of gerontological assessment is attribution of a reaction to old people because it was discovered there. The rosy response bias in evaluating living environments is an example. Incorrect attribution to old age can be avoided by studying wider age ranges and by developing environmental assessment scales that are "age unbiased" in the sense that intelligence tests have been revised to be "gender unbiased" and "ethnicity unbiased."

Data analysis must avoid attributing to the environment what are actually effects of other variables. However, environmental and personal effects may be complementary rather than redundant, and person-environment relationships are important. If the goal is to understand the determinants of residential satisfaction or overall well-being, analyses should derive from a theoretical formulation of direct, indirect, and interactive effects of environmental and personal variables upon outcomes. The goal in determining what contributes to residential satisfaction or well-being is not only to improve theoretical constructs but also to provide sound rationales for programs to improve the living environments of older persons.

REFERENCES

Ackerman, J. O. (1985). Separated, not isolated—As BASIC as administration, backing, and commitment. *The Journal of Long-Term Care Administration, Fall*, 90–94.

American Association of Retired Persons. (1993). *Life-span design of residential environments for an aging population*. Washington, DC: Author.

Baer, W. C. (1976). The evaluation of housing indicators and housing standards. *Public Policy, 24*, 361–393.

Baldwin, L. E. (1984). Retirement communities. In L. Hubbard (Ed.), *Housing options for older Americans*. Washington, DC: American Association of Retired Persons.

Calkins, M. P. (1988). *Design for dementia: Planning environments for the elderly and confused.* Owings Mills, MD: National Health Publishing.

Calkins, M., & Weisman, J. (1992). National Institute on Aging collaborative studies: Special care units for Alzheimer's disease. Therapeutic Environmental Screening Scale (TESS-2+). Unit Observation Checklist: Physical Environment. Manual (Duplicated). School of Architecture and Urban Planning, University of Wisconsin-Milwaukee.

Carp, F. M. (1966). *A future for the aged: Victoria Plaza and its residents*. Austin: University of Texas Press.

Carp, F. M. (1978). Effects of the living environment on activity and use of time. *International Journal of Aging and Human Development, 9*, 75–91.

Carp, F. M. (forthcoming). *Person-environment congruence for psychogenic needs: Effects of residential satisfaction and well-being.*

Carp, F. M., & Carp. A., (1980). Person-environment congruence and sociability. *Research on Aging, 2*, 395–415.

Carp, F. M., & Carp, A. (1981). It may not be the answer, it may be the question. *Research on Aging, 3*, 85–100.

Carp, F. M., & Carp, A. (1982a). Perceived environmental quality of neighborhoods: Development of assessment scales and their relation to age and gender. *Journal of Environmental Psychology, 2*, 295–312.

Carp, F. M., & Carp, A. (1982b). A role for technical environmental assessment in perception of environmental quality and well-being. *Journal of Environmental Psychology, 2*, 171–191.

Carp, F. M., & Carp, A. (1982c). The ideal residential area. *Research on Aging, 4*, 411–439.

Carp, F. M., & Carp, A. (1984). A complementary/congruence model of well-being or mental health for the community elderly. In I. Altman, M. P. Lawton, & J. F. Wohlwill (Eds.), *Elderly people and the environment* (pp. 279–336). New York: Plenum.

Carp, F. M., & Christensen, D. L. (1986a). Technical environmental assessment predictors of residential satisfaction. *Research on Aging, 8*, 269–287.

Carp, F. M., & Christensen, D. L. (1986b). Older women living alone: Technical environmental assessment of psychological well-being. *Research on Aging, 8*, 407–425.

Chen, A., & Newman, S. J. (1987). Validity of older homeowners' housing evaluations. *The Gerontologist, 27*, 309–313.

Christensen, D. L., Carp, F. M., Cranz, G. L., & Wiley, J. A. (1992). Objective housing indicators as predictors of the subjective evaluations of elderly residents. *Journal of Environmental Psychology, 12*, 225–236.

Christenson, M. A. *Lifease*. (Available from author, 2550 University Avenue West, Suite 225, North Court International, Saint Paul, Minnesota 55114)

Coleman, E. A., Barbaccia, J. D., & Croughan-Minihane, M. S. (1990). Hospitalization rates in nursing home residents with dementia. *Journal of the American Geriatrics Society, 38*, 108–112.

Coons, D. H. (1987). *Designing a residential care unit for persons with dementia*. Washington, DC: U.S. Congress, Office of Technology Assessment.

Coons, D. H. (1991). Foreword. In P. E. Sloane & L. J. Mathews, *Dementia units in long-term care* (pp. xi–xii). Baltimore, MD: Johns Hopkins Press.

Czaja, S. J., Weber, R. A., & Nair, S. N. (1993). A human factors analysis of ADL activities: A capacity-demand approach. *Journals of Gerontology: Psychological Sciences, 48*(Special Issue), 44–48.

Gold, D. T., Sloane, P. D., Mathew, L. J., Bledsoe, M. M., & Konanc, D. A. (1991). Special care units: A typology of care settings for memory-impaired older adults. *The Gerontologist, 31*, 467–475.

Grossman, H. D., Weiner, A. S., Salamon, M. J., & Burros, N. (1986). The milieu standard for care of dementia in a nursing home. *Journal of Gerontological Social Work, 9*, 73–89.

Hall, G., Kirschling, M., & Todd, S. (1986, May/June). Sheltered freedom: An Alzheimer's unit in an ICF. *Geriatric Nursing*, 132–137.

Hansen, S., Patterson, M., & Wilson, R. (1988). Family involvement on a dementia unit: The resident enrichment and activity program. *The Gerontologist, 28*, 508–510.

Hiatt, L. (1979, Sept./Oct.). The importance of the physical environment. *Nursing Homes*, 2–10.

Jirovec, R. L., Jirovec, M. M., Bossé, R. (1985). Residential satisfaction as a function of micro and macro environmental conditions among urban elderly men. *Research on Aging, 7*, 601–616.

Kahana, E., Liang, J., & Felton, B. J. (1980). Alternative models of person-environment fit. *Journal of Gerontology, 35*, 584–595.

Kiyak, H. A. (1978). A multidimensional perspective on privacy preferences in institutionalized elderly. In W. E. Rogers & W. H. Ittelson (Eds.), *New directions in environmental design Research: Proceedings of the Ninth Annual Conference of the Environmental Design Research Association* (pp. 79–91). Tucson, AZ: University of Arizona Press.

La Gory, M., Ward, R., & Sherman, S. (1985). The ecology of aging: Neighborhood satisfaction in an older population. *Sociological Quarterly, 26*, 405–418.

Lawton, M. P. (1980). *Environment and aging*. Belmont, CA: Brooks/Cole.

Lawton, M. P. (1981). An ecological view of living arrangements. *The Gerontologist, 21*, 59–66.

Lawton, M. P. (1982). Competence, environmental press and the adaptation of older people. In M. P. Lawton, P. Windley, & T. Byerts (Eds.), *Aging and the environment* (pp. 33–59). New York: Springer.

Lawton, M. P., & Cohen, J. (1974). The generality of housing impact on the well-being of older people. *Journal of Gerontology, 29*, 194–204.

Lawton, M. P., & Nahemow, L. (1979) Social science methods for evaluating the quality of housing for the elderly. *Journal of Architectural Research, 7*, 5–11.

Lawton, M. P., & Simon, B. (1968). The ecology of social relationships in housing for the elderly. *The Gerontologist, 8*, 108–115.

Lemke, S., & Moos, R. H. (1986). Quality of residential settings for the elderly. *Journal of Gerontology, 41*, 268–276.

Maas, M. (1988). Management of patients with Alzheimer's disease in long-term care facilities. *Nursing Clinics of North America, 23*, 57–68.

Mathew, L. J., & Sloane, P. D. (1991). Environmental characteristics of existing dementia units. In P. D. Sloane, L. J. Mathew (Eds.), *Dementia units in long-term care*. Baltimore, MD: Johns Hopkins Press.

Montgomery, J. E., Stubbs, A. C., & Day, S. S. (1980). The housing environment of the rural elderly. *The Gerontologist, 20*, 444–451.

Moos, R. H., & Lemke, S. (1984). Supportive residential settings for older people. In I. Altman, M. P. Lawton, & J. F. Wohlwill (Eds.), *Elderly people and the environment* (pp. 159–190). New York: Plenum.

Moos, R. H., & Lemke, S. (in press). *Group living environments for older adults*. New York: Oxford University Press.

Murray, H. A. (1938). *Explorations in personality*. New York: Oxford University Press.

Nehrke, M. F., Turner, R. R., Cohen, S. H., Whitbourne, S. K., Morganti, J. B., & Hulicka, I. M. (1981). Toward a model of person-environment congruence. *Experimental Aging Research, 7*, 363–379.

Newman, S. J., & Struyk, R. J. (1983). Housing and poverty. *Review of Economics and Statistics, 65*, 243–253.

Newman, S. J., & Struyk, R. J. (1984). An alternative targeting strategy for housing assistance. *The Gerontologist, 24*, 584–592.

Norris-Baker, C., & Scheidt, R. J. (1990). Place attachment among older residents of a "ghost town": A transactional approach. In R. Selby, K. Anthony, J. Choi, & B. Orland (Eds.). *Coming of age*. Oklahoma City, OK: Environmental Design Research Association.

Norris-Baker, C., & Scheidt, R. J. (1991). A contextual approach to serving older residents of economically-threatened small towns. *Journal of Aging Studies, 5*, 333–346.

Norris-Baker, C., & Scheidt, R. J. (in press). Community covenants: An indicator of sustainable small town habitats? In E. Arias & M. Gross (Eds.), *Equitable and sustainable habitats*. Boulder, CO: Environmental Design Research Association.

O'Bryant, S. L., & Wolf, S. M. (1983). Explanations of housing satisfaction of older homeowners and renters. *Research on Aging, 5*, 217–233.

Office of Policy Development and Research. (1980). *Annual Housing Survey*. Washington, DC: Department of Housing and Urban Development.

Ohta, R., & Ohta, B. (1988). Special care units for Alzheimer's disease patients: A critical look. *The Gerontologist, 28*, 803–808.

Pynoos, J., & Cohen, E. (1992a). *Home safety guide for older people*. Washington, DC: Serif Press.

Pynoos, J., & Cohen, E. (1992b). *The perfect fit: Creative ideas for a safe and livable home*. Washington, DC: American Association of Retired Persons.

Pynoos, J., Overton, J., Liebig, P., & Calvert, E. (in press). The delivery of home modifications and repair services. In J. Hyde & S. Lanspery (Eds.), *Housing adaptations to meet changing needs: Research, policy and programs*. Amityville, NY: Baywood.

Scheidt, R. J. (1984). A taxonomy of well-being for small-town elderly: A case for rural diversity. *The Gerontologist, 24*, 84–90.

Scheidt, R. J. (in press). The social ecological approach of Rudolph Moos: Illustrative contributions to housing for the elderly. In P. G. Windley (Ed.), *Handbook on housing and the elderly*. Westport, CT: Greenwood.

Scheidt, R. J., & Norris-Baker, C. (1990). A transactional approach to environmental stress among older residents of rural communities. *Journal of Rural Community Psychology, 11*, 5–30.

Scheidt, R. J., & Windley, P. J. (1982). Well-being profiles of small-town elderly in differing rural contexts. *Community Mental Health Journal, 8*, 257–267.

Scheidt, R. J., Windley, P. J. (1983). The mental health of small-town rural elderly residents: An expanded ecological model. *Journal of Gerontology, 38*, 472–479.

Scheidt, R. J., & Windley, P. J. (1987). Environmental perceptions and patterns of well-being among older Americans in small rural towns. *Comprehensive Gerontology, 1*, 24–29.

Schroeder, F. (1980). Types of American small towns and how to read them. *Southern Quarterly, 19*, 104–135.

Simonson, J. (1981). *Measuring inadequate housing through the use of the Annual Housing Survey.* Washington, DC: U.S. Department of Housing and Urban Development.

Sloane, P. D. Unpublished manuscript, *The TESS 2.* The University of North Carolina at Chapel Hill, School of Medicine, Department of Family Medicine, Chapel Hill.

Sloane, P. D., & Mathew, L. J. (1990, November/December). The therapeutic environment screening scale. *The American Journal of Alzheimer's and Related Disorders Care & Research*, 22–26.

Sloane, P. D., & Mathew, L. J. (1991). *Dementia units in long-term care.* Baltimore, MD: Johns Hopkins Press.

Sloane, P. D., Mathew, L., Desai, J., Weissert, W., & Scarborough, M. (1990). *Specialized dementia units in nursing homes: A study of settings in five states.* Chapel Hill: University of North Carolina.

Steinfeld, E. (1987). Adapting housing for older disabled people. In V. Regnier & J. Pynoos (Eds.), *Housing the aged: Design directives and policy considerations.* New York: Elsevier.

Struyk, R. J. (1977). The housing situation of elderly Americans. *The Gerontologist, 17*, 130–139.

Struyk, R. J., & Soldo, B. J. (1980). *Improving the elderly's housing.* Cambridge, MA: Ballinger.

Struyk, R., & Turner, M. (1984). Changes in the housing situation of the elderly: 1974–79. *Journal of Housing for the Elderly, 2*, 3–20.

Teresi, J. A., Holmes, D., & Monaco, C. (1993). An evaluation of the effects of commingling cognitively and noncognitively impaired individuals in long-term care facilities. *The Gerontologist, 33*, 350–358.

Teresi, J., Lawton, M. P., Ory, M., & Holmes, D. (in press). Measurement issues in chronic care populations: Dementia special care. In D. Holmes, M. Ory, & J. Teresi (Eds.), *Special care units: New models of residential dementia care.* Supplement for *Alzheimer's Disease and Associated Disorders.*

Thompson, M. M. (1992). To the wild west and back again. In F. M. Carp (Ed.), *Lives of career women: Approaches to work, marriage, children* (pp. 71–83). New York: Plenum.

U.S. Congress, Office of Technology Assessment. (1987). *Losing a million minds: Confronting the tragedy of Alzheimer's disease and other dementias* (OTA-BA-323). Washington, DC: U.S. Government Printing Office.

U.S. Congress, Office of Technology Assessment. (1992). *Special care units for people with Alzheimer's and other dementias: Consumer education, research, regulatory, and reimbursement issues* (OTA-H-543). Washington, DC: U.S. Government Printing Office.

Van Nostrand, J. F., Miller, B., & Furner, S. E. (1993). Selected issues of long-term care: Profile of cognitive disability of nursing home residents and the use of informal and formal care by the elderly in the community. In J. F. Van Nostrand, S. E. Furner, & R. Suzman (Eds.), *Health data on older Americans: United States.* Hyattsville, MD: National Center for Health Statistics.

Weisman, G. D., Calkins, M., & Sloane, P. (in press). The environmental context of special care. In D. Holmes, M. Ory, & J. Teresi (Guest Editors), Special care units: New models of residential dementia care. Supplement for *Alzheimer's Disease and Associated Disorders.*

Windley, P. G., & Scheidt, R. J. (1983). Housing satisfaction among rural small-town elderly: A predictive model. *Journal of Housing for the Elderly, 12*, 57–68.

Windley, P. G., & Scheidt, R. J. (1985). Taxonomy and environment–aging interaction: A case for small town diversity. *Journal of Rural Studies, 1*, 297–305.

Windley, P. G., & Scheidt, R. J. (1988). Rural small towns: An environmental context for aging. *Journal of Rural Studies, 4*, 2, 151–158.

CHAPTER 15

Assessing Life Events Among Older Adults

ALEX J. ZAUTRA
DEPARTMENT OF PSYCHOLOGY
ARIZONA STATE UNIVERSITY, TEMPE

AND

GLENN AFFLECK

AND

HOWARD TENNEN
DEPARTMENT OF PSYCHIATRY
UNIVERSITY OF CONNECTICUT SCHOOL OF MEDICINE, FARMINGTON

INTRODUCTION

Why Assess Life Events in Older Adult Populations

Attitudes toward inquiry into the life events of older adults have progressed significantly from the time when one might hear, "Why study events of the aged? Not much change for them, anyway!" This observation is not entirely facetious; older adults as a group report fewer change-producing events on standard life event inventories than do young or middle-aged adults (Murrell, Norris, & Hutchins, 1984). To an extent this may reflect the fact that many items appearing in such inventories include events related to child rearing, employment, and changes in marital status, residence, and friendship patterns; elders do experience divorce, relocation and job loss, but these events are relatively uncommon. Divorce among individuals over 65, for example, occurs at a rate less than 0.2% annually, compared with a rate above 4% among those between 25 and 44 years of age (Hughes, Blazer, & George, 1988). As a result, the appearance of stability characteristics of elders' lives may be somewhat artificial. That is, fewer events among older adults may reflect the fact that commonly used life event inventories do not have sufficient coverage of those experiences that are, in fact, prevalent and influential for elders.

In our review of studies of life stress and the experience of aging more generally, we find four kinds of life experiences that commonly affect older adults (see Hughes, et al., 1988; Murrell, et al., 1984): (a) social losses through death or institutionalization of family and friends, (b) illness events, (c) changes in social roles, such as occur with retirement, becoming disabled, or becoming the caregiver for a disabled family member (Aneshensel, Pearlin, & Schuler, 1993), and (d) shifts in the patterns of everyday life events (Reich & Zautra, 1983). The first three categories fit, interestingly enough, Dohrenwend's (1979) definition of a pathogenic triad: those events that define the character of trauma experienced by soldiers in combat. The fourth category is based on the relatively recent appreciation for the importance of everyday events: The lives of both older adults and younger adults may be characterized not only by major upheavals but also by the patterns of daily life experience, the ebb and flow of smaller life events.

Most inquiries into life events have examined how those events affect emotional and physical well-being. Investigators conceptualize life events as stressors and seek to determine their relationship with such outcomes as depression and other forms of psychopathology and increased vulnerability to illness or injury. Although this rationale for the study of events is sound, it is unnecessarily limited. Events also can signify accomplishments, developmental milestones, and changes for the better in living conditions and family relations. Attention to the positive side of life events promises a more complete understanding of how the life experiences of older adults figure in their psychological well-being (Reich & Zautra, 1988). Furthermore, life event assessments are useful in themselves as ways of depicting the lives of older adults, and studying differences in life course trajectories (Danish, Smyer, & Nowak, 1980) for older adults of different social backgrounds, living conditions, and personality attributes. Similar to Szalai's (1972) interest in time budgets as a means of understanding differences in the quality of life among persons of different social standing, event assessments provide a means of gauging stability and change in the quality of life for different groups of older adults.

This chapter has three broad aims: to identify the most frequently used methods for assessing life events in elders, to examine major methodological problems associated with current assessment practices, and to highlight some of the most promising recent developments in life event assessment, including some that have yet to be applied to older populations. Our goal is to help the reader to evaluate measures and to effectively select instruments from the materials we review.

What Constitutes a Life Event?

Before beginning this review, it is necessary to define what constitutes a life event. This task is not as straightforward as it may appear. There is no universally accepted definition of a life event. The most common definition, taken from the seminal work of Holmes and Rahe (1967), is that a life event is any change in life style routine that prompts a need for adjustment. That change may be desirable or undesirable. Change is a vague criterion, however; events that elicit change can occur at all levels of human behavior, from the irritating changes in one's daily routine occasioned by a flat tire or the loss of a car key to the major social upheavals occurring with the end of Soviet Communism or the flooding of the Mississippi River.

In the past decade, researchers began investigating everyday events in addition to studying the effects of major life changes. Holmes and Holmes (1970) anticipated that the measurement of everyday stress would be useful as an accompaniment to their measures of major life changes. Indeed, this area of research into everyday life continues to show promise. Some interesting developments in this area are reviewed toward the end of this chapter.

There are fewer problems when the criterion of life routine alteration is applied to major events than when it is applied to minor events. When a death in the family occurs, some change can be assumed in survivor life style routine, although the amount of change will vary significantly from one family to the next. However, is "going to lunch with a friend" an event? This experience may or may not represent a change in routine, depending upon the person's frequency of dining out. Space consideration precludes any examination here of relative magnitudes of changes in routines as they may relate to the definition of life event.

Intrapsychic Events. Intrapsychic events such as "became more depressed" introduce further definition difficulties. These events cannot be readily verified by independent observers, introducing ambiguity not only as to whether the event constituted a change, but also as to whether the event ever occurred at all. Moreover, because life events frequently are studied as correlates of affective outcomes such as a change in depressive symptoms, it is wise to exclude from such studies events that describe internal states, in order to reduce overlap of prediction and criterion in the measurement of stress. However, there are occasions when the researcher is interested specifically in those events that define internal states. Such events together fit an established syndrome, such as a major depressive episode or the onset of Alzheimer's disease. In those studies the causal field usually is reversed, and the affective change is studied properly as a cause of observable events and behaviors of the individual and the family. The key to the validity of such studies is the procedures used in confirming the presence of the illness, independent of self-reports of internal state. The other area of uncertainty surrounding intrapsychic events is those events that originate from within the person that are relatively independent of affect, such as ideas, thoughts, new plans, and goals. Verification of the occurrence of these events independent of affective state remains an unfulfilled challenge for the next century in life event research.

Perceived Stress. The assessment of perceived stress gives rise to similar methodological issues. Some researchers have favored assessments of stress perceptions, such as those found in Cohen, Kamark, & Mermelstein's Perceived Stress Scale (1983), because of their focus on the person's response to stress, and not on the stressors themselves. Indeed, Lazarus (1993) has argued persuasively that stress ought to be considered a subset of emotion. The problem one faces in adopting this approach is that of distinguishing individual differences in perceived stress from other correlated conditions. Both antecedent conditions (such as neuroticism) and consequences (such as degree of pain from a chronic illness) may be confounded with measures of perceived stress. As Cook and Campbell (1979) have shown, regression analyses with covariates do not control for all effects of confounds, so it is not possible to rely on post hoc statistical resolution of problems relating to item and construct contamination.

Event measures vary in the degree to which they rely on subjective judgments for assessment of positive or negative levels of change. Included in this review are measures that assess events that are, at least in principle, observable; excluded are assessments based solely on the affective response to events. An exception is made in the discussion of the Life Events and Difficulties (LEDS) scales developed by Brown and Harris (1989). These investigators have developed methods of scoring the average emotional response to events that allow for an assessment of the event's meaningfulness independent of subjective responses.

EVENT INVENTORIES

In Table 15.1, we list 13 frequently used life event inventories. Rather than enumerating a comprehensive list, we have identified those frequently used scales that provide a standard stimulus list of events. Many scales have been revised for use with older adults, as is reflected in scale titles for some of the inventories. The Teri and Lewinsohn (1982) inventories are revised for use with older adults. Krause (1986) has devised a checklist with 77 items, based on the Psychiatric Evaluation Research Inventory (PERI) Life Events Scale, but with revisions for use with older adults. In addition to those measures cited in Table 15.1, there are two minor revisions worthy of note. Davis (1985) modified the Life Events Survey (Sarason, Johnson, & Siegel,1978) to make it applicable to older adults, and Chiriboga (1984) has devised shorter versions of the Hassles and Uplifts scales for older adults.

The inventories vary in their relative comprehensiveness. Some inventories reference only major events; others assess only daily events. The Daily Stress Inventory (Brantley, Waggoner, Jones, & Rappaport, 1987), for example, focuses only on daily stressors, and contains neither desirable events nor major events. The inventories also differ widely in the number of items used to assess health-related life experiences. Although all scales include some probes for additional events not on the list, it is unclear how useful such a strategy is in terms of mobilizing subjects to retrieve information on event occurrences (See Bradburn, Rips, & Shevell, 1987).

TABLE 15.1 Frequently Used Inventories of Life Events

Title	*Number of items*	*Content*	*Subscales available*	*Event ratings available*	*Time frame: frequency rating*
Daily Life Events Inventory (Stone, Kessler, & Haythornthwaite, 1991)	66 items	daily events/mixture of major and minor	work, leisure, family, friends, other	subjective ratings: desirability (1–6 scale), change (1–6 scale), meaningfulness (1–6 scale), control (1–3 scale)	daily: occurence (yes/no)
Daily Stress Inventory (Brantley et al., 1987)	58 items	everyday stressors	none	subjective stressfulness (1–7 scale)	daily: occurence (yes/no)
Geriatric Life Events Schedule (Kahana et al., 1987)	54 items	major events	none	subjective rating: amount of change (0–100 scale)	3-year: occurrence (yes/no)
Hassles and Uplifts Scales (Kanner et al., 1981)	117 hassles 135 uplifts	everyday events, some major events	hassles, uplifts	subjective severity (1–3 scale)	monthly: frequency (0–3 scale)
Checklist of Life Events (Krause, 1986)	77 items	major events	positive life events, negative life events	subjective impact (1–5 scale)	year: occurrence (yes/no)
Life Events and Difficulties Schedule (Brown & Harris, 1989)	40 probes with open-ended inquiry	severe events, on-going difficulties	eight substantive domains indicating change: in role, close ties, personal health, other's health, residence, goal fulfillment, and other dramatic events	interviewer ratings of severity of threat: long-term and short-term (see text)	variable time frame: frequency
Louisville Older Person Event Scale (Murrell et al., 1984)	54 items	major events	health, death, family conflicts, rewards	subjective ratings: change (1–4 scale), desirability (1–7 scale), preoccupation (1–4 scale) reoccurrence (0–7 scale)	1 month to a year: occurrence (yes/no)

Life Events Survey (Sarason, Johnson & Siegel, 1978)	59 items	major and minor events	none	subjective impact (–3 to +3 scale)	6 months: occurrence (yes/no)
Pleasant & Unpleasant Event Schedules for Elderly (Teri & Lewisohn, 1982)	114 pleasant 131 unpleasant	everyday events	mood congruent, mood incongruent	subjective pleasantness/ unpleasantness (0–2 scale)	monthly: frequency (0–2 scale)
PERI Life Events Scales (Dohrenwend, 1979)	102 items	major events	fateful loss, health/ illness, negative role performance, positive role performance	normative ratings of degree of disruption (change) in routine (see text)	1 to 6 months: frequency
Recent Life Changes Questionnaire (Rahe, 1976)	77 items	major events, some everyday events	work, family, personal and social, financial, health	subjective rating of amount of change (0–100 scale)	6 months to 2 years: occurrence (yes/no)
Research Inventory of Major and Small Events for Older Adults (Zautra & Guarnaccia, 1988)	88 major nonhealth, 43 major health; 175 small events, nonhealth; 27 illness symptom events	major and small desirable and undesirable events	13 life domains: immediate family, work, social, recreation, household, financial, crime, transportation, marital and love, extended family, school	normative ratings of major versus small, degree of change, desirability control, and reoccurrence	daily to monthly: frequency (0–2 scale)
UCSF Life Events Questionnaire (Chiriboga, 1984)	125 items	major events	11 dimensions: marriage, family, personal habits, nonfamily, personal, legal, financial, school, health, work, home	none	multiple year: occurrence (yes/no)

The measures were not developed independently. For example, Zautra and Guarnaccia (1988) constructed their measure as a revision of the Small Events Inventory (Zautra, Guarnaccia, & Dohrenwend, 1986) to make it applicable to older adults. Both the Louisville Scale (Murrell et al., 1984) and the PERI Life Events Scale (Dohrenwend, Krasnoff, Askenasy, & Dohrenwend, 1978) were used to construct Zautra and Guarnaccia's (1988) list of major events; the small events were constructed after review of earlier instruments, most notably the Pleasant and Unpleasant Events Schedules (Teri & Lewinsohn, 1982) and the Assessment of Daily Experience (Stone & Neale, 1982), recently renamed The Daily Life Experience Inventory (Stone, Kessler, & Haythorntwaite, 1991). The Recent Life Changes Questionnaire (Rahe, 1976) represents a revision of the original Schedule of Recent Experience developed by Holmes and Rahe (1967).

The time frame for recalling events varies from 3 years or more for the Geriatric Life Events Schedule (Kahana, Kahana, & Young, 1987) to reports on the immediate day's events for the daily event inventories. Some inventories have developed a number of subscales for determining events in specific life domains such as family, friends, work, and leisure; other scales have been constructed across domains in order to assess thematically relevant issues such as interpersonal stress (Zautra, Burleson, Matt, Roth, & Burrows, 1994). In addition to the content subscales, these inventories offer a wide assortment of ways in which to scale events. Some of the most prominent scaling methods are reviewed below.

Event Dimensions

Change. A unifying feature of early life event inventories is that most researchers adopt Holmes and Rahe's (1967) definition of a major event as one that causes a change in the life style routine prompting a need for readjustment. Events were scaled according to degree of readjustment required, using magnitude estimation procedures borrowed from psychophysics (Stevens, 1966). Zautra et al. (1986) used such procedures to define two classes of events, *major* and *small*, selecting an arbitrary designation of 250 magnitude readjustment units as the criterion for a major change.

The use of weights to scale the stressfulness of events is controversial for all but the most crude divisions. There is disagreement, even among experts, on whether and how to assess change. Clearly more needs to be known about the nature of the change for the individual to establish the amount of change associated with the event. Shrout (1981) has demonstrated that the weighting of events per se provides little overall improvement in the score's correlation with criterion measures.

Desirability. Whether the event is a desirable experience, undesirable experience, or both is perhaps the most fundamental attribute of an event. Desirability of an event is currently scored in one of two ways: Ask the individual to rate the event in terms of desirability (e.g., Sarason et al., 1978) or obtain consensus ratings of the event through the use of objective raters. The problems with subjective ratings and estimates are reviewed below. The problems associated with using independent raters stem from the broad range of experiences that may be subsumed under a given event classification. Therefore, an independent rater would have no idea on which side of the ledger to place the response. For example, some inventories continue to ask whether a change has occurred without reference to the direction of the change, for example, "fewer or more arguments with spouse." With relatively minor events the problem can be resolved by rewriting the event to clarify the direction of change. However, the problem is not as easily resolved for major events, because major events (such as retirement) bring with them many changes, some of which may be positive and some negative. Later in this chapter, we describe recent developments in the measurement of major events that provide a potential solution to determining desirability.

Another way to estimate desirability is to obtain profiles of an individual's plans and goals independent of event ratings and to match event occurrence with the degree to which it furthers or disrupts ongoing projects. Work along these lines in the area of daily events has begun (Campbell, Chew, & Scratchley, 1991) and may provide a way of estimating the desirability of events in everyday life.

There is now substantial evidence that desirable events that fit with a person's goals and plans are qualitatively different from those events that disrupt or change ongoing plans, goals, and activities. Individual differences in the number of desirable events typically predict subjective ratings of quality of life but contribute less to the prediction of psychological distress than does the number of undesirable events (Thoits, 1983; Zautra & Reich, 1983; Zautra, Reich, and Guarnaccia, 1990). Correlations between desirable events and measures of psychological well-being are nearly always positive (Reich & Zautra, 1988). Thus, desirable events appear to define a different class of life experience. This argues for separate scales of positive and negative life experiences rather than rating events along a continuum from desirable to undesirable.

Controllability of Events. In addition to change and desirability, controllability is considered an important dimension along which events are scored. Uncontrollable events are thought to provoke the greatest psychological upset (Thoits, 1983). Dohrenwend, Raphael, Schwartz, Stueve, & Skodol (1993) have developed methods of assessing whether an event is "fateful." Fateful events are those that occur independent of the behavior of the person and are therefore uncontrollable by that person. The aim of determining degree of fatefulness is not simply to provide a rating for each event, but to allow for clear causal inferences about the effects of the event on psychological and physical health by being able to separate presumed causal events from their effects. Among older adults, death and illness of family members are generally considered fateful events. Personal injury and illness are also, in principle, fateful; however, those illnesses and the treatments prescribed can influence outcomes such as well-being directly, rather than through their life stress effects.

Controllable events tend to be more desirable. Zautra and Reich (1980) used consensus ratings of events as either "origin" or "pawn," and later developed lists of events for older adults that they called "demands" and "desires" (Reich, Zautra, & Hill, 1987), where the central distinctions between the events were the degree of control the person exercised over their occurrence (origin vs. pawn) and the source of the need generated (desire vs. demand).

Person-Environment Fit: Event Congruence. Another perspective on the meaning of life events has been offered by life span developmental researchers, who attempt to discern the degree to which events are consistent with developmental level and social norms. Neugarten (1976) proposed that a socially prescribed timetable exists for the occurrence of major events such as marriage, retirement, illness, and loss of family members. Events that fit the normative patterns are more likely to elicit ready adaptation than are those experienced "off-time," which may be perceived as more stressful changes.

There are many ways in which events can be evaluated for their degree of fit—social norms provide only one context from which to judge an event's congruence. Fit with a person's plans, with his or her history and expectation for future events may also be part of an assessment of event ecology. Indeed, Lowenthal, Thurnher, and Chiriboga (1975) have shown that the nonoccurrence of expected desirable events can be an important source of dissatisfaction.

Perfect congruence may not be optimal for adjustment. Some degree of incongruence may be desirable for psychological growth, provided the disruption produced by the events are within the range of tolerable effects (Danish, et al., 1980; Kahana, 1975; Lawton & Nahemow, 1973).

Goodhart and Zautra (1984) illustrated an event congruence approach through the analysis of life events from a community sample of older adults. They constructed age-related norms for the occurrence of 60 life events and found non-normative events to have a greater impact on elders' ratings of quality of life than normative events. The evaluation of event congruence with personal, social, and developmental norms is likely to receive increased attention in future studies of older adults.

Recurrent Versus New Events. An implicit feature of an event's perceived change and controllability is whether it is unforeseen or a part of a pattern of events. Adaptation may occur more readily for recurrent events than for new events. The person who has experienced an event previously is more likely to have established effective coping strategies. Recurrent events are also more predictable, allowing for anticipatory coping. On the other hand, recurrent events increase a sense of helplessness when they are unwanted and lead to lower self-esteem and greater vulnerability to future stressful events. Thus, they may signify chronic strains (Avison & Turner, 1988) or what Brown and Harris (1989) call "ongoing difficulties."

Major events are seldom evaluated in terms of degree of recurrence, but elderly individuals commonly experience some stressors repeatedly. The death of close friends or family members happens repeatedly for some elders, and major illness downturns are common for those with chronic illnesses like arthritis. Eysenck (1983) hypothesized "stress inoculation effects," and Guarnaccia (1990) found evidence that experience with death of a spouse may lessen the impact of other deaths for older adults. Erdal (1992) found, however, that recurrent arthritis downturns continued to adversely affect well-being among chronically ill elders in comparison to healthy controls, even after accounting for baseline differences in well-being.

Degree of Threat. Brown and his colleagues (e.g., Brown & Harris, 1989) have developed methods for rating contextual threat associated with a major life event. Through extensive probing, interviewers record a detailed account of the events as experienced. They present information about the event to a group of raters who assess the degree of threat to the average person in a similar circumstance. Their ratings reflect assessments of "short-term" and "long-term" threat (Brown & Harris, 1989, p.25), depending upon the length of time the threat to self is expected to last. Other investigators, instead of using independent raters, have employed subjective ratings from which to assess the person's reaction to the event. Brown and Harris (1989) obtained both subjective and expert ratings of events to identify the individual's most meaningful events avoiding sole reliance on a subjective reaction when determining the stressfulness of an event. Many researchers using these scoring procedures have related events to psychological and physical health outcomes. The use of expert ratings of threat has proven useful in distinguishing events that have little emotional impact from those that have a considerable impact.

METHODOLOGICAL ISSUES IN THE MEASUREMENT OF EVENTS

Issues in Item Construction

Zautra, Guarnaccia, Reich, & Dohrenwend (1988) recommended that researchers apply the following criteria for construction of items in event inventories in order to reduce confounding with other variables that are likely to be important antecedents and consequences of events:

1. The event ought to be observable, so that it is, in principle at least, verifiable.
2. The event should have a discrete beginning, rather than refer to an event as a change of "more than or less than" quality.
3. The event should be able to be rated reliably as desirable or undesirable by independent judges.

4. The event should signify a change in ongoing activities in keeping with the original definition of a life event.

Criteria such as these have not been applied systematically in the construction of event inventories, and problems of confounding continue to plague the field as a result (French, Knox, & Gekoski, 1992). As Kasl (1992) notes, it is critical for the analysis of the effects of life events that the assessment of events be made as independently as possible from the respondent's affective response. To accomplish this task, the researcher would do well to accept as events only those experiences that are discrete, observable occurrences, even if that means leaving out intrapsychic events.

The assessment of illness as an event is particularly troublesome because many aspects of illness, such as pain and fatigue, require subjective description. French et al. (1992) report considerable confounding in the relation between life events and illness due to contamination of events described in checklists with illness outcomes and a failure to account for individual differences in the history of illness prior to event occurrence. These problems cannot be resolved easily. If such events are simply deleted from event inventories, the investigator would lose important information. The use of prospectively designed studies can aid in the interpretation of how illness events influence subsequent health and mental health. For example, Larsen and Kasimatis (1991) examined daily patterns of physical symptoms across time to see if personality would affect the relation between changes in physical symptoms and mood. Based on the physiology of the disease, the researcher also may be able to distinguish properly between health events that are signs of the illness and those clearly independent of the syndrome.

Confounding with Subjective States

As already stated, events that refer to subjective states often overlap with study outcomes. Dohrenwend, Dohrenwend, Dodson and Shrout (1984) had 371 clinical psychologists rate the degree to which items on the original Hassles Scale (Kanner, Coyne, Schaefer, & Lazarus, 1981) were likely to be symptoms of a psychological disorder. This expert panel identified a third of the items as more likely than not to be a symptom of a psychological disorder. It was this scale and others like it that were claimed to be superior to major life events scales because they were more likely to be correlated with outcomes such as depression and anxiety.

The problems of confounding extend beyond scale content to include the use of subjective ratings of dimensions such as those just reviewed: stressfulness, undesirability, controllability, degree of threat, and event resolution. Ratings of the affective impact of events are, at least in part, reflective of the person's response to the event, and not of the occurrence of the event per se. A person's emotional state at the time of the rating, as well as a propensity toward negative affectivity (Watson & Clark, 1984), are likely to lead to endorsements of negative subjective states.

The debate continues as to the validity of stress response measures, given the potential for confounding with antecedent conditions, such as psychopathology, and with consequences of interest to the researcher, such as psychological adjustment. Green (1986) provides a useful commentary on these issues, suggesting that investigators should measure all aspects of the life stress process, including subjective responses to events, in a way that keeps the components of the process separate.

Redundancy

Monroe (1982) points out that event items often overlap, with multiple items assessing the same experience. Items can be linked, as in "car breaks down" and "had an automobile repair expense," or they may describe a pattern of events that always or nearly always co-occur, for example, "marital infidelity" and "marital conflict." Investigators sometimes build redundancy into a scale in a misguided attempt to improve reliability. The best inventories may actually have low α reliabilities. It is preferable for event inventories to count each event only once. If each event is selected to be independent of every other event, however, the resulting items on the scale are generally uncorrelated.

Comprehensiveness

Whereas no list of events can be exhaustive, event measures vary considerably in their degree of comprehensiveness. Through the use of open-ended probing for additional events not on the investigator's list, it is possible to survey more fully the life experiences of older adults. Failure to assess an event is a more serious shortcoming when assessing experiences than when assessing other constructs because each item is expected to be unique in its coverage of a salient person-environment transaction. Most checklists of life events emphasize stressors and present relatively fewer desirable events for respondents to endorse. Yet older adults report 3 times more desirable events than undesirable events (Zautra et al., 1990). Indeed, a comprehensive assessment of the quality of a person's life is not possible without attending to both categories of events. The costs of excluding positive events extend to statistical treatment of the data. Stressful events often include some desirable as well as undesirable aspects. Relocation is an example of such a stressor. Correlations between relocation and an outcome such as anxiety would be attenuated if the move could also be shown to lead to positive events, which are inversely correlated with the same outcome.

Reliability of Event Reports

There is little doubt that the original method of assessing life events by asking subjects to recall experiences over the past 6 months to a year from a checklist of events does not provide an accurate estimate of the events that have occurred, even if major events are being assessed (Jenkins, Hurst, & Rose, 1979). There is a sizable drop-off in the total number of events reported with retrospective recall intervals greater than a month or so. Raphael, Cloitre, and Dohrenwend (1991) found that subjects reported twice as many major events over a year's period when asked to report events each month, than when those same subjects reported over the entire year, retrospectively. There were four times as many health problem events reported at monthly intervals compared with expected levels from reports of the retrospective year. In contrast, Brown and Harris (1989) report high levels of accuracy over a year for severe events when using their intensive interviewing methods. Respondents also may be more likely to deny threatening events as a means of regulating current affects. Further, some subjects may "telescope": misremember the date of occurrence of events as closer to the present than in reality (Bradburn et al., 1987).

Reproducibility of Events: Accuracy in Reports

Test-retest correlations tend to be moderately high when examining total scores of life event inventories. Raphael et al., (1991) found correlations of .5 to .6 between total events reported over a year compared with the sum of monthly reports over the same time period. Monthly test-retest reliabilities for small events such as hassles (Kanner et al., 1981) and pleasant events (MacPhillamy & Lewinsohn, 1982) have ranged from .7 to .8. For both major and daily events, test-retest correlations may be artificially high, as simple reporting biases would lead to higher correlations, and because correlations between total scores do not guarantee that the same events are being reported.

Raphael et al. (1991) investigated the concordance between events reported at monthly interviews for a year and those reported retrospectively for the same period. Of events reported during one of the monthly interviews and/or at the year retrospective review, only 25% were reported in both. Over 60% of the events were reported only during the monthly interviews. Only a small portion of these discordant results could be resolved through review of respondent's descriptions of events. Concordance was also 1.13 times greater for each 30 days closer to the retrospective review. These figures are not at all encouraging for the investigator who wishes to obtain information about events that occurred more than a month prior to the assessment.

Level of Agreement Between Raters

Interrater reliability estimated from agreement obtained between respondent and a confidant appears to depend greatly on the nature of the events being reported. For daily experiences appearing on the Assessment of Daily Experiences (Stone & Neale, 1982), only modest concordance was obtained between husbands' and wives' reports of events experienced by the husbands (r=.31). More meaningful events were more likely to be reported by both, suggesting that lack of concordance arises because the confidant cannot have full knowledge of the activities of the target person (Stone et al., 1991). Concordance between psychiatric patients and their relatives on major events has ranged from a low of 22% to a high of 81% agreement, increasing with a more detailed inquiry into the nature of the event (Brown & Harris, 1989). These findings should promote caution in the use of event lists to establish the occurrence of a single life event, unless additional probes are included to prompt greater recall.

Problems in Intracategory Variability

One of the greatest threats to the validity of life event scales as measures of life stress is the considerable variability in the degree of change associated with any particular event (Dohrenwend et al.,1993). For example, for an older adult the loss associated with the death of a friend may be very major or very minor, depending upon whether the person was an integral member of the person's social network. Dohrenwend et al. (1993) report that the amount of change reported by respondents experiencing several events within a category often varies as much as the amount of change reported between categories of events. For example, variability in estimates of change as a function of the institutionalization of a close friend may be as great as variability in estimated degree of change in that experience and an event in a completely different domain, such as retirement.

The problems of intracategory variability in amount of change are relatively less severe with minor events, which reflect relatively small changes in routine. Yet the measurement of daily life experience is not immune to these problems. Small events can have symbolic meaning, particularly when they occur within an area of personal vulnerability. Lazarus, Kanner, & Folkman (1980) provide the poignant example of a disabled person in the following passage: "The shoelace might break, but a major part of the psychological stress created thereby, is the implication that one cannot control one's life, that one is helpless in the face of the most stupid of trivialities" (p.26).

Subject ratings of stressfulness and undesirability provide a potential solution, but at the cost of potential confounding with criteria when the study is directed toward the examination of outcomes such as mental health and symptoms of psychological disturbance. It is common for individuals experiencing both distress and health problems to display what is called *effort after meaning*, an attempt to identify causes for their distress. Events may be reported erroneously, and subjective accounts given retrospectively are even more likely to be biased. For studies employing a prospective design, the use of subjective ratings is less problematic, although the potential for contamination with outcomes is still significant.

RECENT METHODOLOGICAL ADVANCES IN THE STUDY OF MAJOR LIFE EVENTS

Because of the many threats to reliability and validity associated with the assessment of life events, many investigators have chosen to focus on a single major life event that can be verified independently. Events such as spousal bereavement, retirement, institutionalization of a close family member, and stroke may be examined in depth through the design of interview and questionnaire methods that identify personality features, social situational factors, and important dimensions of the experience that contribute to the event's impact on those who experience it. By utilizing carefully matched controls, differences between those with and without the experience may be examined as well. Ryff and Essex (1992) studied the experience of relocation in this manner; Phifer, Kaniasty, & Norris (1988) examined the effect of a major flood on the health and well-being of 200 older adults in a prospectively designed study.

The study of a single life experience has been successful because it provides in-depth information on the nature of the life event as experienced by the respondent. Often, however, the researcher is interested in an assessment of the full range of an individual's experiences, not just the impact of single events. Indeed, the co-occurrence of two or more major stressors itself may be an important datum in attempting to understand the person's adjustment difficulties. Two distinct approaches have been offered to solve the problems of reliability and validity in life event reports, while at the same time allowing for the assessment of multiple life events. These approaches reflect shared distrust in checklist methods, but diverge in their use of subjective and other contextual information in judging the magnitude of the event.

Life Events and Difficulties Schedule (LEDS)

The first of these approaches, developed by George Brown and his colleagues (e.g., Brown & Harris, 1989), relies on ratings of *contextual threat* made from information gathered in a semistructured interview covering 40 events in eight domains, including major changes in social role and health for self or close family members, changes in residence or other change in contact with close friends or relatives, forecasts of change, goal-oriented changes, and dramatic events like an automobile accident (see Table 15.1). The interviewer probes events informally, but with a lengthy series of questions in mind about what led to and followed the event, as well as what were the circumstances surrounding its occurrence, and whether the event was construed as positive and/or threatening to current adjustment. Two forms of threat are rated by consensus of expert judges from the verbal descriptions provided by the interviewer: *short-term* and *long-term threat*. Short-term threat refers to the threat on the day of the event or soon afterward. Long-term threat refers to the threat implied a week after the event. For example, an uncomplicated childbirth would be rated as low on long-term threat but high on short-term threat. Ratings of threat reflect the respondent reaction to the event, and the personal and social context surrounding its occurrence, and not how threatening the event would be for people in general.

There are many advantages to this approach to measuring the stress of life events. Because events are described in detail, intraevent variability is greatly reduced. Brown and Harris (1989) report excellent interjudge reliability. The informal, yet persistent, probing interviewing methods attempt to follow the natural flow or sequence of events, which is likely to enhance recall (Bradburn et al., 1987), and reduce self-protective biases in the reporting of negative events. In a comparison between the use of a checklist of events and the LEDS method, 26% of those events rated as severe by the LEDS were not reported on a checklist. Further, Brown and Harris (1989) report 80% agreement on event occurrence between the subject and a close relative when using the LEDS methodology, which is substantially higher than that found with standard life event inventories.

There are two potential shortcomings of this method. First, researchers often cannot afford its cost. The LEDS is expensive in terms of administration and scoring time, and extensive training is needed to learn the scoring system. The second problem is methodological. Contextual scoring of threat relies in part on background variables such as personal history and social circumstances. As a consequence, the scores on threat are not independent of the background variables. Researchers interested in distinguishing between such potential background variables and current ratings would find the next approach, offered by Dohrenwend et al. (1993), more appealing.

The Structured Event Probe and Narrative Rating Method (SEPARATE)

Dohrenwend et al. (1993) identified three classes of variables in the study of life stress processes: life events, ongoing situations, and personal dispositions. To keep the assessment of life events separate from the other two classes of variables, and to circumvent the problems of reliability and validity in event reports, the authors have introduced a method of event probes and expert ratings within a more highly standardized set of interview procedures than is used in the LEDS. This method begins with a checklist of events, uses detailed probes of the events identified by the respondent, and elicits a detailed narrative about the antecedents of the event and what was involved in the actual experience. Different probes are used for different events and are applied systematically. For example, determination of whether an event was life threatening is not probed in the case of loss events but is probed for personal injury and illness events. Event descriptions are abstracted and rated by two judges. Those ratings are normative, based on what would be considered "normal" for the "average" person.

The events may be rated on several different dimensions, including desirability, magnitude of change, and fatefulness. Contextual factors such as the person's income and marital status are expunged from event narratives to keep the ratings of the event independent of personal or social characteristics. Separate subjective appraisals of the events are also taken on dimensions such as perceived control, degree of change in social domains, and desirability.

The Dohrenwend et al. (1993) approach has been applied in only a few studies thus far, and there are insufficient data on the reliability and improvements in validity provided by the method compared to a checklist alone. Nevertheless, the method is a promising alternative to the LEDS. The procedures are fairly well standardized, requiring relatively less expertise and training for interviewers and for raters. The method also promises to keep the ratings of events separate from context. Like the LEDS, the approach does require extensive interviewing time with the subject. It would be valuable to examine in future studies how well subjective ratings of degree of positive and negative changes associated with major life events compare with expert ratings of the magnitude of change for those same events.

THE STUDY OF EVERYDAY LIFE EVENTS

There are several advantages to the study of everyday life events as opposed to major life experiences. Everyday events cast experience in smaller, less heterogenous units. Because they occur and recur more frequently, the researcher can design prospective studies of their effects over many repeated intervals. Tennen, Suls, and Affleck (1991) enumerated several of the most promising reasons for studying everyday events. The first is purely descriptive: to chronicle daily life as a useful starting point from which to develop theoretical formulations. A second promise lies in the ability to test new models of how major events influence well-being. Do major life events affect well-being in part by influencing everyday affairs (Kanner, et al., 1981; Caspi, Bolger, & Eckenrode, 1987)? This hypothesis is best articulated by Felner and associates (Felner, Rowlison, & Terre, 1986; Rowlison & Felner, 1988), who view major events as initiators of a transitional process that ultimately alters everyday life. Thus, the death of a spouse is not only a significant loss, but also disrupts established recreational patterns, formerly shared responsibilities, and day-to-day social relations.

Tennen et al. (1991) noted an interesting variant of this formulation in the literature on depression. Although depression is associated with major events (Brown & Harris, 1989), depressive episodes can often be precipitated by seemingly mundane events (Paykel, 1978). For someone who has recently experienced a major life event, an argument with a co-worker may serve as the trigger for a depressive episode. Day (1981) also reports evidence of such triggers for schizophrenic episodes. Examining people's daily lives thus affords the opportunity to examine the indirect yet significant contributions of major events to well-being and to determine which small events are most hazardous for whom.

Finally, some questions about the impact of life events can be answered only by studying individuals from day to day. For example, how do daily stressors affect mood beyond the day of their occurrence? If daily stress precedes physical illness, what is the time lag for this effect? Indeed, each illness that may be triggered by stressful daily events may have a different incubation time, from a few days to a week or longer. Only through frequent assessment is it possible to capture delayed effects of stress on physical health (Zautra et al., 1988).

These are only some of the questions that demand daily inquiry. Another set of questions relate to the study of patterns in experience and behavior. Daily event studies can determine when and how individuals habituate to events (Bolger et al., 1989). They allow us to examine the frequency of change in the adaptation to events (Campbell et al., 1991; Larsen, 1987), and individual differences in reactivity to stressful events (Bolger & Schilling, 1991; Affleck, Tennen, Urrows, & Higgins, in press). Most clearly, daily event studies allow us to investigate temporal processes that are obscured in cross-sectional studies, and lead us to consider time as a psychological variable (Larsen, 1991).

Advances in the Conduct of Daily Event Studies

Stone et al., (1991) discussed many methodological and procedural issues facing researchers who wish to undertake daily event studies. Among other options available to the daily events researcher, they evaluated several methods for recording events (e.g., experience sampling techniques, open-ended diaries, checklists, telephone interviewing). In Table 15.1, we listed those inventories most frequently used, with modification, to study everyday life events. Investigators have also used open-ended probes of daily experiences to elicit events (e.g., Epstein, 1979). Bolger and Schilling (1991), for example, asked subjects to report stressors in each of nine categories with open-ended inquiries about "overload" at home and at work, and about family demands. Csikszentmihalyi and Graef (1980) used a beeper device that subjects carried with them throughout the day. When the beeper signalled, subjects identified their immediate activity, thoughts, and feelings. A related procedure for the investigation of daily life is the time budget (Szalai, 1972). A person is provided a time schedule for a given day and asked to enter the activities in which they engaged during the 24-hour period, broken into 15-minute segments.

Potential problems exist with each of these methods, depending upon their uses. Time-budget methods do not distinguish between ongoing daily activities and events that typically have been viewed as a change in routine (although if multiple days were reported, it is conceivable that changes could be rated). Some existing checklists contain events that are essentially changes in internal states, and some lists do not distinguish between major and small events. In the interest of brevity, item specificity may be sacrificed. Open-ended formats for event elicitation have several distinct advantages in studies of event perception; however, they may be less useful than lists for obtaining estimates of small event frequency, due to individual differences in verbal response rates. One compromise between a desire to be comprehensive while using a standard stimulus set and a wish to reduce labor-intensive demands of the lengthy inventories is to familiarize participants with the events lists prior to data collection. Participants could be mailed the event schedule and asked to review the items, before each assessment. Another approach is to focus on a subset of the most salient life events, such as interpersonal events or physical symptoms, rather than attempt to account for all daily life events. Doing so enhances the feasibility of sampling within days comprehensively, within a given life domain.

Within-Day Assessments. Of particular interest to daily event researchers are innovative techniques for assessing experiences more than once a day. Most investigators who use end-of-the day diaries to summarize that day's events find that the strongest associations between daily events, physical symptoms, and emotional well-being are same-day associations; lagged relations denoting the effect of events on next-day outcomes are typically far weaker (Affleck et al., in press). This raises the possibility that within-day reports may capture causal sequences not detectable otherwise.

Within-day data collection procedures have often involved signalling participants in some way—either through electronic pagers or watch alarms—that it is time for them to record data. Obviously, without a way to monitor compliance with these requests, the investigator is in the dark about adherence to the data collection schedule. With the availability of programmable hand-held computers that allow "time-stamping" of responses, it is now possible to overcome this limitation of within-day assessment practices. Several investigators, including the second and third authors, in a recently initiated study of daily life with fibromyalgia pain, have established the feasibility of using computerized diaries to gather information from participants many times a day (Haythornthwaite, Anderson, & Moore, 1992; Paty, Kassel, & Shiffman, 1992; Totterdell & Folkard, 1992). As Stone et al. (1991) note, information can be conveyed in less time with computerized diaries than with traditional paper-and-pencil methods, and complex "responding trees" can be presented in a more user-friendly format. Because computerized diaries can be programmed to allow subjects some say over the timing of the data recording request, they appear less likely to disrupt daily life than other signalling techniques.

Idiographic Studies of Daily Events

Investigators of life events in both elderly and younger populations typically have sought answers to nomothetic questions: are there lawful relations between event occurrence and other variables across individuals? The dominant approach of asking nomothetic questions has led to an ignorance of the unique insights to be gained from the idiographic study of life events, as it has in other areas of the literature on stress and adaptation (Brantley & Jones, 1993; Tennen et al., 1991). Whereas the nomothetic approach pursues relations across individuals, the idiographic approach examines relations within individuals across situations or across time (Michela, 1990).

There are at least three advantages to using within-person, idiographic methods to investigate daily life events. First, a within-person design obviates the between-person differences in stable dispositions or situations that confound interpretations of correlations between life events and adaptational outcomes. Second, within-person designs can establish temporal sequences, which, in turn, strengthen causal inferences (West & Hepworth, 1991).

Findings from a study of daily events reported prospectively by individuals with rheumatoid arthritis (Tennen & Affleck, in press) illustrate well the first benefit of within-person designs. Each participant reported the occurrence of desirable and undesirable events for 75 consecutive days using the Daily Life Experience Inventory (Stone & Neale, 1982; Stone et al., 1991). The between-persons correlation between the total number of desirable and undesirable events reported on the 75 daily diaries was .50: Individuals who experienced more undesirable events apparently experienced more desirable events. However, three factors—gender, work outside the home, and children living at home—accounted fully for this association. The moderately high association was due to the fact that women who work outside the home and have children living at home experience more events altogether.

A question that cannot be answered by between-persons analysis is how desirable and undesirable events change in concert across days of an individual's life. When the event reports were disaggregated and all sources of between-person confounding eliminated, nearly two-thirds of the individuals displayed a significant inverse correlation between desirable and undesirable events from day to day. Most important, no single individual evinced the significant positive correlation between desirable and undesirable events obtained from the between-person analysis. These divergent findings underscore the unique insights that can be gained from using idiographic, within-person methods of analysis. They highlight the fact that both the magnitude and direction of associations can change when questions are framed at the between-persons versus within-person level, and that one cannot draw within-person inferences from between-persons relations.

Other findings from this study (Affleck et al., in press) illustrate how within-person analysis can establish temporal sequences and strengthen causal inferences. In addition to supplying daily reports of events, participants rated their mood disturbance and their pain intensity using standard scales. Time series regression equations furnished "stress reactivity" coefficients for each individual, reflecting the extent to which that person's undesirable daily events on a given day were accompanied by increased mood disturbance or pain the following day. These analyses controlled for serial dependencies in each individual's pain and mood daily series and established the temporal precedence of events by controlling for events occurring the following day. At the between-persons level, individuals who experienced more undesirable daily events were more emotionally distressed and suffered more intense pain over the period of daily reporting. But the within-person analysis revealed widespread individual differences in the relations of events with next-day emotional or physical distress. Some individuals' pain and mood were indeed reactive to changes in daily events, others' mood and pain were unrelated to daily stressors, and still others showed improvements in pain and mood following an increase in undesirable events.

Unique Methodological Challenges of Idiographic Daily Event Studies

Investigator and Participant Burden. The promise of time-intensive studies of daily life experiences among the elderly cannot be fulfilled without appreciating the methodological challenges posed by these studies (see Stone et al., 1991; Tennen & Affleck, in press). As Tennen and Affleck (in press) note, this method imposes major burdens on both participants and researchers. For participants, it means a willingness to undergo weeks or months of daily monitoring and to submit their data on a daily basis in order to assure compliance. This requires uncommon dedication and an openness toward sharing the intimate details of one's daily life. For investigators it means an almost obsessive monitoring of the data collection process and the willingness to wait patiently for data to accumulate.

Data Management and Statistical Analysis. A second challenge noted by Tennen and Affleck (in press) involves managing and analyzing an extraordinarily complex data set, comprising what may amount to thousands of person-days of data, accessing these data when necessary, and keeping track of what constitutes a separate study for each individual in the sample. This in itself is a demanding task requiring that the investigator learn new data management and data analytic approaches.

Examples of within-person data analytic strategies for daily event studies are proliferating in the literature, but researchers face a confusing and often intimidating evaluation of alternatives. The ultimate question for most investigators will be how each participant's daily event series maps onto other serially measured variables, such as mood or physical symptoms. Some investigators have used a *target-control period* strategy (Stone, Reed, & Neale, 1987) whereas others have used what West and Hepworth (1991) call a *concomitant time series* approach. The first tactic is appropriate when one is interested in the consequences of an uncommonly stressful day. Symptoms or mood on the target day and following days are compared with those occurring during a period set off by a control day characterized by low stress. Unfortunately, the use of restrictive criteria to designate target and control periods excludes many, sometimes most, subjects from the final analysis.

The concomitant time series approach poses a different question: what is the relationship of stressors on each day with mood or symptoms on that day or following days? West and Hepworth (1991) reviewed several alternatives for the concomitant time series analysis of daily event data and recommended a three-step strategy that begins with idiographic time series modelling, moves to the identification of individual differences and commonalities in the idiographic findings, and ends with an account of sources of interindividual variation in intraindividual relations. The interested reader can consult West and Hepworth (1991) for an informative integration of time series modelling and meta-analysis procedures for accomplishing these steps.

For numerous conceptual and statistical reasons, West and Hepworth (1991) criticize the common practice of pooling data across subjects and days to model a within-person association for the sample as a whole (Cutrona, 1986; Marco & Suls, 1993; Michela, 1990). Most important, pooled models obscure likely individual differences in the deterministic components (trend, cyclical, and autoregressive parameters) of the time series. Nonetheless, pooling data across subjects may be the only choice for within-person analysis when the number of time points per individual is too small to ensure the reliability of idiographic statistics. Jaccard and Wan (1993) demonstrated how between-person variance can be removed from pooled data sets through least-squares dummy variable analysis in order to isolate within-person relations. Hierarchical linear modelling (Bryk & Raudenbush, 1987) affords another option for pooled data analysis and has the advantage of being able to incorporate individual differences in slopes and intercepts. Bolger and Schilling (1991) use an adaptation of this strategy for their within-person analysis of linkages between daily events and mood. Kenny and Zautra (in press) present an alternative approach using latent variables and structural equation modelling for data sets with relatively short series (4 time periods or more) and many subjects (100 or more).

Measurement Reactivity. Finally, there is the potentially serious threat to validity posed by the possible reactive effects of intensive self-monitoring (Tennen and Affleck, in press). The most obvious threat, well known to behavior therapists who use it to therapeutic advantage and reflected in debriefing sessions with subjects who participated in a daily study of individuals with rheumatoid arthritis (Affleck et al., in press), is that people might change their behavior as they detect contingencies between events and states. Perhaps the most serious threat to validity is that the very task of asking people to become self-focused may create or cement the very linkages we then "discover." An emerging experimental (Croyle & Uretsky, 1987; Salovey & Birnbaum, 1989) and field study (Larsen & Cowen, 1988) literature suggests that self-focused attention may forge linkages between stress, symptoms, and emotions that might not generalize to situations in which subjects are left free to ignore their negative experiences each day. This potential problem underscores the need to compare self-monitors with appropriate contrast groups at the beginning and end of an intensive diary study.

SUMMARY AND RECOMMENDATIONS

The evidence we have reviewed indicates that the assessment of life events provides valuable data on both the major challenges to adaptation and also the ups and downs of everyday life that pervade the lives of older adults. Numerous advances in measurement and conceptualization of stress have been made since the first Schedule of Recent Experience (Holmes & Rahe, 1967) was published. We did encounter some neglect of these advances in the literature, with some authors continuing to employ outdated instruments, and showing little knowledge or sophistication about the methodological issues involved in the assessment of events. To the extent possible, we hope that our review may raise consciousness among those researchers who are interested in assessment of life events, and provide direction toward advances in the measurement of events.

Clearly, there are many choices available among methods for the examination of the lives of older adults. These range from in-depth probes of the antecedents and consequences of major life events to investigations into small changes in routine within a single day. The selection of instruments and design for study depends on the research question. The many years of experience among investigators in this field does provide a sobering view of what can be attained in retrospective assessments. Distortions in reporting due to memory loss and variability in the meaning of events classified in the same category must be addressed. The problems of confounded measurement of events when perceptions of stress and other response-based appraisals are employed continue to plague the field. Athough such measurements may be quite appropriate in some studies the points raised in this review should encourage more thoughtfulness in the selection of such measures in future research.

Recommendations for "best" measures are tempered by the understanding that investigators do not always have the same aims in mind. Nevertheless, there are some general principles that researchers might follow in making their choices. Event measures should be comprehensive in scope, relatively free of confounding with variables assessing antecedents and consequences of events, and constructed for use with the appropriate age group. Although it often is useful to assess subjective responses to events, we urge that such assessments be taken in a way that assures independence between the reporting of events and reactions to them. A number of response scales have been used with success to assess subjective ratings of many qualities of life experience including desirability, cause, control, and stressfulness. These scales may be used productively, provided the researcher does not comingle scores on these subjective measures with estimates of degree of stress as estimated by the actual occurrence of life events. Experience suggests that the best estimates of life stress for use in identifying individual differences and change in levels over time are those that derive from indicators of the occurrences themselves, and not from reactions to events.

It is demanding of time and labor to use extensive probes to verify the occurrence of major events and clarify their meaning. Nevertheless, such attention to detail often is necessary to score the degree of stress associated with a single major life experience. Of the two approaches described in this review, the Structural Event Probe and Narrative Rating Method (SEPARATE) would appear to offer the best hope of quantifying the extent of negative change associated with a life event in a way that keeps the scoring of the event separate from those variables that might affect the impact of the event on the person's health and mental health.

In-depth probes of everyday events are not as crucial since any single small event is expected to have a relatively modest impact. More important to the examination of everyday life events is the use of measurements that are comprehensive because the quantitative estimates of degree of stress are likely to depend on counts and frequencies more than ratings. Positive events should be included in order to obtain a full appraisal of the quality of everyday life's events. As mentioned earlier, failure to include positive events in the assessment can also lead to underestimates of the impact of negative events. There are few empirical studies of recall bias with small events, but one month is suggested as an outside limit on the time frame for recall of such events. Indeed, devices that allow for sampling of events daily, and even within days, are preferable to retrospective accounts extending over a week or more.

The inquiry into events continues to hold considerable promise in the study of the lives of older adults. Advances in the design and analysis of daily events instruments have opened a new chapter in life event research. The improvements offered in the assessment of major life experiences are also likely to prompt new discoveries concerning the impact of events such as spousal bereavement, retirement, and severe illness and injury events. It is hoped that this review may serve as a reference to guide those interested in advancing our understanding of the lives of older adults through the study of life event processes.

REFERENCES

Affleck, G., Tennen, H., Urrows, S., & Higgins, P. (in press). Person and contextual features of stress reactivity: Individual differences in relations of undesirable daily events with mood disturbance and chronic pain intensity. *Journal of Personality and Social Psychology.*

Aneshensel, C. S., Pearlin, L. P., & Schuler, R. H. (1993). Stress, role captivity, and the cessation of caregiving. *Journal of Health and Social Behavior, 34*, 54–70.

Avison, W. R., & Turner, R. J. (1988). Stressful life events and depressive symptoms: Disaggregating the effects of acute stressors and chronic strains. *Journal of Health and Social Behavior, 29*, 253–264.

Bolger, N., DeLongis, A., Kessler, R. C., & Schilling, E. A. (1989). Effects of daily stress on negative mood. *Journal of Personality and Social Psychology, 57*, 808–818.

Bolger, N., & Schilling, E. A. (1991). Personality and the problems of everyday life: The role of neuroticism in exposure and reactivity to daily stressors. *Journal of Personality, 59*, 3, 355–386.

Bradburn, N. M., Rips, L. J., & Shevell, S. K. (1987). Answering autobiographical questions: The impact of memory and inference on surveys. *Science, 236*, 157–161.

Brantley, P., & Jones, G. (1993). Daily stress and stress-related disorders. *Annals of Behavioral Medicine, 15*, 17–26.

Brantley, P. J., Waggoner, C. D., Jones, G. N., & Rappaport, N. B. (1987). A daily stress inventory: Development, reliability, and validity. *Journal of Behavioral Medicine, 10*, 61–74.

Bryk, A. S., & Raudenbush, S. W. (1987). Application of hierarchical linear models to assessing change. *Psychological Bulletin, 101*, 147–158.

Brown, G. W., & Harris, T. O. (1989). *Life events and illness*. New York: Guilford.

Campbell, J., Chew, B., & Scratchley, L. (1991). Cognitive and emotional reactions to daily events: The effects of self-esteem and self-complexity. *Journal of Personality, 50*, 473–506.

Caspi, A., Bolger, N., & Eckenrode, J. (1987). Linking person and context in the daily stress process. *Journal of Personality and Social Psychology, 52*, 184–195.

Chiriboga, D. A. (1984). Social stressors as antecedents of change. *Journal of Gerontology, 39*, 468–477.

Cohen, S., Kamark, T., & Mermelstein. (1983). A global measure of perceived stress. *Journal of Health and Social Behavior, 24*, 385–396.

Cook, T. D., & Campbell, D. T. (1979). *Quasi-experimentation: Design and analysis issues for field settings* (pp. 295–320). Chicago: Rand McNally.

Croyle, R. T., & Uretsky, M. (1987). Effects of mood on self-appraisal of health status. *Health Psychology, 6*, 239–253.

Csikszentmihalyi, M., & Graef, R. (1980). The experience of freedom in daily life. *American Journal of Community Psychology, 8*, 410–414.

Cutrona, C. E. (1986). Behavioral manifestations of social support: A microanalytic investigation. *Journal of Personality and Social Psychology, 51*, 201–208.

Danish, S. J., Smyer, M. A., & Nowak, C. A. (1980). Developmental intervention: Enhancing life-event processes. *Life-Span Development and Behavior, 3*, 339–366.

Davis, G. R. (1985). Developmental patterns of stress and coping: Middle age and older adulthood. *Dissertation Abstracts International, 46*, 10A. (University Microfilms No. 85–21, 580)

Day, R. (1981). Life events and schizophrenia: The "triggering" hypothesis. *Acta Psychiatrica Scandinavica, 64*, 97–122.

Dohrenwend, B. P. (1979). Stressful life events and psychopathology: Some issues of theory and methods. In J. Barrett, R. M. Ross, & G. L. Klerman (Eds.), *Stress and mental disorder* (pp. 1–15). New York: Raven.

Dohrenwend, B. S., Dohrenwend, B. P., Dodson, M., & Shrout, P. E. (1984). Symptoms, hassles, social support and life events: The problem of confounded measures. *Journal of Abnormal Psychology, 93*, 220–230.

Dohrenwend, B. S., Krasnoff, L., Askenasy, A. R., & Dohrenwend, B. P. (1978). Exemplification of a method for scaling life events. The PERI Life Events Scale. *Journal of Personality and Social Psychology, 19*, 205–229.

Dohrenwend, B. P., Raphael, K. G., Schwartz, S., Stueve, A., & Skodol, A. (1993). The structured event probe and narrative rating method for measuring stressful life events.

In L. Goldberger & S. Breznitz (Eds.), *Handbook of stress* (2nd ed., pp. 174–199). New York: Free Press.

Epstein, S. (1979). The stability of behavior: I. On predicting most of the people much of the time. *Journal of Personality and Social Psychology, 37*, 1097–1126.

Erdal, K. (1992). The psychological impact of illness downturns: A comparison of new versus chronic conditions. Unpublished masters thesis, Arizona State University, Tempe.

Eysenck, H. J. (1983). Stress, disease, and personality: The "inoculation effect." In C. L. Cooper (Ed.), *Stress research* (pp. 121–146). New York: Wiley.

Felner, R. D., Rowlison, R. T., & Terre, L. (1986). Unraveling the Gordian knot of life change events: A critical examination of crisis, stress, and transitional frameworks for prevention. In S.M. Auerbach & A.L. Stolberg (Eds.), *Children's life crisis events: Prevention intervention strategies* (pp. 39–63). New York: McGraw-Hill.

French, S. L., Knox, V. J., & Gekoski, W. L. (1992). Confounding as a problem in relating life events to health status in elderly individuals. *American Journal of Community Psychology, 20*, 2.

Goodhart, D. E., & Zautra, A. J. (1984). Assessing quality of life in the community: An ecological approach. In W. A. O'Connor & B. Lubin (Eds.), *Ecological approaches to clinical and community psychology*, 251–290. New York: Wiley.

Green, B. L. (1986). On the confounding of "hassles" stress and outcome. *American Psychologist, 41*, 714–719.

Guarnaccia, C. A. (1990). An alternative perspective on the effects of conjugal bereavement on future losses: Stress inoculation. Unpublished doctoral dissertation, Arizona State University, Tempe.

Haythornthwaite, J., Anderson, D., & Moore, L. (1992). Social and behavioral factors associated with episodes of inhibitory breathing. *Journal of Behavioral Medicine, 15*, 573–588.

Holmes, R. S., & Holmes, T. H. (1970). Short-term intrusions into the life style routine. *Journal of Psychosomatic Research, 11*, 213–218.

Holmes, T. H., & Rahe, R. H. (1967). The social readjustment scale. *Journal of Psychosomatic Research, 11*, 213–218.

Hughes, D. A., Blazer, D. G., & George, L. K. (1988). Age differences in life events: A multivariate controlled analysis. *International Journal of Aging and Human Development, 27*, 3, 207–220.

Jaccard, J., & Wan, C. (1993). Statistical analysis of temporal data with many observations: Issues for behavioral medicine data. *Annals of Behavioral Medicine, 15*, 41–50.

Jenkins, C. D., Hurst, M. W., & Rose, R. M. (1979). Life changes: Do people really remember? *Archives of General Psychiatry, 36*, 379–384.

Kahana, E. A. (1975). A congruence model of person-environment interaction. In M. P. Lawton, R. G. Windley, & T. O. Byerts (Eds.), *Theory development in environment and aging*. New York: Springer Publishing.

Kahana, E. F., Kahana, B., & Young, R. (1987). Influences of diverse stress on health and well-being of community aged. In A. M. Fowler (Ed.), *Post traumatic stress: The healing journey*. Washington, DC: Veterans Administration.

Kasl, S. V. (1992). Stress and health among the elderly: Overview of issues. In M. L. Wykle, E. Kahana, & J. Kowal (Eds.), *Stress and health among the elderly* (pp. 5–34). New York: Springer.

Kanner, A. D., Coyne, J. C., Schaefer, C., & Lazarus, R. S. (1981). Comparison of two modes of stress measurement: Daily hassles and uplifts versus major life events. *Journal of Behavioral Medicine, 4*, 1–39.

Kenny, D., & Zautra, A. J. (in press). The trait-state-error model for multiwave data. *Journal of Consulting and Clinical Psychology.*

Krause, N. (1986). Stress and sex differences in depressive symptoms among older adults. *Journal of Gerontology, 41*, 727–731.

Larsen, R. J. (1987). The stability of mood variability: A spectral analytic approach to daily mood assessments. *Journal of Personality and Social Psychology, 52*, 1195–1204.

Larsen, R. J. (1991, August). Issues in the study of daily events. In H. Tennen (Chair), *Daily events and experiences: Research challenges and directions.* Symposium conducted at the meeting of the American Psychological Association, San Francisco.

Larsen, R., & Cowan, G. (1988). Internal focus of attention and depression: A study of daily experience. *Motivation and Emotion, 12*, 237–249.

Larsen, R. J., & Kasimatis, M. (1991). Day-to-day physical symptoms: Individual differences in the occurrence, duration, and emotional concomitants of minor daily illnesses. *Journal of Personality, 59*, 387–424.

Lawton, M. P., & Nahemow, L. (1973). Ecology and the aging process. In C. Eisdorfer & M.P. Lawton (Eds.), *The psychology of adult development and aging* (pp. 619–674). Washington, DC: American Psychological Association.

Lazarus, R. S. (1993). Why we should think of stress as a subset of emotion. In L. Goldberger & S. Breznitz (Eds.), *Handbook of stress* (2nd ed. pp. 21–39). New York: Free Press.

Lazarus, R. S., Kanner, A. D., & Folkman, S. (1980). Emotions: A cognitive-phenomenological analysis. In R. Plutchik & H. Kellerman (Eds.), *Theories of emotion. Vol. 1: Emotion: theory, research and experience.* New York: Academic Press.

Lowenthal, M. F., Thurnher, M., & Chiriboga, D. (1975). *Four stages of life.* San Francisco: Jossey-Bass.

MacPhillamy, D. J., & Lewinsohn, P. M. (1976). *Manual for the Pleasant Events Schedule.* Unpublished manuscript, University of Oregon.

MacPhillamy, D. J., & Lewinsohn, P. M. (1982). The Pleasant Events Schedule: Studies on reliability, validity, and scale intercorrelation. *Journal of Consulting and Clinical Psychology, 50*, 363–380.

Marco, C., & Suls, J. (1993). Daily stress and the trajectory of mood: Spillover, response assimilation, contrast, and chronic negative affectivity. *Journal of Personality and Social Psychology, 64,* 1053–1063.

Michela, J. (1990). Within-person correlational design and analysis. In C. Hendrick and M. Clark (Eds.), *Research methods in personality and social psychology*, 279–311. Newbury Park, CA: Sage.

Monroe, S. M. (1982). Life events assessment: Current practices, emerging trends. *Clinical Psychology Review, 2*, 435–453.

Murrell, S. A., Norris, F. H., & Hutchins, G. L. (1984). Distribution and desirability of life events in older adults: Population and policy implications. *Journal of Community Psychology, 12*, 301–311.

Neugarten, B. L. (1976). Adaptation and the life cycle. *The Counseling Psychologist, 6*, 16–20.

Paty, J., Kassel, J., & Shiffman, S. (1992). Assessing stimulus control of smoking: The importance of base rates. In M. DeVries (Ed.), *The experience of psychopathology* (pp. 347–352). Cambridge, England: Cambridge University Press.

Paykel, E. S. (1978). Contribution of life events to causation of psychiatric illness. *Psychological Medicine, 8,* 245–253.

Phifer, J. F., Kaniasty, K. Z., & Norris, F. H. (1988). The impact of natural disaster on the health of older adults: A multiwave prospective study. *Journal of Health and Social Behavior, 29,* 65–78.

Raphael, E. G., Cloitre, M., & Dohrenwend, B. P. (1991). Problems of recall and misclassification with checklist methods of measuring stressful life events. *Health Psychology, 10,* 62–74.

Rahe, R. H. (1976). Epidemiological studies of life change and illness. *International Journal of Psychiatry in Medicine, 6,* 133–146.

Reich, J. W., & Zautra, A. J. (1983). Demands and desires in daily life: Some influences on well-being. *American Journal of Community Psychology, 11,* 41–57.

Reich, J. W., & Zautra, A. J. (1988). Direct and stress-moderating effects of positive life experiences. In L.H. Cohen (Ed.), *Life events and psychological functioning: Theoretical and methodological issues* (pp. 149–181). Newbury Park: Sage.

Reich, J. W., Zautra, A. J., & Hill, J. (1987). Activity, event transactions, and quality of life in older adults. *Psychology and Aging, 2,* 116–124.

Rowlison, R. T., & Felner, R. D. (1988). Major life events, hassles, and adaptation in adolescence: Confounding in the conceptualization and measurement of life stress and adjustment revisited. *Journal of Personality and Social Psychology, 55,* 432–444.

Ryff, C. D., & Essex, M. J. (1992). The interpretation of life experience and well-being: The sample case of relocation. *Psychology and Aging, 7,* 507–517.

Salovey, P., & Birnbaum, D. (1989). Influence of mood on health-relevant cognitions. *Journal of Personality and Social Psychology, 57,* 539–551.

Sarason, I. G., Johnson, J. H., & Siegel, J. M. (1978). Assessing the impact of life changes: Development of the Life Experiences Survey. *Journal of Consulting and Clinical Psychology, 48,* 932–946.

Shrout, P. E. (1981). Scaling of stressful life events. In B. S. Dohrenwend & B. P. Dohrenwend (Eds.), *Stressful life events and their contexts* (pp. 29–47). New York: Prodist.

Stevens, S. S. (1966). A metric for the social consensus. *Science, 151,* 530–541.

Stone, A. A., Kessler, R. C., & Haythornthwaite, J. A. (1991). Measuring daily events and experiences: Decisions for the researcher. *Journal of Personality, 59,* 575–607.

Stone, A. A., & Neale, J. M. (1982). Development of a methodology for assessing daily experiences. In A. Baum & J. Singh (Eds.), *Environment and health* (pp. 49–83). Hillsdale, NJ: Erlbaum.

Stone, A. A., Reed, B. R., & Neale, J. M. (1987). Changes in daily event frequency precede episodes of physical symptoms. *Journal of Human Stress, 13,* 70–74.

Szalai, A. (Ed.). (1972). *The use of time.* The Hague: Mouton.

Tennen, H., & Affleck, G. (in press). Daily processes in coping with chronic pain: Methods and analytic strategies. In M. Zeidner & N. Endler (Eds.), *Handbook of coping.* New York: Wiley.

Tennen, H., Suls, J., & Affleck, G. (1991). Personality and daily experience: The promise and the challenge. *Journal of Personality, 59,* 313–337.

Teri, L., & Lewinsohn, P. (1982). Modification of the Pleasant and Unpleasant Events

Schedules for use with the elderly. *Journal of Consulting and Clinical Psychology, 50*, 444–445.

Thoits, P. A. (1983). Dimensions of life events that influence psychological distress: An evaluation and synthesis of the literature. In H. B. Kaplan (Ed.), *Psychosocial stress: Trends in theory and research* (pp. 33–103). New York: Academic Press.

Totterdell, P., & Folkard, S. (1992). In situ repeated measures of affect and cognitive performance. *Behavior Research Methods, Instruments, and Computers, 24*, 545–553.

Watson, D., & Clark, L. A. (1984). Negative affectivity: The disposition to experience aversive emotional states. *Psychological Bulletin, 96*, 465–490.

West, S. G., & Hepworth, J. T. (1991). Statistical issues in the study of temporal data: Daily experiences. *Journal of Personality, 59*, 609–662.

Zautra, A. J., Burleson, M. H., Matt, K. S., Roth, S., & Burrows, L. (1994). Interpersonal stress, depression, and disease activity in rheumatoid arthritis and osteoarthritis patients. *Health Psychology, 13*, 1–10.

Zautra, A. J., & Guarnaccia, C. A. (1988 November). *Research inventory of major and small life events for older adults*. Paper presented at 41st annual meeting of the Gerontological Society of America, San Francisco, CA.

Zautra, A. J., Guarnaccia, C. A., & Dohrenwend, B. P. (1986). Measuring small events. *American Journal of Community Psychology, 19*, 54–71.

Zautra, A. J., Guarnaccia, C. A., Reich, J. W., & Dohrenwend, B. P. (1988). The contribution of small events to stress and distress. In L. H. Cohen (Ed.), *Life events and psychological functioning: Theories and methodological issues* (pp. 123–148). Newbury Park: Sage.

Zautra, A. J., & Reich, J. W. (1980). Positive life events and reports of well-being: Some useful distinctions. *American Journal of Community Psychology, 8*, 657–669.

Zautra, A., & Reich, J.W. (1983). Life events and perceptions of life quality: Developments in a two factor approach. *Journal of Community Psychology, 11*, 121–132.

Zautra, A. J., Reich, J. W., & Guarnaccia, C. A. (1990). Some everyday life consequences of disability and bereavement for older adults. *Journal of Personality and Social Psychology, 59*, 550–561.

CHAPTER 16

Multidimensional Assessment Instruments: Present Status and Future Prospects

LINDA K. GEORGE
DEPARTMENT OF PSYCHIATRY
DUKE UNIVERSITY MEDICAL CENTER, DURHAM

INTRODUCTION

Assessment tools vary widely in scope. Multidimensional assessment instruments are the most ambitious in that regard: The purpose of such tools is to generate information about the major dimensions of life experience, yielding a valid "snapshot" of the whole person. As this definition implies, multidimensional assessment tools are intended to provide information at two levels. First, information is gathered about multiple salient dimensions of well-being, with each dimension viewed as important in its own right. Second, the comprehensiveness of the dimensions examined is expected to yield an accurate picture of the functioning and well-being of the whole person.

The originators and advocates of multidimensional assessment tools typically note two advantages to their use. The most frequently noted advantage is examination of the "whole" person. Although the need for assessing discrete areas of functioning and well-being is uniformly acknowledged, comprehensive information about the individual is also valuable. As noted below, arguments that the quality of both research and practice are enhanced when information is available about the whole person can be marshalled. The second theme that pervades the literature on multidimensional assessment is the need to understand the relationships among dimensions of functioning. Two examples illustrate the importance of this theme. First, older individuals often compensate for deficits in one dimension of well-being by using assets in other life domains. For example, a physically disabled individual may be able to sustain community residence and enjoyment of life with the help of social support provided by family and friends. Another individual, with similar disability but lacking social support, may require institutional placement. Thus, the consequences of impairment in one dimension of well-being often cannot be understood without knowledge of other dimensions. Second, interventions (defined in the broadest sense to include formal and informal, as well as narrow and broad, services) may have an impact on multiple life dimensions. For example, provision of congregate meals, intended to improve nutritional status, has been shown to benefit participants socially as well as nutritionally. In the absence of multidimensional assessment, the far-ranging and often unintended consequences of interventions would not be observed.

Conceptual Foundations of Multidimensional Assessment Instruments

In the understandable struggle to demonstrate the psychometric adequacy of multidimensional assessment instruments, too little attention has been paid to their differing conceptual underpinnings. Stated bluntly, selection of a specific instrument implies acceptance of the developers' view of the salient dimensions of human existence. Similarly, choice of an assessment tool also implies acceptance of the way each dimension of functioning is conceptualized. There now are several multidimensional assessment instruments with high-quality psychometric properties. It is less often recognized that the conceptual foundations of these instruments vary widely in terms of the hypothesized dimensions of well-being, the ways that specific dimensions are conceptualized, and the degree to which subjective versus objective data are elicited.

Another important conceptual issue is the intended target population(s). Some instruments were designed to assess functioning in later life; others are more broadly applicable to the adult population. Some measures were developed solely for use with community residents; a few were designed for use in long-term care facilities; even fewer apply to both community and institutional populations. Some assessment tools can be used only if study participants are capable of providing valid self-report data; others assume that information will be provided by sources other than the study participant; a few make provisions for both self-report or informant data. These differences in instrument design reflect different conceptualizations of (as well as pragmatic constraints on the measurement of) functioning and well-being. Because of the relative neglect of this issue, special attention will be paid to the theoretical underpinnings of the multidimensional assessment instruments reviewed here.

Appropriate Uses of Multidimensional Assessment Instruments

One of the strengths of multidimensional assessment tools is the claim that they are useful for both research and practice (e.g., Kane & Kane, 1981). Multidimensional assessment instruments have been used for three primary types of research problems: needs assessment, quality of life determinations, and outcome measurement in intervention studies. For the first two research traditions, the major attraction of multidimensional assessment tools is their breadth. Thus, if an investigator wants to understand the full range of potential service needs of older adults, an appropriately broad assessment tool is required. Similarly, quality of life is typically viewed as encompassing the well-being of the whole person in multiple dimensions. Multidimensional assessment instruments are used in intervention studies to capture the full range of changes that can be generated by intervention. As noted above, interventions can have ripple effects, intended or unintended and positive or negative, on dimensions of functioning other than the one that is the focus of intervention. Multidimensional assessment tools also are especially useful for studies in which the intervention is broad and nonspecific (e.g., residential relocation).

In the field of gerontology, multidimensional assessment tools have been identified as especially useful for three practice purposes: planning and targeting services, providing clinicians with a holistic view of older clients, and as screening instruments. For purposes of planning services, multidimensional assessment tools provide information about the broad range of functional dimensions relevant to service provision (e.g., social services as well as health care). For targeting services, an imperative given limited resources, multidimensional assessment can identify subgroups most in need of services and discriminate between those older persons who are and are not able to compensate for deficits in functioning via resources in other dimensions. For providing services to individuals, it has been suggested that, if clinicians can obtain broad-based information about their clients in a systematic and economical way, they can act as informal gatekeepers or case managers, providing those services for which they are responsible and referring clients for other appropriate services. Beyond the referral function, information about multiple dimensions of functioning may increase clinicians' abilities to provide the full range of services that clients need. Multidimensional assessment also may be useful for screening, identifying dimensions of functioning in which more in-depth assessment is likely to be cost effective.

A REVIEW OF SELECTED MULTIDIMENSIONAL ASSESSMENT INSTRUMENTS

In this section, six multidimensional assessment instruments are reviewed. Several criteria were used in selecting them. First, and of top priority, these six instruments are among those used most frequently; information about their psychometric properties is generally available. Thus, this set of instruments is proposed as a kind of "top echelon" of available tools. Second, these instruments were designed for multiple target populations—for both older adults and for adults of all ages, for institutional as well as community residents, for both populations capable of self-report and those for whom data must be obtained from informants. Third, and finally, the conceptual foundations and scope, as well as the intended uses, vary widely for these instruments.

The OARS Methodology

The oldest and most frequently used multidimensional assessment tool is the Older Americans Resources and Services (OARS) Methodology, developed and refined by investigators at Duke University (Pfeiffer, 1975a; Duke University Center for the Study of Aging and Human Development, 1978; Fillenbaum, 1988). The OARS Methodology includes two major instruments: the Multidimensional Functional Assessment Questionnaire (MFAQ) and the Services Assessment Questionnaire (SAQ). Only the MFAQ is considered here. The MFAQ was designed to measure multiple dimensions of functional status among older adults. Subsequent research by other investigators suggests that it can be used with adults of all ages.

The MFAQ measures functional status in five dimensions: social resources, economic resources, mental health, physical health, and self-care capacity (activities of daily living [ADLs]). The questionnaire consists of 70 questions answered by the respondent, 10 questions about the respondent to be an answered by an informant (if available), and 14 questions about the respondent answered by the interviewer. Most questions are applicable to either community or institutional residents. Alternate questions are provided for the few items that are not universally applicable. In addition, an abbreviated version of the MFAQ may be administered to a knowledgeable informant if the respondent is incapable of being interviewed. The MFAQ elicits both objective and subjective data in each of the five dimensions. Of necessity, however, the informant interview is restricted to objective information. The MFAQ was designed to be administered as an interview. Duke investigators continue to advocate the interview format, although Morris and Boutelle (1985) report successful self-administration of the MFAQ with intact older adults.

Initially, the MFAQ was used to generate interviewer-rated summary impairment ratings for all five dimensions. The summary ratings have a common metric: a scale that ranges from *excellent functioning* (1) to *totally impaired* (6). Subsequently, computerized algorithms for the summary ratings were developed (George, Landerman, & Fillenbaum, 1982).

Although the MFAQ is most identifiable when used in its entirety, several discrete scales were extracted from the MFAQ: (a) the Short Portable Mental Status Questionnaire (SPMSQ), a 10-item cognitive impairment screen (Pfeiffer, 1975b); (b) the Short Psychiatric Evaluation Schedule (SPES), a 15-item scale that includes common symptoms of functional mental disorders (Pfeiffer, 1979); and (c) two scales measuring instrumental activities of daily living (IADL) and physical activities of daily living (ADL) based on the pioneering work of Lawton and Brody (1969).

More recently, the entire MFAQ was subjected to psychometric analysis to identify subscales in all five dimensions (George et al., 1982). Exploratory factor analysis, confirmatory factor analysis, and multidimensional scaling techniques were used to identify subscales and assess their reliabilities. The analyses generated eleven subscales: three in the social resources section (Frequency of Social Interaction, Availability of Emotional and Instrumental Social Support, and Perceived Quality of Social Relationships); one in the economic resources section (Perceived Adequacy of Financial Status); five in the mental health section (the SPMSQ, Sleep Problems, Energy vs. Fatigue, Trust vs. Suspiciousness, and Life Satisfaction); one in the physical health section (Self-Perceptions of Health); and the two ADL subscales (Physical ADL and Instrumental ADL). George et al. suggest that these subscales adequately represent all the functional dimensions except physical health. Duke investigators have never advocated an abbreviated form of the MFAQ. But use of the eleven subscales with a few additional questions measuring demographic factors and income would reduce the size of the MFAQ by approximately half.

The development and initial psychometric evaluation of the MFAQ was based on three samples: (a) a 10% probability sample of community residents age 65 and older in Durham County, N.C. (n=997), (b) a sample of persons age 65 and older presenting at a geriatric clinic with multiple problems (n=98), and (c) a 20% probability sample of all nursing and rest home residents age 65 and older in Durham County (n=102). The community and institutional samples were of sufficient quality to provide norms for both summary ratings and items. Initial reliability and validity data were obtained from those samples. Interrater reliability coefficients ranged from .67 to .87 across the five dimensions of functioning (Fillenbaum & Smyer, 1981). A test-retest reliability trial indicated that, over a 5-week interval, 91% of the MFAQ item responses were identical. Two strategies were used for assessing validity. First, summary ratings for four of the five dimensions were compared to independent ratings by relevant professionals (social resources ratings were not included). Kendall's τ coefficients for the four summary ratings ranged from .60 for physical health to .83 for ADL. Second, comparisons of the three samples demonstrated the expected gradient for all five summary ratings: community residents exhibited best functioning, institutional residents exhibited the most impairment, and the clinic sample was intermediate.

Recent refinements of the MFAQ included reliability assessment. First, and most obvious, use of the computer algorithm for generating the summary ratings ensures absolute reliability. Given the absence of interviewer ratings, interrater reliability is not an issue, and meaningful comparisons across studies are ensured. Internal consistency reliability information also is available for the 11 subscales: alphas range from .52 to .87. (George & Fillenbaum, 1985).

Since its development, the MFAQ has been used by many investigators, several of whose studies provide important documentation about its properties. First, the MFAQ has been used in its entirety in two major studies: the General Accounting Office's longitudinal study of the well-being of older adults in Cleveland, Ohio (Comptroller General, 1977a; 1977b) and the Statewide Survey of Virginia's Older Adults (McAuley, Arling, Nutty, & Bowling, 1980). Those two studies, both based on probability samples of large numbers of older adults, provide additional norms for MFAQ items and summary ratings. Second, the mental health section of the MFAQ has received substantial attention. The SPMSQ has been tested as a measure of both cognitive impairment and organic brain disease. It appears that the SPMSQ is one of several useful screens for current cognitive status, but its utility as a diagnostic tool is questionable (Dalton,Pederson, Blom, & Holmes, 1987; Fillenbaum, 1980; Haglund and Schuckitt, 1976; Smyer, Hofland, & Jonas, 1979; Wolber, Romaniuk, Eastman, & Robinson, 1984). The SPES also has been examined in several studies, including administration to a large sample of Swedish twins, aged 26–86 (Gatz, Pederson, & Harris, 1987). Several investigators report identification of subscales similar to those reported in the recent refinement of the MFAQ (Gatz et al., 1987; Liang, Levin, & Krause, 1989; Haug, Belgrave, & Gratton, 1984). These studies also provide internal consistency reliability estimates for the subscales. In all cases, the reliability estimates are very high (.75 and higher).

Comprehensive Assessment and Referral Evaluation (CARE)

The CARE has a long and complex history. The original version of the CARE was developed by Gurland and colleagues for a cross-national study (United States and United Kingdom) of mental hospital admissions (Gurland et al., 1977). Later research focused on older adults in the two countries—both community-dwelling and institutionalized elderly (e.g., Gurland et al., 1979; Gurland et al., 1983). The sample for the study of mental hospital admissions had an upper age limit of 59, but the later studies and subsequent refinements were based on samples of older adults.

Originally, the CARE included 1,500 items and required 1.5-2 hours to administer. The CARE subsequently received substantial psychometric refinement, generating five new versions of differing lengths and designed for different populations and research uses (Gurland & Wilder, 1984). This review will focus on the three versions of the CARE that have been most frequently used and have received the most psychometric attention: CORE-CARE, SHORT-CARE, and IN-CARE.

The CORE-CARE. CORE-CARE consists of 314 items that comprise 22 scales: Cognitive Impairment, Depression/Demoralization, Subjective Memory Problems, Somatic Symptoms, Heart Disorder, Stroke Effects, Cancer, Respiratory Symptoms, Arthritis, Leg Problems, Sleep Disorders, Hearing Disorders, Vision Disorders, Hypertension, Ambulation Problems, Activity Limitations, Service Utilization, Financial Hardship, Dissatisfaction with Neighborhood, Fear of Crime, Social Isolation, and Retirement Dissatisfaction (Golden, Teresi, & Gurland, 1984). These subscales convey a great deal about the conceptual underpinnings of the instrument. The scope is quite comprehensive. The vast majority of the scales, however, address physical and mental health issues—and the scales conform more closely to diagnostic categories than is typical of most multidimensional tools.

The developers of CORE-CARE have carefully documented its psychometric properties. The reliability and validity assessments are based on data obtained from two probability samples of elderly community residents in New York City (*N*=445) and London (*N* = 396). Interrater reliabilities across the 22 scales range from .59 to .87 (Golden et al., 1984). Internal consistency coefficients for the 22 scales also are high; alphas range from .72 to .95.

Three strategies were used to examine validity. Construct validity was addressed by comparing CORE-CARE scale scores to (a) independent interviews with family members and (b) independent diagnostic and global ratings performed by clinicians and researchers. Correlations between CORE-CARE scale scores and family ratings ranged from .30 to .70; those between scale scores and professional ratings ranged from .40 to .75 (Teresi, Golden, Gurland, Wilder, & Bennett, 1984). Concurrent validity for the activity limitations and cognitive impairment scales was established by demonstrating that they were strongly related to two variables obtained from family members: inconvenience resulting from the older persons' limitations and plans for institutional placement (Teresi, Golden, & Gurland, 1984). Longitudinal data covering a 1-year interval were available for some sample members, permitting examination of predictive validity. First, impressive cross-time stability was observed for several scales, including Hearing, Vision, Cognitive Impairment, Health Problems, Activity Limitations, and Service Utilization. Second, several scales, as measured at Time 1, were significant predictors of mortality one year later: Cognitive Impairment, Depression, Sleep Problems, Somatic Symptoms, Health Problems, Ambulation Problems, and Activity Limitations (Teresi et al., 1984). The validity data are incomplete: Not all of the 22 scales were included in the validity analyses, and no cutpoints are provided for the scale scores. The last issue is important because the scales vary widely in metric. Relative to many assessment tools, however, the validity data for CORE-CARE are impressive.

CORE-CARE has been used in a variety of subsequent studies, yielding additional reliability estimates. Cohen and Rajkowski (1982) used CORE-CARE in a study of older single-room occupancy hotel (SRO) residents. Internal consistency reliability coefficients in that sample ranged from .28 to .89, although only two scales had alphas of less than .60. In a sample of 704 Hispanic elderly in Los Angeles County, internal consistency coefficients for the 22 scales ranged from .49 to .94 (Lopez-Aqueres, Kemp, Plopper, Staples, & Brummel-Smith, 1984). Holmes et al. (1989) used CORE-CARE in a study of 269 functionally impaired elderly residing in 53 Israeli kibbutzim. They report reliability coefficients ranging from .59 to .93 for 14 of the 22 scales.

The SHORT-CARE. SHORT-CARE is an abbreviated form of CARE, in both scope and length (Gurland, Golden, Teresi, & Challop, 1984). It includes six scales from CORE-CARE (Cognitive Impairment, Depression/Demoralization, Subjective Memory Problems, Somatic Symptoms, Sleep Disorders, and Activity Limitations), plus additional items that are used for diagnostic purposes. SHORT-CARE focuses on three issues: dementia, depression, and disability.

Items from the six CORE-CARE scales are rearranged to yield three new scales: Depression/Demoralization, Dementia, and Disability. The additional items, unique to SHORT-CARE, are used with scale items, to generate what Gurland et al. call "operational diagnoses" for pervasive depression and pervasive dementia. SHORT-CARE scales and diagnoses were developed using the samples of community-dwelling older adults in the United States and United Kingdom described above.

Reliability and validity assessment was performed separately for the SHORT-CARE scales and operational diagnoses. For the scales, interrater reliability coefficients were quite high (.94 for depression, .76 for dementia, and .91 for disability). Internal consistency reliability coefficients for the three scales were .75, .64, and .81, respectively. Internal reliability coefficients for the two diagnoses are .90 for depression and .88 for dementia. SHORT-CARE validity was assessed using the same general strategies described above for the CORE-CARE. Validity coefficients for both the scales and diagnoses are acceptable, although they are somewhat higher for the diagnoses.

Gurland and colleagues (Gurland et al., 1988) later used SHORT-CARE in a randomized clinical trial of treatment of systolic hypertension among older adults. In that study, internal consistency reliability coefficients ranged from .51 to .84 at baseline and from .64 to .84 at follow-up interviews a year later. Interrater reliability estimates ranged from .66 to .96. Spagnoli, Foresti, MacDonald, & Williams (1986) used the SHORT-CARE Dementia and Depression scales in a study of nursing home residents in Milan, Italy. They report interrater reliability coefficients of .96 and .83 for Dementia and Depression, respectively. Spagnoli and colleagues also performed validity analyses, comparing scale scores for dementia and depression with clinical assessments. They report good sensitivity and excellent specificity and positive predictive values for both scales. The cutpoints they used for these assessments, however, are unclear.

The SHORT-CARE is interesting because it is more than simply an abbreviated version of CORE-CARE. Gurland and colleagues' clinical orientation is especially obvious in SHORT-CARE's operational diagnoses. As is true of the CORE-CARE scales, SHORT-CARE's scales and diagnoses lack cutpoints. The authors note that this is a problem, but prefer to let cutpoint decisions be made by each investigator. They demonstrate that the choice of cutpoint involves trade-offs (e.g., of sensitivity for specificity). Nonetheless, the absence of standard cutpoints makes comparisons difficult across studies and populations.

IN-CARE. IN-CARE is designed for assessing older adults in institutional settings. I have found only one description of IN-CARE by its developers (Gurland et al., 1979). Because it was written before the published CARE revisions in 1984, I am not sure that description applies to the most recent version of IN-CARE. As described in Gurland et al. (1979), IN-CARE is a hierarchical instrument designed to accommodate populations in which significant proportions of members cannot report information for all or some of the scales in CORE-CARE. IN-CARE begins with a screen that covers several topics: cognitive impairment, current health, self-care capacity, reasons for admission, and the ability to follow simple commands. Performance on the screening interview leads to one of four protocols: an extended interview; a shorter interview, focused on physical health and psychiatric symptoms (for those who are cognitively intact, but too frail to tolerate the full interview); a performance test of ADL-related tasks (given to those too impaired to be interviewed but capable of following simple commands); or cessation of testing. The reliability and validity data accompanying for the 1979 description of IN-CARE are difficult to interpret because of the instrument's hierarchical form.

IN-CARE has been used in some recent research. In a comparison of demented nursing home residents who were and were not placed in special care units, Holmes et al. (1990) report that alphas for the IN-CARE scales range from .59 to .95. In a study evaluating the effectiveness of a nursing intervention in long-term care facilities, Teresi et al. (1993) report internal consistency reliability coefficients of .56 to .98 for the affect scales, .63 to .89 for the behavior scales, and .63 to .70 for the chart review measure.

Despite the limited information available, IN-CARE is an interesting instrument. Its hierarchical format offers one strategy for maximizing the information available from frail and/or impaired older adults. It is not clear, however, that IN-CARE should be used exclusively for institutional populations. Although the percentage is lower than in institutions, a nontrivial proportion of community-dwelling older adults are too impaired to participate in traditional interviews. This leads to questions about CORE-CARE and SHORT-CARE as well: It is not clear, based on available publications, how data are obtained from or about respondents with severe cognitive or physical impairments.

Multilevel Assessment Instrument (MAI). The Multilevel Assessment Instrument (MAI) was developed by Lawton and associates at the Philadelphia Geriatric Center (Lawton, Moss, Fulcomer, & Kleban, 1982). The MAI measures functioning in seven dimensions: Physical Health, Cognition, ADL, Time Use, Social Interaction, Personal Adjustment (which includes both mental health symptoms and life satisfaction), and Perceptions of the Environment. Each dimension includes both objective and subjective questions. Each dimension yields a summary rating scale ranging from *worst functioning* (1) to *best functioning* (5) and subscales. The subscales can be scored by hand or by computer. The full-length MAI includes 135 items and requires 50 minutes, on average, for administration.

Lawton et al. (1982) credit the OARS MFAQ as the springboard for the MAI. Their conceptualization of the salient dimensions of functioning and well-being differ somewhat from those in the MFAQ: Several MFAQ dimensions have been disaggregated into discrete domains (e.g., cognition is separated from other mental health issues), and two MAI dimensions—time use and environmental perceptions—are not in the MFAQ. Unlike the MFAQ, however, the MAI does not include an economic resources dimension, although it includes a single item measuring income.

Three criterion groups were used in refining and testing the psychometric properties of the MAI. One group consisted of older adults living independently in the community: 253 older adults living in 5 census tracts in Philadelphia and 173 tenants from 11 public housing sites in Philadelphia. The second group consisted of 99 older adults who were receiving high-intensity in-home services from a family services or homemaker agency. The third group included 65 older adults who were waiting for admission to nursing homes. Although these samples do not generate population norms, they are heterogeneous and appropriate for psychometric assessment of the MAI.

Reliability testing of the MAI was extensive. Interrater reliability was tested for the summary rating scales of the seven dimensions. Results indicated that 95% of the paired ratings exhibited no difference or only 1-point difference; intraclass correlations ranged from .58 to .88. Test-retest reliability was assessed over a 3-week interval and ranged from .73 to .95 for the seven dimensions. Internal consistency reliability for the seven domains is high; alphas ranged from .71 to .93. Validity was assessed using two primary strategies. First, correlations between the criterion variable and ratings for the seven domains ranged from .05 to .54. Second, MAI scores correlated from .23 to .69 with the independent and blinded ratings of experts. Reliability and validity information also is available for the subscales within the seven dimensions (Lawton et al., 1982).

Lawton et al. (1982) offer four forms of the MAI: the full version, to which all information presented above applies; a middle version (38 items); a short version (24 items); and a "best item" for each of the seven dimensions. The middle and short versions generate scores for the seven domains in the full MAI. Reliability and validity data for those forms differ surprisingly little from those for the full MAI. I am not impressed with single-item approaches to assessment, even when the single item is the best item. But the middle and short forms of the MAI appear quite useful; scope is retained while length is abbreviated, with little evidence of high psychometric costs.

Like most multidimensional assessment tools, the MAI lends itself to extraction of specific scales. The major impact of the MAI on research to date appears to be in the use of extracted scales (e.g., Lawton, Kleban, Moss, Rovine, & Glicksman, 1989; Pruchno, Kleban, Michaels, & Dempsey, 1990; Young & Kahana, 1989). Given its quality, however, I view the MAI as an attractive multidimensional assessment instrument.

Iowa Self-Assessment Inventory (ISAI). The Iowa Self-Assessment Inventory is one of the shortest multidimensional assessment tools available. It was developed by Morris and Buckwalter (1988), who wanted their instrument to have several characteristics: (a) it would be brief, (b) it could be self-administered, and (c) it would focus exclusively on subjective perceptions of well-being. The ISAI has been revised (Morris et al., 1990; Morris, Buckwalter, Cleary, Gilmer, & Andrews,1992); the current form includes a 5-item section eliciting demographic characteristics and 56 items tapping seven domains: Economic Resources, Emotional Balance, Physical Health, Trusting Others, Mobility, Cognitive Status, and Social Support. The ISAI is easily administered and scored and takes only 15 minutes, on average, to complete.

Several samples were used for the development, refinement, and psychometric assessment of the ISAI. Two primary samples were used to refine the instrument to its current form: 1,153 older adults recruited from community service sites and 420 respondents recruited later from similar service programs. These are samples of convenience and their results cannot be viewed as population norms. Moreover, the authors acknowledge that their samples included few urban residents and very few nonwhites (Morris et al., 1990).

Factor analysis was used to reduce the original 120-item ISAI to its present form and to create subscales that are empirically homogeneous and conceptually clear. Psychometric assessment to date has been limited. Internal consistency reliability coefficients for the seven scales are high: alphas range from .74 to .86. Test-retest reliability information has not been reported. Of most concern is the limited information concerning validity. At this point, the only claims to validity are expected correlations between ISAI scale scores and demographic variables (Morris et al., 1990).

The ISAI is an instrument in progress. To date, its originators have focused on its development and refinement, rather than applications demonstrating its utility. The ISAI is applicable to only the most functional members of the older population. The exclusively subjective nature of the scales also limits its uses. On the other hand, ISAI developers have devoted 5 years to its development. We must hope that they will demonstrate the unique role that this kind of multidimensional assessment tool offers to aging research and practice.

Medical Outcomes Study (MOS) Measures. The Medical Outcomes Study is a large, quasi-experimental research project, designed to examine the impact of variations in physician practice styles and differing models of health care delivery on patient outcomes (Tarlov et al., 1989). In addition to more traditional outcomes, such as mortality and lab results, MOS investigators wished to examine patient-centered outcomes including functional capacity and perceptions of health. This led to the development of the MOS measures, a set of instruments of varying lengths, conceptualized to elicit information about 12 dimensions of functioning and well-being: Physical Functioning, Mobility, Role Functioning, Social Functioning, Psychological Distress/Well-Being, Cognitive Functioning, Health Perceptions, Health Distress, Energy/Fatigue, Sleep, Pain, and Physical/Psychophysiologic Symptoms.

There are four primary MOS measures: the full, 149-item MOS Functioning and Well-Being Profile (MOSFWBP), which includes 35 scales and eight summary indices; the 113-item MOS Functioning and Well-Being Profile—Core Subset (MOSFWBP-C), which contains 20 scales and four summary indexes; the 36-item MOS Short Form (SF-36), which generates 8 scale scores; and the MOS 6-item General Health Survey, which includes one item each from six dimensions in the MOSFWBP (Stewart et al., 1992; Ware & Sherbourne, 1992). Although MOS developers originally proposed a 20-item short form, they now recommend the SF-36 instead (Ware & Sherbourne, 1992; McHorney, Ware, & Raczek, 1993; McHorney, Ware, Rogers, Raczek, & Lu, 1992). Two MOS measures will be reviewed here: the MOSFWBP and the SF-36.

The sampling scheme for the MOS is very complex; it involves five stages, ranging from selection of geographic sites and health care settings to specific physicians and their patients (Rogers et al., 1992). For our purposes, it is sufficient to note that more than 11,000 patients (adults aged 18 and older) participated in the screening stage and approximately 3,000 completed the baseline assessment; a smaller subset of patients, sampled to represent specific health conditions, were assessed longitudinally. It should be kept in mind that all study participants were patients in the health care system.

Psychometric assessment of the MOSFWBP was extensive and complex; detailed information is available elsewhere (Hays & Stewart, 1990, 1992). In brief, internal consistency reliability coefficients for the scales in the MOSFWBP range from .63 to .98. Validity assessments included predictive validity, multitrait scaling, and, especially, construct validity assessment. The primary focus of the validity assessment was determination of the major dimensions underlying MOSFWBP items. The investigators conclude that two primary constructs underlie the item pool: Physical Health and Mental Health.

The SF-36 assesses eight dimensions of functioning and well-being: Physical Limitations, Role Limitations due to Physical Health Problems, Social Functioning, Pain, Psychological Distress/Well-being, Role Limitations due to Emotional Problems, Energy and Fatigue, and General Health Perceptions. It also includes a single item tapping respondents' perceptions of change in health (Ware & Sherbourne, 1992). Validity assessment of the SF-36 is based on analysis of criterion groups determined by type (physical vs. mental) and severity of illness. Results reported by McHorney et al. (1993) support the ability of the SF-36 subscales to discriminate among patient groups in a meaningful manner. Another validity study (McHorney et al., 1992) compares the short and long forms of the MOS and COOP charts, which yield functional status ratings based on review of medical records (e.g., Nelson, Wasson, & Kirk, 1987), again with criterion groups used as the basis of assessment. Results indicate that the long form of the MOS performs better than both the SF-36 and the Dartmouth Primary Care Cooperative Information (COOP) charts.

The MOS is receiving substantial attention as a new approach to multidimensional functional assessment. Information to date is impressive but incomplete regarding its validity and testing characteristics, although its developers are refreshingly explicit concerning limitations and the costs of using the short rather than long form of the MOS (lower validity and poorer performance in longitudinal analyses). Information also is lacking about the degree to which MOS scales perform equally as well for older adults as for young and middle-aged adults—age norms are not available. It also is important that the conceptual foundations of the MOS be recognized; more than most multidimensional assessment tools, the MOS focuses specifically on illness.

Minimum Data Set (MDS). The Omnibus Budget Reconciliation Act of 1987 (OBRA) mandated the development of a national resident assessment tool for use in nursing facilities. In response to this congressional mandate, the Health Care Financing Administration convened a panel of experts to develop and test such an assessment tool, resulting in the Minimum Data Set (MDS) for Resident Assessment and Care Screening (Morris et al., 1990). A two-stage field test was performed. Analysis of data from the first-stage MDS resulted in substantial revision of the instrument to reduce length and increase reliability. Interestingly, the major article describing the development of the MDS, which provides the revised MDS in its entirety, has reliability coefficients for some of the scales in the original version but provides no information about reliability of the revised MDS beyond the statement that it is "much improved." Validity information is not presented.

The MDS is organized in 16 sections that presumably represent its conceptual underpinnings: identification and background information, cognitive patterns, communication/hearing patterns, vision patterns, physical functioning and structural problems (including ADLs), continence, psychological well-being, mood and behavior problems, activity pursuit patterns, disease diagnoses, health conditions, oral/nutritional status, oral/dental status, skin condition, medication use, and special treatments and procedures. The MDS clearly focuses primarily on illness; psychosocial dimensions of functioning are largely ignored. The MDS is designed to be completed by a health care provider, typically a nurse. It requires about 90 minutes for completion.

The MDS is one component of a larger, two-part system, called the Resident Assessment Instrument, that is designed to meet OBRA requirements. The MDS is the primary screening and assessment tool. The other component of the system consists of Resident Assessment Protocols (RAPs; Morris et al., 1991), which are used to identify problems in need of treatment and link those problems to care plan guidelines and goals. Specific MDS items trigger the need for RAPs. This review is limited to the MDS per se.

Given the impetus for its development, it is not surprising that the MDS has had little psychometric assessment beyond the ability of nursing staff to complete the assessment forms reliably. However, it has already become, by federal mandate, a major assessment and data collection tool for nursing home populations. Its research potential is less clear. Moreover, its most likely contribution to aging research may be its provision of a database of nursing home patients rather than an assessment tool that is used in other research projects. Research based on the MDS database is already available (e.g., Riter & Fries, 1992; Ensberg, Paletta, Galecki, Dacko, & Fries, 1993). The potential of a very large MDS database has already generated divergent reviews from the research community. Kane (1990) praises the potential value of the database for both research and practice, whereas Teresi and Holmes (1992) are less enthusiastic about its research potential because of important methodological limitations of both the MDS itself and, especially, the uncontrolled conditions under which it is used. For the moment, my evaluation is closer to that of Teresi and Holmes. In its present form, the MDS is suitable for some research purposes, especially those that focus on service utilization. If it is to be useful for other research purposes, however, careful psychometric assessment is required. Beyond the instrument itself, the MDS database must be used with great caution: The overall quality of the data and the comparability of data from different nursing homes remains unclear and suspect.

Selecting a Multidimensional Assessment Instrument

As the above reviews demonstrate, several high-quality multidimensional assessment tools are available to the gerontological research and practice communities. These instruments offer users a variety of conceptualizations of the salient dimensions of functioning and well-being, tools of varying lengths and complexity, and tools with varying, but usually satisfactory, evidence of psychometric adequacy. In this section, major issues of concern when selecting a multidimensional assessment instrument are briefly considered.

Evidence of reliability and validity is always a major issue in selection of measurement tools. Reflecting my selection criteria in choosing instruments to be reviewed, the psychometric adequacy of the six instruments considered here is quite high. With the exception of the MDS, all of the instruments reviewed are of good to excellent reliability. Validity data are available—and satisfactory—for most measures as well. Validity data for the OARS MFAQ, various versions of the CARE, and MAI are quite impressive. A large quantity of validity data have been described by the developers of the MOS, especially for its full form. But I do not find MOS validity analyses, based primarily on multidimensional scaling techniques, as compelling as the predictive and criterion group validity strategies that figured prominantly in the validity assessments of the OARS MFAQ, CARE instruments, and MAI. Both the ISAI and MDS are more recent measures for which the absence of validity data appears to reflect the state of instrument development to date. If those measures are to gain respect in the research community, rigorous validity analyses will be needed.

Sensitivity to change is the one psychometric property upon which all six measures can be faulted. Information about sensitivity to change is scant or nonexistent for all six multidimensional assessment tools. Several of the measures have been used in longitudinal studies in which change is observed over time. But such evidence tells us little about the magnitude of change in the individual that is needed to generate changes in scale scores of the various instruments. The lack of documentation regarding sensitivity to change is especially troublesome for investigators who wish to select a multidimensional assessment tool as the outcome measure in an intervention study.

A major factor that should be used in selecting a multidimensional assessment measure is its conceptual foundation. The six instruments reviewed above differ widely in the number, discreteness, and content of the dimensions of functioning assessed. The OARS MFAQ has the smallest number of dimensions, although the availability of multiple scales within the five dimensions offers the investigator a number of more fine-grained and discrete measures, if desired. In contrast, the CORE-CARE, full MOS battery, and MDS have large numbers of dimensions that measure highly specific facets of functioning. They also tend to be more clinically oriented measures than the OARS MFAQ, MAI, and ISAI. In general, the clinically oriented measures focus on narrowly defined dimensions that correspond to diagnostic or syndromal classification systems. In contrast, the OARS MFAQ and MAI focus more specifically on functioning per se, with little attempt to link functioning to etiologic or diagnostic issues. Ironically, although the clinically oriented tools measure larger numbers of discrete areas of functioning, they are not more conceptually comprehensive than the tools that measure fewer functional dimensions. Indeed, I judge the OARS MFAQ and MAI to be the most comprehensive in terms of eliciting information about the full range of salient dimensions of functioning. Both of those measures are superior to the others in measuring social functioning. Beyond that, the OARS MFAQ includes a solid battery measuring both objective economic resources and perceptions of their adequacy and the MAI includes a dimension that elicits information about perceptions of the environment within which the respondent functions.

Another important conceptual difference among multidimensional assessment instruments is the degree to which they focus on relatively objective data about the respondent, subjective perceptions of the respondent, or both. The ISAI is restricted to subjective perceptions of well-being. Because it was designed to be completed by nursing staff in long-term care facilities, the MDS focuses almost exclusively on objective data. The other instruments include both objective and subjective data, although it appears that only the OARS MFAQ and MAI were constructed specifically to include paired objective and subjective measures of the same facets of functioning. In both the CARE and MOS instruments, many of the subjective items are used specifically for assessing clinical concepts such as depression, demoralization, and psychological distress. Psychosocial research has long documented that the relationships between objective data and subjective perceptions of the same phenomena are typically modest. Therefore, investigators should carefully consider the degree to which they desire objective data, subjective perceptions, or both when selecting a multidimensional assessment tool.

Finally, practical considerations play a critical role in selection of a multidimensional assessment measure. From a practical point of view, the options open to investigators are most limited when they wish to study the full range of functional status in the older population (i.e., both physically robust and physically frail, both cognitively intact and cognitively impaired, or both community and institutional residents). Two of the instruments reviewed here are quite limited with regard to the proportion of the older population with which they can be used. By design, the ISAI is applicable only to cognitively intact older adults. Also by design, the MDS is applicable only to institutional residents. There is no evidence that the MOS measures, or parts of them, can be administered to proxy informants when respondents are too cognitively impaired to participate in an interview. The OARS MFAQ, MAI, and CARE instruments offer more options in this regard. The MFAQ includes special instructions for use with nursing home residents and persons too cognitively impaired to provide reliable self-report data. In addition, the reliability and validity assessments performed by developers of the OARS included data from nursing home residents and severely cognitively impaired older persons. Both the overall ratings and discrete scales in the MFAQ include coding instructions that accommodate these variations in administration. Similar options are available with the MAI. A different approach was used for the CARE: a separate instrument, the IN-CARE, was developed for use with institutional residents. Although the IN-CARE is an interesting and apparently high-quality instrument, it does not generate scores comparable to those yielded by the CORE-CARE or SHORT-CARE. Consequently, it is not clear that the CARE can be used to generate comparable information about community and institutional residents.

UNRESOLVED ISSUES AND FUTURE PROSPECTS

Although several high-quality multidimensional assessment instruments are available, important issues remain unresolved. In addition, multidimensional assessment tools have had less impact on research and practice than might have been expected or hoped.

Although many methodological issues have been addressed well by the developers of multidimensional assessment instruments, one way of better understanding their strengths and weaknesses has been ignored: administering several instruments to the same sample. For example, Andrews and Withey (1976) administered multiple measures of subjective well-being to the same samples, generating specific information about how the various measures "stack up" against each other. This kind of "head-to-head" comparison has not been performed with multidimensional assessment tools. There are understandable reasons for this omission. Most important, because multidimensional assessment instruments are long and time consuming, there would be significant practical problems in conducting a study in which several tools are administered to the same subjects. Nevertheless, valuable information would be gained by empirical comparisons of instruments such as the OARS MFAQ, MAI, CARE, and MOSFWBP.

Investigators often use combinations of discrete scales in lieu of a single multidimensional assessment tool. Opting for combinations of scales from multiple sources rather than a single multidimensional assessment instrument is ultimately an uninformed decision, however. Information is unavailable about the costs and benefits of using a variety of scales versus use of a multidimensional functional assessment tool. Again, the time and financial resources required have undoubtedly been obstacles to such comparative studies.

Although additional information is always desirable, I do not believe that methodological concerns are the major reason that multidimensional assessment instruments are used infrequently. The primary issue, I think, is that the developers and advocates of multidimensional assessment have failed to convince researchers and practitioners that the investments of professional time and energy required to administer such instruments are worth the payoff. Bluntly, we haven't made a compelling case for the widespread use of multidimensional assessment tools. Logical and abstract arguments abound concerning the benefits of multidimensional assessment. But compelling data are lacking. To date, we have not demonstrated that researchers cannot afford to neglect any major dimension of functioning. And we certainly have not convinced clinicians and practitioners that they can better serve older patients and clients if they use standardized multidimensional assessment. I know from personal experience that suggesting to clinicians that an instrument requiring 45–60 minutes to administer might be used as a screening tool to trigger in-depth clinical evaluation of problems generates groans rather than excitement. When clinicians use the term "screening tool," they want an instrument that takes 5 minutes, not an hour.

One of the characteristics of the multidimensional assessment tools reviewed here is that they are based on self-report data (of respondents or of an informed proxy). The only exception to this statement is one of the four forms of IN-CARE, which focuses on performance of ADL-related tasks in response to simple commands. During the past few years, interest in performance-based rather than self-report measures of functioning has increased dramatically (e.g., Guralnik, Branch, Cummings, & Curb, 1989; Reuben & Siu, 1990; Mahurin, DeBettignies, & Pirozzolo, 1991; Tinetti, 1986; Klein & Bell, 1982). Guralnik et al. (1989) suggest that performance-based measures may have several advantages over self-report measures: patient acceptability, validity, reliability, and sensitivity to change. Although this issue is relevant to only certain dimensions of functioning, especially ADL capacity, preferences for performance measures could lead investigators away from multidimensional assessment tools that include only self-report data.

Although definitive evidence remains unavailable, studies that include head to head comparisons fail to find performance measures superior to self-report data (Myers, Holliday, Harvey, & Hutchinson, 1993; Reuben, Siu, & Kimpau, 1992). As Myers and colleagues note, however, the central issue is not the overall superiority of performance versus self-report measures but rather delineation of the research and clinical purposes for which each measurement strategy is best suited. For example, self-report measures may be more acceptable to research subjects and better reflect the experience of impaired functioning among cognitively intact respondents, whereas performance measures may be a preferred strategy for use with cognitively impaired respondents. Continuing efforts to better understand the relative advantages and disadvantages of performance versus self-report measures will probably be a major focus of research during the next few years.

Semantic problems also seem to muddy the waters when researchers and clinicians discuss comprehensive assessment. Researchers tend to equate comprehensive assessment with multidimensional assessment tools. For clinicians, the term connotes in-depth diagnostic assessment by health professionals with specialized training and experience. (For a cogent and thoughtful review of geriatric assessment from a clinical perspective, see Cohen & Feussner, 1989). An example of this semantic difference can be seen in the editorial by Calkins (1985), written in response to a paper about the OARS Methodology (George & Fillenbaum, 1985). Calkins' editorial usefully explicates the convergences and divergences between multidimensional assessment, as that term is typically used, and geriatric assessment as linked to the medical model.

In all areas—research, policy, and practice—time pressures are an obstacle to use of multidimensional assessment tools. Research teams argue about what can be included in their data collection efforts item by item. Policy makers want to define poverty, disability, and other important concepts using the fewest items possible. Under existing reimbursement systems, clinicians must see multiple patients per hour to make a living—a problem likely to be exacerbated in an era of managed care. These pressures lead to "bare bones" data collection for which multidimensional assessment tools are poor candidates. The developers of such tools often respond by offering very abbreviated versions of their instruments, sometimes offering one best item for each dimension. The desire to provide abbreviated instruments is understandable, but the methodological quality of some of these "mini" tools is questionable. By definition, they lack the comprehensiveness that is the hallmark of multidimensional assessment.

Several high-quality multidimensional assessment tools are available, but availability does not ensure use or growth of knowledge based on those tools. If multidimensional assessments are to secure a productive place in gerontological research and practice, efforts are required to demonstrate that their benefits equal or exceed their costs. This is the next step for advocates of multidimensional assessment instruments; it is both a vital and an urgent one.

REFERENCES

Andrews, F. M., & Withey, S. B. (1976). *Social indicators of well-being*. New York: Plenum.

Calkins, E. (1985). OARS methodology and the "medical model." *Journal of the American Geriatrics Society, 33*, 648–649.

Cohen, C., & Rajkowski, H. (1982). What's in a friend? Substantive and theoretical issues. *The Gerontologist, 22*, 261–266.

Cohen, H. J., & Feussner, J. R. (1989). Comprehensive geriatric assessment: Mission not yet accomplished. *Journals of Gerontology: Medical Sciences, 44*, M175–M177.

Comptroller General. (1977a). *The well-being of older people in Cleveland, Ohio*. Washington, DC: U.S. General Accounting Office.

Comptroller General. (1977b) *Home health—The need for a national policy to better provide for the elderly*. Washington, DC: U.S. General Accounting Office.

Dalton, J. E., Pederson, S. L., Blom, B. E., & Holmes, N. R. (1987). Diagnostic errors using the Short Portable Mental Status Questionnaire with a mixed clinical population. *Journal of Gerontology, 42*, 512–514.

Duke University Center for the Study of Aging and Human Development. (1978). *Multidimensional functional assessment: The OARS Methodology* (2nd ed.). Durham. NC: Author.

Ensberg, M. D., Paletta, M. J., Galecki, A. T., Dacko, C. L., & Fries, B. E. (1993). Identifying elderly patients for early discharge after hospitalization for hip fracture. *Journals of Gerontology: Medical Sciences, 48*, M187–M195.

Fillenbaum, G. G. (1980). Comparison of two brief tests of organic brain impairment, the MSQ and the Short Portable MSQ. *Journal of the American Geriatrics Society, 28*, 381–384.

Fillenbaum, G. G. (1988). *Multidimensional functional assessment of older adults*. Hillsdale, NJ: Erlbaum.

Fillenbaum, G. G., & Smyer, M. A. (1981). The development, validity, and reliability of the OARS Multidimensional Functional Assessment Questionnaire. *Journal of Gerontology, 36*, 428–434.

Gatz, M., Pederson, N. L., & Harris, J. (1987). Measurement characteristics of the mental health scale from the OARS. *Journal of Gerontology, 42*, 332–335.

George, L. K., & Fillenbaum, G. G. (1985). The OARS Methodology: A decade of experience in geriatric assessment. *Journal of the American Geriatrics Society, 33*, 607–615.

George, L. K., Landerman R., & Fillenbaum, G. G. (1982). *Developing measures of functional status and service utilization: Refining and extending the OARS Methodology*. Durham, NC: Duke University Center for the Study of Aging and Human Development.

Golden, R. R., Teresi, J. A., & Gurland, B. J. (1984). Development of indicator scales for the Comprehensive Assessment and Referral Evaluation (CARE) Interview Schedule. *Journals of Gerontology, 39*, 138–146.

Guralnik, J. M., Branch, L. G., Cummings, S. R., & Curb, J. D. (1989). Physical performance measures in aging research. *Journals of Gerontology: Medical Sciences, 44*, M141–M146.

Gurland, B., Copeland, J., Kelleher, M., Kuriansky, J., Sharpe, L., & Dean, L. (1983). *The mind and mood of aging: The mental health problems of the community elderly in New York and London*. New York: Haworth.

Gurland, B., Cross, P., Defiguerido, J., Shannon, M., Mann, A. H., Jenkins, R., Bennett, R., Wilder, D., Wright, H., Killeffer, E., Godlove, C., Thompson, P., Ross, M., & Deming, W. E. (1979). A cross-national comparison of the institutionalized elderly in the cities of New York and London. *Psychological Medicine*, *9*, 781–788.

Gurland, B., Golden, R. R., Teresi, J. A., & Challop, J. (1984). The SHORT-CARE: An efficient instrument for the assessment of depression, dementia, and disability. *Journal of Gerontology*, *39*, 166–169.

Gurland, B., Kuriansky, J., Sharpe, L., Simon, R., Stiller, P., & Birkett, P. (1977). The Comprehensive Assessment and Referral Evaluation (CARE): Rationale, development, and reliability. *International Journal of Aging and Human Development*, *8*, 9–42.

Gurland, B. J., Teresi, J., Smith, W. M., Black, D., Hughes, G., & Edlavitch, S. (1988). Effects of treatment for isolated systolic hypertension on cognitive status and depression in the elderly. *Journal of the American Geriatrics Society*, *36*, 1015–1022.

Gurland, B. J., & Wilder, D. E. (1984). The CARE interview revisited: Development of an efficient, systematic, clinical assessment. *Journal of Gerontology*, *39*, 129–137.

Haglund, R. M. J., & Schuckitt, M. A. (1976). A clinical comparison of tests of organicity in elderly patients. *Journal of Gerontology*, *31*, 654–659.

Haug, M., Belgrave, L. L., & Gratton, B. (1984). Mental health in the elderly: Factors in stability and change. *Journal of Health and Social Behavior*, *25*, 100–115.

Hays, R. D., & Stewart, A. L. (1990). The structure of self-reported health in chronic disease patients. *Psychological Assessment: A Journal of Consulting and Clinical Psychology*, *2*, 22–30.

Hays, R. D., & Stewart, A. L. (1992). Construct validity of the MOS health measures. In A.L. Stewart & J. E. Ware, Jr. (Eds.), *Measuring functioning and well-being* (pp. 325–344). Durham, NC: Duke University Press.

Holmes, D., Teresi, J., Holmes, M., Bergman, S., King, Y., & Bentur, N. (1989). Informal versus formal supports for impaired elderly people: Determinants of choice on Israeli kibbutzim. *The Gerontologist*, *29*, 195–202.

Holmes, D., Teresi, J., Weiner, A., Monaco, C., Ronch, J., & Vickers, R. (1990). Impacts associated with special care units in long-term care facilities. *The Gerontologist*, *30*, 178–183.

Kane, R. L. (1990). Standardized assessment as a means rather than an end. *The Gerontologist*, *30*, 291–292.

Kane, R. A., & Kane, R. L. (1981). *Assessing the elderly*. Lexington, MA: Lexington Books.

Klein, R. M., & Bell, B. (1982). Self-care skills: Behavioral measurement with Klein-Bell ADL Scale. *Archives of Physical Medicine and Rehabilitation*, *63*, 335–338.

Lawton, M. P., & Brody, E. M. (1969). Assessment of older people: Self-maintaining and instrumental activities of daily living. *The Gerontologist*, *9*, 179–186.

Lawton, M. P., Kleban, M. H., Moss, M., Rovine, M., & Glicksman, A. (1989). Measuring caregiver appraisal. *Journals of Gerontology: Psychological Sciences*, *44*, P61–P71.

Lawton, M. P., Moss, M., Fulcomer, M., & Kleban, M.H. (1982). A research and service-oriented multilevel assessment instrument. *Journal of Gerontology*, *37*, 91–99.

Liang, J., Levin, J. S., & Krause, N. M. (1989). Dimensions of the OARS mental health measures. *Journals of Gerontology: Psychological Sciences, 44*, P127–P138.

Lopez-Aqueres, W., Kemp, B., Plopper, M., Staples, F. R., & Brummel-Smith, K. (1984). Health needs of Hispanic elderly. *Journal of the American Geriatrics Society, 32*, 191–198.

Mahurin, R. K., DeBettignies, B. H., & Pirozzolo, F. J. (1991). Structured assessment of independent living skills: Preliminary report of a performance measure of functional abilities in dementia. *Journals of Gerontology: Psychological Sciences, 46*, P58–P66.

McAuley, W. J., Arling, G., Nutty, C. L., & Bowling, C. A. (1980). *Final report of the statewide survey of older Virginians*. Richmond, VA: Virginia Center on Aging.

McHorney, C. A., Ware, J. E. Jr., & Raczek, A. B. (1993). The MOS 36-item Short-Form Health Survey (SF-36): II. Psychometric and clinical tests of valdidity in measuring physical and mental health constructs. *Medical Care, 31*, 247–263.

McHorney, C. A., Ware, J. E. Jr., Rogers, W., Raczek, A. E., & Lu, J. F. R. (1992). The validity and relative precision of MOS short- and long-form health status scales and Dartmouth COOP charts. *Medical Care, 30*, MS253–MS265.

Morris, J. N., Hawes, C., Fries, B. E., Phillips, C. D., Mor, V., Katz, S., Murphy, K., Drugovitch, M. L., & Friedlob, A.S. (1990). Designing the National Resident Assessment Instrument for Nursing Homes. *The Gerontologist, 30*, 293–307.

Morris, J. N., Hawes, C., Murphy, K., Nonemaker, S., Phillips, C., Fries, B. E., & Mor, V. (1991). *Resident Assessment Instrument training manual and resource guide*. Natick, MA: Eliot Press.

Morris, W. W., & Boutelle, S. (1985). Multidimensional functional assessment in two modes. *The Gerontologist, 25*, 638–643.

Morris, W. W., & Buckwalter, K. C. (1988). Functional assessment of the elderly: The Iowa Self-Assessment Inventory. In C. F. Waltz & O. L. Strickland (Eds.), *Measurement of nursing outcomes, Vol. 1: Measuring client outcomes* (pp. 328–351). New York: Springer.

Morris, W. W., Buckwalter, K. C., Cleary, T. A., Gilmer, J. S., & Andrews, P. H. (1992). The development and use of the Iowa Self-Assessment Inventory (ISAI). In B. Vellas & J. L. Albarede (Eds.), *Facts and research in gerontology*, (pp. 203–209). New York: Springer.

Morris, W. W., Buckwalter, K. C., Cleary, T. A., Gilmer, J. S., Hatz, D. L., & Studer, M. (1990). Refinement of the Iowa Self-Assessment Inventory. *The Gerontologist, 20*, 243–248.

Myers, A. M., Holliday, P. J., Harvey, K. A., & Hutchinson, K.S. (1993). Functional performance measures: Are they superior to self-assessments? *Journals of Gerontology: Medical Sciences, 48*, M196–M206.

Nelson, E. C., Wasson, J., & Kirk, J. (1987). Assessment of function in routine clinical practice: Description of the COOP chart method and preliminary findings. *Journal of Chronic Disease, 40*, (Suppl.), 55S–78S.

Pfeiffer, E. (Ed.) (1975a). *Multidimensional functional assessment: The OARS Methodology* (1st ed.). Durham, NC: Duke University Center for the Study of Aging and Human Development.

Pfeiffer, E. (1975b). A Short Portable Mental Status Questionnaire for the assessment of organic brain deficit in elderly patients. *Journal of the American Geriatrics Society, 23*, 433–441.

Pfeiffer, E. (1979). A Short Psychiatric Evaluation Schedule: A new 15-item monotonic scale indicative of functional psychiatric disorder. In Bayer Symposium VII, *Brain function in old age* (pp. 228–236). New York: Springer.

Pruchno, R. A., Kleban, M. H., Michaels, E. J., & Dempsey, N. P. (1990). Mental and physical health of caregiving spouses: Development of a causal model. *Journals of Gerontology: Psychological Sciences, 45*, P192–P199.

Reuben, D. B., & Siu, A. L. (1990). An objective measure of physical function of elderly outpatients: The Physical Performance Test. *Journal of the American Geriatrics Society, 38*, 1105–1112.

Reuben, D. B., Siu, A. L., & Kimpau, S. (1992). The predictive validity of self-report and performance-based measures of function and health. *Journals of Gerontology: Medical Sciences, 47*, M106–M110.

Riter, R. N. & Fries, B. E. (1992). Predictors of the placement of cognitively impaired residents on special care units. *The Gerontologist, 32*, 184–190.

Rogers, W. H., McGlynn, E. A., Berry, S. H., Nelson, E. C., Perrin, E., Zubkoff, M., Greenfield, S., Wells, K. B., Stewart, A. L., Arnold, S. B., & Ware, J. E., Jr. (1992). Methods of sampling. In A. L. Stewart & J. E. Ware, Jr. (Eds.), *Measuring functioning and well-being* (pp. 27–47). Durham, NC: Duke University Press.

Smyer, M. A., Hofland, B. F., & Jonas, E. A. (1979). Validity study of the Short Portable Mental Status Questionnaire. *Journal of the American Geriatrics Society, 27*, 263–269.

Spagnoli, A., Foresti, G., MacDonald, A., & Williams, P. (1986). Dementia and depression in Italian geriatric institutions. *International Journal of Geriatric Psychiatry, 1*, 15–23.

Stewart, A. L., Sherbourne, C. D., Hays, R. D., Wells, K. B., Nelson, E. C., Kamberg, C. J., Rogers, W. H., Berry, S. H., & Ware, J. E., Jr. (1992). Summary and discussion of MOS measures. In A. L. Stewart and J. E. Ware, Jr. (Eds.), *Measuring functioning and well-being* (pp. 345–372). Durham, NC: Duke University Press.

Tarlov, A. R., Ware, J. E., Jr., Greenfield, S., Nelson, E. C., Perrin, E., & Zubkoff, M. (1989). The medical outcomes study: An application of methods for monitoring the results of medical care. *Journal of the American Medical Association, 262*, 925–930.

Teresi, J. A., Golden, R. R., & Gurland, B. J. (1984). Concurrent and predictive validity of indicator scales developed for the Comprehensive Assessment and Referral Evaluation Interview Schedule. *Journal of Gerontology, 39*, 159–165.

Teresi, J. A., Golden, R. R., Gurland, B. J., Wilder, D. E., & Bennett, R. G. (1984). Construct validity of indicator scales developed from Comprehensive Assessment and Referral Evaluation Interview Schedule. *Journal of Gerontology, 39*, 147–157.

Teresi, J. A., & Holmes, D. (1992). Should MDS data be used for research? *The Gerontologist, 32*, 148–151.

Teresi, J., Holmes, D., Benenson, E., Monaco, C., Barrett, V., Ramirez, M., & Koren, M. J. (1993). A primary care nursing model in long-term care facilities: Evaluation and impact on affect, behavior, and socialization. *The Gerontologist, 33*, 667–674.

Tinetti, M. E. (1986). Performance-oriented assessment of mobility problems in elderly patients. *Journal of the American Geriatrics Society, 34*, 119–126.

Ware, J. E., Jr., & Sherbourne, C. D. (1992). The MOS 36-item Short-Form Health Survey (SF-36) I. Conceptual framework and item selection. *Medical Care, 30*, 473–483.

Wolber, G., Romaniuk, M., Eastman, E., & Robinson, C. (1984). Validity of the Short Portable Mental Status Questionnaire with elderly psychiatric patients. *Journal of Consulting and Clinical Psychology, 52*, 712–713.

Young, R. F., & Kahana, E. (1989). Specifying caregiver outcomes: Gender and relationship aspects of caregiver strain. *The Gerontologist, 29*, 660–666.

Index

M

N

www.ingramcontent.com/pod-product-compliance
Lightning Source LLC
LaVergne TN
LVHW011904200926
848484LV00002B/529